T0198197

Emergencies in the Older Adult

Editors

ROBERT S. ANDERSON Jr
PHILLIP D. MAGIDSON
DANYA KHOUJAH

EMERGENCY MEDICINE CLINICS OF NORTH AMERICA

www.emed.theclinics.com

Consulting Editor
AMAL MATTU

May 2021 • Volume 39 • Number 2

ELSEVIER

1600 John F. Kennedy Boulevard • Suite 1800 • Philadelphia, Pennsylvania, 19103-2899

http://www.theclinics.com

**EMERGENCY MEDICINE CLINICS OF NORTH AMERICA Volume 39, Number 2
May 2021 ISSN 0733-8627, ISBN-13: 978-0-323-77662-2**

Editor: Joanna Collett

Developmental Editor: Axell Purificacion

Emergency Medicine Clinics of North America (ISSN 0733-8627) is published quarterly by Elsevier Inc., 360 Park Avenue South, New York, NY, 10010-1710. Months of issue are February, May, August, and November. Business and Editorial Offices: 1600 John F. Kennedy Boulevard, Suite 1800, Philadelphia, PA 19103-2899. Customer Service Office: 6277 Sea Harbor Drive, Orlando, FL 32887-4800. Periodicals postage paid at New York, NY, and additional mailing offices. Subscription prices are $100.00 per year (US students), $359.00 per year (US individuals), $926.00 per year (US institutions), $220.00 per year (international students), $462.00 per year (international individuals), $986.00 per year (international institutions), $100.00 per year (Canadian students), $423.00 per year (Canadian individuals), and $986.00 per year (Canadian institutions). International air speed delivery is included in all *Clinics'* subscription prices. All prices are subject to change without notice. **POSTMASTER:** Send address changes to *Emergency Medicine Clinics of North America*, Elsevier Periodicals Customer Service, 11830 Westline Industrial Drive, St. Louis, MO 63146. Customer Service (orders, claims, online, change of address): Elsevier Periodicals **Customer Service, 11830 Westline Industrial Drive, St. Louis, MO 63146. Tel: 1-800-654-2452 (U.S. and Canada); 314-453-7041 (outside U.S. and Canada). Fax: 314-453-5170. E-mail: journalscustomerservice-usa@elsevier.com (for print support);** journalsonlinesupport-usa@elsevier.com (for online support).

Reprints. For copies of 100 or more of articles in this publication, please contact the Commercial Reprints Department, Elsevier Inc., 360 Park Avenue South, New York, NY 10010-1710. Tel.: 212-633-3874; Fax: 212-633-3820; E-mail: reprints@elsevier.com.

Emergency Medicine Clinics of North America is covered in *MEDLINE/PubMed (Index Medicus), Current Contents/Clinical Medicine, EMBASE/Excerpta Medica, BIOSIS, SciSearch, CINAHL, ISI/BIOMED,* and *Research Alert.*

Printed in the United States of America.

Contributors

CONSULTING EDITOR

AMAL MATTU, MD
Professor and Vice Chair of Academic Affairs, Department of Emergency Medicine, University of Maryland School of Medicine, Baltimore, Maryland, USA

EDITORS

ROBERT S. ANDERSON Jr, MD
Departments of Emergency Medicine and Internal Medicine, Maine Medical Center, Portland, Maine, USA

PHILLIP D. MAGIDSON, MD, MPH
Assistant Professor, Department of Emergency Medicine, Department of Medicine, Division of Geriatric Medicine and Gerontology, Johns Hopkins School of Medicine, Baltimore, Maryland, USA

DANYA KHOUJAH, MBBS, MEHP
Attending Physician, Emergency Medicine, MedStar Franklin Square Medical Center, Adjunct Volunteer Assistant Professor, Department of Emergency Medicine, University of Maryland School of Medicine, Baltimore, Maryland, USA

AUTHORS

ROBERT S. ANDERSON Jr, MD
Departments of Emergency Medicine and Internal Medicine, Maine Medical Center, Portland, Maine, USA

KIMBERLY BAMBACH, MD
Department of Emergency Medicine, The Ohio State University Wexner Medical Center, Columbus, Ohio, USA

LEAH BRIGHT, DO
Physician, Associate Program Director, Emergency Medicine Department, Johns Hopkins Hospital, Baltimore, Maryland, USA

ROBERT M. BROWN, MD
Attending Physician and Visiting Professor, Department of Emergency Medicine, Virginia Tech Carilion School of Medicine, Carilion Roanoke Memorial Hospital, Roanoke, Virginia, USA

CHRISTOPHER R. CARPENTER, MD, MSc
Professor, Department of Emergency Medicine, Emergency Care Research Core, Washington University School of Medicine in St. Louis, St Louis, Missouri, USA

NICOLE CIMINO-FIALLOS, MD
Assistant Medical Director, Department of Emergency Medicine, Meritus Medical Center, Hagerstown, Maryland, USA

DREW CLARE, MD
Assistant Professor of Emergency Medicine, University of Florida, Jacksonville, Florida, USA

DEBRA EAGLES, MD, MSc
Assistant Professor, Department of Emergency Medicine, School of Epidemiology and Public Health, University of Ottawa, Associate Scientist, Ottawa Hospital Research Institute, Ottawa, Ontario, Canada

KAMI M. HU, MD, FAAEM, FACEP
Assistant Professor, Departments of Emergency Medicine and Internal Medicine, University of Maryland School of Medicine, Baltimore, Maryland, USA

WENNIE HUANG, PharmD, BCPS
Department of Surgery, Division of Emergency Medicine, Duke University Hospital, Durham, North Carolina, USA

DANYA KHOUJAH, MBBS, MEHP
Attending Physician, Emergency Medicine, MedStar Franklin Square Medical Center, Adjunct Volunteer Assistant Professor, Department of Emergency Medicine, University of Maryland School of Medicine, Baltimore, Maryland, USA

STEPHEN Y. LIANG, MD, MPHS
Divisions of Emergency Medicine and Infectious Diseases, Washington University School of Medicine, St Louis, Missouri, USA

PHILLIP D. MAGIDSON, MD, MPH
Assistant Professor, Department of Emergency Medicine, Department of Medicine, Division of Geriatric Medicine and Gerontology, Johns Hopkins School of Medicine, Baltimore, Maryland, USA

SARA MANNING, MD
Assistant Professor, Department of Emergency Medicine, University of Maryland School of Medicine, Baltimore, Maryland, USA

BONNIE MARR, MD
Physician, Palliative Care Department, Johns Hopkins Hospital, Baltimore, Maryland, USA

ASHLEY N. MARTINELLI, PharmD, BCCCP
Clinical Pharmacy Specialist, Emergency Medicine, Department of Pharmacy, University of Maryland Medical Center, Baltimore, Maryland, USA

MICHAEL McGARRY, MD
Emergency Physician, Department of Emergency Medicine, Northwest Medical Center, Margate, Florida, USA

ELIZABETH A. PONTIUS, DPT
Maine Medical Center, Portland, Maine, USA

LUNA RAGSDALE, MD, MPH
Department of Surgery, Division of Emergency Medicine, Duke University Hospital, Emergency Department, Durham VA Health Care System, Durham, North Carolina, USA

TONY ROSEN, MD, MPH
Department of Emergency Medicine, Weill Cornell Medical College, NewYork-Presbyterian Hospital, New York, New York, USA

MARY MORGAN SCOTT, MD
Department of Medicine, Washington University School of Medicine in St. Louis, St Louis, Missouri, USA

CHRISTINA L. SHENVI, MD, PhD
Assistant Professor, Department of Emergency Medicine, The University of North Carolina at Chapel Hill, Chapel Hill, North Carolina, USA

NICOLE SORIA, MD
Attending Physician, Emergency Medicine, Assistant Medical Director, US Acute Care Solutions, Mercy Health West Hospital, Volunteer Assistant Professor, Geriatric Division, Department of Family and Community Medicine, University of Cincinnati, Cincinnati, Ohio, USA

LAUREN T. SOUTHERLAND, MD, FACEP
Associate Professor, Department of Emergency Medicine, The Ohio State University Wexner Medical Center, Columbus, Ohio, USA

RYAN SPANGLER, MD
Assistant Professor, Department of Emergency Medicine, University of Maryland School of Medicine, Baltimore, Maryland, USA

REBECCA THEOPHANOUS, MD
Department of Surgery, Division of Emergency Medicine, Duke University Hospital, Durham, North Carolina, USA

JAMES P. WOLAK, MD
Department of Psychiatry, Maine Medical Center, Portland, Maine, USA; Assistant Professor of Psychiatry, Tufts University School of Medicine, Boston, Massachusetts, USA

KORIE L. ZINK, MD, MS
Emergency Medicine Resident Physician, Johns Hopkins University, Baltimore, Maryland, USA

Contents

> Geriatric emergency medicine has emerged as a subspecialty of emergency medicine over the past 25 years. This emergence has seen the development of increases in training opportunities, care delivery strategies, collaborative best practice guidelines, and formal geriatric emergency department accreditation. This multidisciplinary field remains ripe for continued development in the coming decades as the aging US population parallels a call from patients, health care providers, and health systems to improve the delivery of high-value care. This article educates emergency medicine practitioners and highlights high-value care practice trends to inform and prioritize decision-making for this unique patient population.

> Geriatric trauma patients will continue to increase in prevalence as the population ages, and many specific considerations need to be made to provide appropriate care to these patients. This article outlines common presentations of trauma in geriatric patients, with consideration to baseline physiologic function and patterns of injury that may be more prevalent in geriatric populations. Additionally, the article explores specific evidence-based management practices, the significance of trauma team and geriatrician involvement, and disposition decisions.

> In 30 years, adults 65 and older will represent 20% of the US population, with increased medical comorbidities leading to higher rates of critical illness and mortality. Despite significant acute illness, presenting symptoms and vital sign abnormalities may be subtle. Resuscitative guidelines are a helpful starting point but appropriate diagnostics, bedside ultrasound, and frequent reassessments are needed to avoid procrustean care that may worsen outcomes. Baseline functional status is as important as underlying comorbid conditions when prognosticating, and the patient's personal wishes should be sought early and throughout care with clear communication regarding prospects for immediate survival and overall recovery.

Delirium is common in older emergency department (ED) patients. Although associated with significant morbidity and mortality, it often goes unrecognized. A consistent approach to evaluation of mental status, including use of validated tools, is key to diagnosing delirium. Identification of the precipitating event requires thorough evaluation, including detailed history, medication reconciliation, physical examination, and medical work-up, for causes of delirium. Management is aimed at identifying and treating the underlying cause. Meaningful improvements in delirium care can be achieved when prevention, identification, and management of older delirious ED patients is integrated by physicians and corresponding frameworks implemented at the health system level.

Chronic brain failure, also known as dementia or major neurocognitive disorder, is a syndrome of progressive functional decline characterized by both cognitive and neuropsychiatric symptoms. It can be conceptualized like other organ failure syndromes and its impact on quality of life can be mitigated with proper treatment. Dementia is a risk factor for delirium, and their symptoms can be similar. Patients with dementia can present with agitation that can lead to injury. Logic and reason are rarely successful when attempting to redirect someone with advanced dementia. Interactions that offer a sense of choice are more likely to succeed.

Older adults are susceptible to serious illnesses, including atrial fibrillation, congestive heart failure, pneumonia, and pulmonary embolism. Atrial fibrillation is the most common arrhythmia in this age group and can cause complications such as thromboembolic events and stroke. Congestive heart failure is the most common cause of hospital admission and readmission in the older adult population. Older adults are at higher risk for pulmonary embolism because of age-related changes and co-morbidities. Pneumonia is also prevalent and is one of the leading causes of death.

When older adults experience acute coronary syndrome (ACS), they often present with what are considered "atypical" symptoms. Because their symptoms less often match the expected presentation of ACS, older patients can have delayed time to assessment, to performance of an electrocardiogram, to diagnosis, and to definitive management. Unfortunately, it is this very group of patients who are at the highest risk for having ACS and for complications from ACS. This article aims to outline presentation, outcomes, and potential solutions of underrecognition of ACS in the older adult population.

Ryan Spangler and Sara Manning

Care of geriatric patients with abdominal pain can pose significant diagnostic and therapeutic challenges to emergency physicians. Older adults rarely present with classic signs, symptoms, and laboratory abnormalities. The incidence of life-threatening emergencies, including abdominal aortic aneurysm, mesenteric ischemia, perforated viscus, and other surgical emergencies, is high. This article explores the evaluation and management of several important causes of abdominal pain in geriatric patients with an emphasis on high-risk presentations.

Nicole Soria and Danya Khoujah

Older adults are frequently seen in the emergency department for genitourinary complaints, necessitating that emergency physicians are adept at managing a myriad of genitourinary emergencies. Geriatric patients may present with acute kidney injury, hematuria, or a urinary infection and aspects of how managing these presentations differs from their younger counterparts is emphasized. Older adults may also present with acute urinary retention or urinary incontinence as a result of genitourinary pathology or other systemic etiologies. Finally, genital complaints as they pertain to older adults are briefly highlighted with emphasis on emergent management and appropriate referrals.

Mary Morgan Scott and Stephen Y. Liang

Infections in elderly patients can prove diagnostically challenging. Age-related factors affecting the immune system in older individuals contribute to nonspecific presentations. Other age-related factors and chronic conditions have symptoms that may or may not point to an infectious diagnosis. Delay in administration of antimicrobials can lead to poor outcomes; however, unnecessary administration of antimicrobials can lead to increased morbidity and contribute to the emergence of multidrug-resistant organisms. Careful clinical assessment and consideration of patient history and risk factors is crucial. When necessary, antimicrobials should be chosen that are appropriate for the diagnosis and deescalated as soon as possible.

Ashley N. Martinelli

Increasing prescription drug use trends in the United States affects patients across all ages, but especially the geriatric patient. As patients age, they are at increased risk for adverse events owing to natural changes in body composition and organ function, increased sensitivity to medications, and a higher chance of adverse events from drug–drug interactions and polypharmacy. Falls are common and can increase morbidity and mortality. To mitigate falls, it is imperative to have a comprehensive approach to screening home medication lists, be aware of and avoid high-risk medications, and deprescribe agents that are potentially inappropriate for this patient population.

Elder abuse affects many older adults and can be life threatening. Older adults both in the community and long-term care facilities are at risk. An emergency department visit is an opportunity for an abuse victim to seek help. Emergency clinicians should be able to recognize the signs of abuse, including patterns of injury consistent with mistreatment. Screening tools can assist clinicians in the diagnosis of abuse. Physicians can help victims of mistreatment by reporting the abuse to the appropriate investigative agency and by developing a treatment plan with a multidisciplinary team to include a safe discharge plan and close follow-up.

The rehab services of Physical Therapy, Occupational Therapy, and Speech Language Pathology (PT/OT/SLP) are areas of emerging practice in the emergency department (ED). These specialty consult services can provide ED physicians with valuable, nuanced assessments for the older adults that will assist in determining a safe discharge plan. PT and OT interventions in the ED have been shown to decrease hospital admissions and readmissions, increase patient satisfaction, and decrease cost. Rehab specialists provide physicians with an expanded scope of management options that can greatly enhance the care of patients in the ED.

Each emergency department (ED) visit represents a crucial transition of care for older adults. Systems, provider, and patient factors are barriers to safe transitions and can contribute to morbidity and mortality in older adults. Safe transitions from ED to inpatient, ED to skilled nursing facility, or ED back to the community require a holistic approach, such as the 4-Ms model—what matters (patient goals of care), medication, mentation, and mobility—along with safety and social support. Clear written and verbal communication with patients, caregivers, and other members of the interdisciplinary team is paramount in ensuring successful care transitions.

The incorporation of palliative care to address the needs of the older adult is a vital part of emergency medicine. Recognizing the trajectory of chronic diseases in older adults and the myriad of medical diseases amenable to palliative care is paramount. Early involvement of palliative care should be considered the cornerstone to overarching management of the older adult presenting to the emergency department.

EMERGENCY MEDICINE CLINICS OF NORTH AMERICA

SERIES OF RELATED INTEREST

Orthopedic Clinics
https://www.orthopedic.theclinics.com/

THE CLINICS ARE NOW AVAILABLE ONLINE!
Access your subscription at:
www.theclinics.com

Foreword

Emergencies in the Geriatric Patient

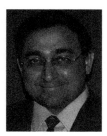

Amal Mattu, MD
Consulting Editor

Any clinician who has spent time working in the emergency department (ED) in recent years knows that our patients are getting older. During my last shift, 11 out of the 25 patients I cared for were over the age of 65, three of whom were over the age of 75, and one of the patients was over the age of 90. Care of these patients was challenging: each of them brought with them a host of prior medical problems, significant risks for polypharmacy, and sometimes vague complaints. Evaluations were sometimes further confounded by hearing problems, memory issues, and altered mental status.

There is no surprise that elderly patients routinely receive more extensive workups in the ED, partly because of the difficulty in obtaining an accurate, reliable history and physical examination. Despite these extensive workups, elderly patients suffer a higher rate of morbidity and mortality from similar diseases experienced by younger patients.[1,2] Complicating matters further, the elderly are prone to experiencing specific diseases that in and of themselves are associated with higher rates of mortality, including myocardial infarction, stroke, aortic dissection or rupture, mesenteric ischemia, and so on. Just as pediatricians often preach that children are not simply little adults, so we should understand that elderly patients are not simply old adults. There are so many special considerations in this group of patients that they deserve their own curriculum, just as children do.

Emergency Medicine Clinics of North America has strongly endorsed the need for focused curricula in geriatric emergency medicine for many years. We have made a point of including geriatric emergency topics sprinkled into many of the issues, and we have also had specific geriatric-themed issues, the last one in August 2016. In our current issue, we once again present another update on care of elderly in the ED.

Emergency Medicine Clinics of North America is honored to have 3 true experts in geriatric emergency medicine bring us some critical updates in this field. Drs Anderson and Magidson both have combined practices in emergency medicine and

Emerg Med Clin N Am 39 (2021) xiii–xiv
https://doi.org/10.1016/j.emc.2021.02.002
0733-8627/21/© 2021 Published by Elsevier Inc.

emed.theclinics.com

geriatrics, and Dr Khoujah is a national- and international-level educator in geriatric emergencies. They have combined their knowledge and expertise, and together they have assembled an outstanding group of authors who will update our knowledge on geriatric emergencies. The issue begins with basic epidemiologic information that will help the novice physician understand the true scope of the problems we face in caring for elderly patients in the ED. Then, the focus shifts to many of the life-threatening conditions, including trauma, vascular disease (acute coronary syndrome, stroke), abdominal emergencies, and infections. Vitally important articles are also provided on 2 conditions that unfortunately seem to be increasing in prevalence—elder abuse and polypharmacy. Finally, articles pertaining to transitions of care and end-of-life care round out the issue.

It is incumbent on every emergency clinician—physicians, physician assistants, nurse practitioners, and nurses—to learn about and understand the special issues that relate to elder patients in our EDs. Traditional emergency medicine training curricula simply do not address these issues adequately, and the result is that critical health conditions can be misdiagnosed, and critical psychosocial issues are missed. This issue of *Emergency Medicine Clinics of North America* will serve as an invaluable addition to the training of every type of clinician that is involved in emergency care of elderly patients. Our sincere thanks go to the Guest Editors and the authors for their time and commitment to this important issue.

Amal Mattu, MD
Department of Emergency Medicine
University of Maryland School of Medicine
110 South Paca Street
6th Floor, Suite 200
Baltimore, MD 21201, USA

E-mail address:
amattu@som.umaryland.edu

REFERENCES

1. Spangler R, Pham TV, Khoujah D, et al. Abdominal emergencies in the geriatric patient. Int J Emerg Med 2014;7:43.
2. Caterino JM. Evaluation and management of geriatric infections in the emergency department. Emerg Med Clin N Am 2008;26:319–43.

Preface

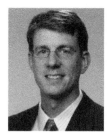 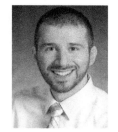 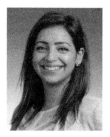

Robert S. Anderson Jr, MD Phillip D. Magidson, MD, MPH Danya Khoujah, MBBS, MEHP
Editors

We are excited to bring you this geriatric-focused issue of *Emergency Medicine Clinics of North America*. The authors have done a thorough job of interpreting the literature and distilling important concepts so you can be prepared for your next shift (or hospital meeting). While education in our field correctly trains us for the next trauma or airway disaster, the realities of our shifts are often quite different. Chief complaints that fill our days often include "weak and dizzy," "fall," "confusion," "dementia with behaviors," and so forth. The reality is that most of us are inundated with geriatric patients for whom our training, our environment, and our team can sometimes seem ill prepared.

There are 3 themes we hope our readers will encounter and incorporate into their own practices:

1. "I did not know that": Age-specific clinical pearls to improve medical decision making and care for older adults in all emergency settings. Older adults can and should receive individualized care outside of academic centers and geriatric-specific emergency departments (EDs).
2. "Who should I call?": Taking care of older patients is a team sport. Our colleagues upstairs have been playing this way for years; it is past time the ED does as well. Successful care of the older adults includes involvement of nurse case managers, pharmacists or pharmacy technicians, social workers, rehabilitation specialists, including physical, occupational, and speech therapists, geriatricians, and palliative care providers to name a few. Get to know these team members in your system and invite them into the ED.
3. "What's next?": Fortunately, a robust community of geriatric experts has laid the groundwork for all of us. There are many resources for the physician searching for reliable geriatric education, EDs looking for specific toolkits, and systems attempting a rehaul of the entirety of their geriatric emergency care. The American College of Emergency Physician's Geriatric Emergency Department Accreditation program is a wonderful example. Other examples referenced in the issue include the Institute for Healthcare Improvement's 4 M's Age-Friendly Health System's

Emerg Med Clin N Am 39 (2021) xv–xvi
https://doi.org/10.1016/j.emc.2021.02.001
0733-8627/21/© 2021 Published by Elsevier Inc.

Initiative and the Geriatric Emergency Department Collaborative. Pick what resonates with your needs and bring it to your practice and your group.

With all the stresses of our work, our sincere hope is that taking care of older adults in your busy ED should not be one of them. Please enjoy this issue of *Emergency Medicine Clinics of North America*. Learn some things, strive to meet new people in your health system, and make plans for improvement in your clinical practice.
Best wishes.

Robert S. Anderson Jr, MD
Departments of Emergency Medicine and
Internal Medicine
Maine Medical Center
22 Bramhall Street
Portland, ME 04102, USA

Phillip D. Magidson, MD, MPH
Department of Emergency Medicine
Division of Geriatric Medicine
and Gerontology
Johns Hopkins University School
of Medicine
A1 East Suite 150
4940 Eastern Avenue
Baltimore, MD 21224, USA

Danya Khoujah, MBBS, MEHP
Department of Emergency Medicine
University of Maryland School of Medicine
Department of Emergency Medicine
MedStar Franklin Square Medical Center
9000 Franklin Square Dr
Baltimore, MD 21237, USA

E-mail addresses:
anderr3@mmc.org (R.S. Anderson)
pmagidson@jhmi.edu (P.D. Magidson)
dkhoujah@gmail.com (D. Khoujah)

Twitter: @DanyaKhoujah (D. Khoujah)

Trends in Geriatric Emergency Medicine

Phillip D. Magidson, MD, MPH[a,b,*], Christopher R. Carpenter, MD, MSc[c]

KEYWORDS

- Geriatrics • Emergency medicine • Older adults • Geriatric screening tools

KEY POINTS

- The US population is aging and with this, there will be increasing use of the emergency department by older adults.
- In the emergency department, older adults have longer lengths of stay, require more resources, and are more likely to be admitted with associated functional decline compared with their younger counterparts.
- Formal geriatric emergency department guidelines and subsequent accreditation standards aimed at improving care provided to older adults in the ED exist and are valuable resource for clinicians and health system administrators alike.
- Numerous screening instruments are available for the evaluation of older adults and geriatric-specific syndromes including falls, dementia, delirium, and elder abuse.

INTRODUCTION

The American Geriatrics Society was created in 1942 when visionary medical leaders understood that scientific advances would catalyze historically unprecedented growth in the proportion of aged adults in the next century. Although experts projected three-fold increases in the demand for geriatrics care between 2000 and 2030, most medical schools lacked divisions or departments of geriatrics in the late twentieth century.[1] The John A. Hartford Foundation recognized that caring for an aging world would become the responsibility of all specialties rather than a handful of geriatricians. In response, they provided seed funding to emergency medicine in the 1990s that supported early research around the unique challenges of older adult care in the

[a] Department of Emergency Medicine, Johns Hopkins University School of Medicine, 4940 Eastern Avenue, A1 East, Suite 150, Baltimore, MD 21224, USA; [b] Department of Medicine, Division of Geriatric Medicine and Gerontology, Johns Hopkins University School of Medicine, 4940 Eastern Avenue, A1 East, Suite 150, Baltimore, MD 21224, USA; [c] Department of Emergency Medicine, Emergency Care Research Core, Washington University in St. Louis School of Medicine, Campus Box 8072, 660 South Euclid Avenue, St Louis, MO 63110, USA
* Corresponding author. Department of Emergency Medicine, Johns Hopkins University School of Medicine, 4940 Eastern Avenue, A1 East, Suite 150, Baltimore, MD 21224.
E-mail address: pmagidson@jhmi.edu
Twitter: @GeriatricEDNews (C.R.C.)

Emerg Med Clin N Am 39 (2021) 243–255
https://doi.org/10.1016/j.emc.2020.12.004
0733-8627/21/© 2021 Elsevier Inc. All rights reserved.

emergency department (ED) and ultimately catalyzed the subspecialty of geriatric emergency medicine (**Fig. 1**).

Over the next two decades, the Society for Academic Emergency Medicine (SAEM) and American College of Emergency Physicians (ACEP) created geriatric emergency medicine interest groups. Members of these ACEP and SAEM subgroups subsequently published the concept of a geriatric emergency department followed by quality indicators, resident core competencies, research priorities, and more textbooks.[2–6] Self-described geriatric EDs (GEDs) began to appear in 2009 with increasing frequency. Unfortunately, the actual geriatric attributes of these EDs varied considerably.[7] As the US population ages and the demand for high-value, low-cost care continues to rise, emergency medicine leaders will need to develop innovative, evidence-based practices for the care of older adults.[8] However, the anticipated insolvency of Medicare by 2026 combined with a paucity of high-quality clinical research demonstrating inarguable benefit or cost-effectiveness will inevitably create tension between early innovators and health care system leaders seeking pragmatic solutions.[9–11] As this history merges with present health care financing challenges, the subspecialty of geriatric emergency medicine will inevitably play a large part in the next articles of emergency medicine.

EPIDEMIOLOGY

According to the US Census Bureau, adults 65 years of age and older will outnumber children younger than 18 by 2034 for the first time in history.[12] Furthermore, between 2016 and 2060, the US population will increase about 25%. However, the population growth of those greater than or equal to 65 years of age is expected to increase by 92%, those greater than or equal to 85 years of age by 198%, and those greater than or equal to 100 years of age by nearly 620%.[13] The country's EDs have already begun to appreciate these changing demographics.

Between 2007 and 2017, the total number of ED visits increased by nearly 19%, whereas those by patients greater than or equal to 65 years of age increased by 28%.[14,15] As the rate of growth of older adults outpaces the US population, the number of visits by this demographic is certain to rise. This rise in older adults seen in the ED will further strain many already overcrowded and underresourced departments, hospitals, and health care systems.

Older adults present to the ED with higher acuity and require more resources during their ED visits compared with younger adults.[16–18] Moreover, compared with younger patients, the length of stay for older adults in the ED is significantly longer by 20%.[19] When it comes to hospitalization, older adults are nearly seven times more likely to be admitted to the hospital and five times more likely to be admitted to the intensive care unit compared with patients younger than the age of 65.[16]

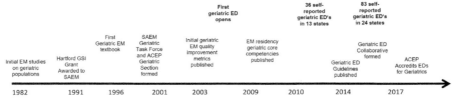

Fig. 1. Geriatric emergency medicine historical timeline. ACEP, American College of Emergency Physicians; AGS, American Geriatrics Society; EM, emergency medicine; ENA, Emergency Nurses Association; GSI, geriatrics for specialty initiative; SAEM, Society for Academic Emergency Medicine.

Despite increased levels of acuity, resource use, and higher need for hospitalization in the older adult population, nearly 20% of these patients present to the ED with a specific self-care problem, such as those related to cognitive and functional impairments or difficulties with activities of daily living.[20,21] Many of these self-care issues are overlooked or otherwise not considered by ED clinicians who are focused on time-sensitive disease and injury because the traditional emergency model has been to focus on one problem per patient, whereas frail older adults sometimes require a more holistic approach.[22]

ACCREDITATION AND CARE MODELS

In response to many of these unique and unmet needs, a collaborative effort among ACEP, American Geriatric Society, Emergency Nurses Association, and SAEM led to the creation of GED guidelines designed to measurably improve care of older adults.[23] These guidelines highlight six domains for quality improvement: (1) staffing and administration, (2) transitions of care, (3) education of ED staff, (4) quality improvement, (5) equipment and supplies, and (6) geriatric-specific policies and procedures. The subsequent endorsement of these guidelines by multiple emergency medicine organizations worldwide helped to accelerate the development of unique geriatric emergency care models and the more formal recognition of GEDs by health care systems. The development of these specific GEDs has increased considerably since the publication of the aforementioned guidelines with a 2018 paper having identified a total of 83 self-identified GEDs.[7,24] These guidelines and the subsequent acceleration in GEDs convinced ACEP to begin formal accreditation of hospitals' efforts to implement geriatric quality improvement efforts into their EDs. GED accreditation is additional evidence of the emergence of unique needs of older adult care and further drives the dissemination of evidence-based geriatric emergency care and practice recommendations. It is hoped these recommendations will offer meaningful benefit to not only emergency medicine practitioners (EMPs), hospitals, health systems, and their community but also to older adult patients.[25]

The development of the GED accreditation process, coupled with the GED guidelines published in 2014, have provided guidance, models, metrics, and motivation for hundreds of health care systems to improve care of older adults seen in the ED at the local level. This local innovation has helped to tailor care models specific to individual ED needs and the communities they serve. These care models may include a separate physical space for older adults, a geriatric champion on the ED staff, geriatric practitioners within the ED, or an ED-based observation unit focused on the care of older adults.[26] As of January 2021, a total of 212 EDs received ACEP accreditation.[27]

SCREENING TOOLS

An important component of the GED guidelines and ACEP accreditation criteria is a process for identifying age-related vulnerabilities. ED research has consistently demonstrated that neither nurses nor EMPs proactively identify or document dementia, delirium, falls, malnutrition, depression, or other vulnerabilities.[28–33] Identifying these issues is essential for GEDs because these problems are associated with increased (and perhaps preventable) risk of ED return visits, hospital admissions, and patient dissatisfaction. In response, numerous screening instruments exist to improve care of older adults. Some have been developed specifically for the ED, whereas others, not developed specifically for older adults seen in the ED, have been used in that setting. However, most of these screening instruments are imperfect to identify either high-risk (likelihood ratio+ >10) or low-risk (likelihood ratio- <0.10) subsets despite decades of research.[34] Many theories exist as to why such instruments yield suboptimal accuracy. For example, in deriving vulnerability assessment instruments, such as the Identification of Seniors At Risk, investigators likely need to consider various issues, such as the process of care, ability to identify confounding geriatric syndromes in the ED, standardized definitions of outcomes, pragmatic capacity to predict complex outcomes after brief ED evaluation, and adherence to diagnostic accuracy reporting standards.[35,36] Pragmatically, neither patients nor clinicians tolerate paralysis by analysis while awaiting instruments that are more accurate. Today's ED practitioners still need to make treatment and disposition decisions for patients, so they must rely on imperfect screening instruments while researchers strive to derive better instruments (**Fig. 2**).[37] **Table 1** summarizes some of the most common screening tools currently used.

EDUCATION/WORKFORCE PREPARATION

With a primary focus on the diagnosis, treatment, and disposition of patients suffering from time-sensitive disease or injury, EMP evaluation and management of older adults presenting with geriatric syndromes may be suboptimal.[66–68] Reasons for this are likely multifactorial but the paucity of geriatric-specific education has been historically recognized as one contributing factor.[69,70] Consequently, many emergency medicine residency graduates report discomfort managing geriatric patients leading to the development of core competencies within geriatric emergency care.[4,71]

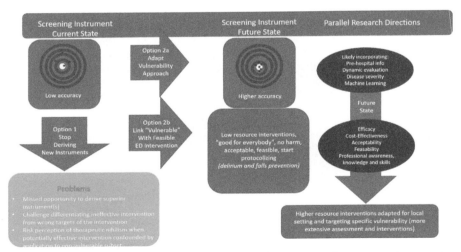

Fig. 2. A growing appreciation for the importance of geriatric syndrome screening counterbalanced by the recognition of current instrument imperfections quantified in **Table 1** leaves geriatric EDs confronting two paths forward for "vulnerability" screening. Option 1 would cease efforts to derive more accurate instruments than currently exist. Alternatively, Option 2a would adapt prior methods to derive "vulnerability" instruments that incorporate pre-ED data, dynamic re-evaluations throughout ED episode of care, social and system factors, and current disease severity, perhaps using disruptive innovation, such as machine learning. Option 2b could occur simultaneously with 2a, while responding to risk identified by currently available instruments with widely available and generally acceptable interventions. (*Modified from* Carpenter CR, Mooijaart SP. Geriatric Screeners 2.0: Time for a Paradigm Shift in Emergency Department Vulnerability Research. J Am Geriatr Soc. 2020:1-4; with permission.)

Table 1
Geriatric ED screening instruments

Domain	Studied Specifically in the ED	Pearls and/or Pitfalls
Falls		
Timed Get Up and Go[38] Graded tool for fall risk assessment	Yes	Quick to complete (less than a minute); however, LR+ only 0.99 and LR- 1.04 for patients in the ED.[39]
Chair test Graded tool to assess strength and endurance	Yes	Quick to complete (less than a minute); however, recent evidence suggests poor accuracy (LR+ 1.02 and LR- 0.92) for patients in the ED.[39]
Hendrich II Fall Risk Model[40] Graded risk factor model used to assess risk for falls	Yes	Get Up and Go test is a component of this tool; originally designed as an inpatient fall risk tool with questionable utility in the ED.[41] ED-based sensitivity/specificity unavailable.
Carpenter Tool[42,43] Scale that identifies risk for fall within 6 mo	Yes	Identifies low-risk, not high-risk with LR+ of 2.38 and LR- of 0.11 at score >1. Awaits external validation.
Delirium		
bCAM[44,45] Binary screen for delirium	Yes	Found to have LR+ of 20 and LR- of 0.17. When performed with the DTS, LR+ 19.52 and LR- 0.19.[46]
DTS[47] Binary screen for delirium	Yes	Found to have LR+ of 2.18 and LR- of 0.04. When performed with the bCAM LR+ of 19.52 and LR- of 0.19 in the ED.[46]
4 ATs[48] Graded score for identification of delirium or cognitive impairment	Yes	Rapidly performed in the ED LR+ of 3.23 and LR- of 0.22.[49]
Elder Abuse		
Elder abuse suspicion index Binary screen that may raise the concern for abuse	No	Short, 6-question screening tool (completed in <2 min) with LR+ 1.88 and LR- 0.71.[50]
Hwalek-Sengstock Elder Abuse Screening Test Adjunctive survey to supplement clinical concern for abuse	No	External validated tool that may identify elders who would benefit from protective services.[51,52] ED-based sensitivity/specificity unavailable.
Elder Assessment Instrument Unscored survey	Yes	Lengthy, 41-question, survey that has been used in the ED settings.[53,54] ED-based sensitivity/specificity unavailable.

(continued on next page)

Table 1
(continued)

Domain	Studied Specifically in the ED	Pearls and/or Pitfalls
Functional capacity		
Katz Index of Independence in Activities of Daily Living Graded score for patient independence	No	Well established tool that can identify those patients at risk of not being able to complete ADL in the community.[55] There are no formal reliability or validity studies in ED settings.
Vulnerability		
Triage Risk Assessment Tool Binary tool used to predict future increased risk of negative outcomes	Yes	5-questions derived to predict multiple outcomes, including 30-d any adverse outcome (LR+ 1.3, LR- 0.67).[56]
ISAR Binary tool used to predict negative outcomes	Yes	A 6-question tool originally designed for deployment in the ED.[57] Prognostic accuracy suggests ISAR is not consistently able to predict risk of ED returns, functional decline, readmissions, or adverse outcomes.[56] For example, LR+ 1.3, LR- 0.56 for any adverse outcome at 30-d.[56]
Frailty		
CFS[58,59] Overall health summary of patient, single score	Yes	Applicability to ED, given it comments more on the likelihood of death or institutionalization, is less obvious.[60] Area under the curve for 30-d mortality and hospitalizations was 0.81 and 0.72, respectively.[61] In ED, CFS reliability >0.86 for all age groups.[62]
Edmonton Frail Scale Graded scale to identify frail older adults	No	Validated tool for use by nongeriatricians in various settings; however, not studied in the ED.[63]
FRAIL Scale Graded scale to identify frail older adults	No	Validated study that can help clinicians identify patients at risk for decline in health functioning long-term and outside of the ED setting.[64] ED-based sensitivity/specificity unavailable.
Dementia		
AMT-4 Binary evaluation for abnormal cognition	Yes	Only validated in European EDs. LR+ 7.7, LR- 0.31.[65]
Caregiver AD8 Binary assessment for cognitive impairment	Yes	Less accurate but the only instrument not requiring patient participation and most sensitive for highly educated. LR+ 2.5, LR- 0.39.[65]
Ottawa 3DY Binary evaluation for cognitive dysfunction	Yes	Less accurate than AMT-4, LR+ 2.3, LR- 0.17.[65]

Abbreviations: ADL, activities of daily living; AMT-4, Abbreviated Mental Test-4; bCAM, Brief Confusion Assessment Method; CFS, Clinical Frailty Scale; DTS, delirium triage screen; ISAR, Identification of Seniors At Risk; LR, likelihood ratio.

Efforts are underway to improve residents' knowledge, attitudes, and ability to care for this patient population with some success.[72,73] The development of continued graduate medical education opportunities has also increased in recent years, specifically geriatric emergency medicine fellowships. These programs represent another important step in the professional maturation of geriatric emergency care, offering senior residents and residency graduates opportunities for enhanced clinical and research training.[74]

Nursing education within geriatric emergency care has also evolved as the number of older adults presenting to the ED increases. The Geriatric Emergency Nurses Education Course has become one of the cornerstone educational modules for ED nurses seeking additional geriatric training. Introduced in 2004, this course has been shown to increase nurses' knowledge of geriatric concepts, self-rated ability to care for those with geriatric syndromes, and the use of geriatric assessment tools.[75,76]

More resources have become available over the past decade to assist in the education of emergency nurses caring for older adults.[77] In fact, as a component of GED accreditation offered by ACEP, a nursing champion with demonstrable geriatric-specific education must be identified.[25] Nonetheless, many emergency nurses identify inadequate geriatric training as a barrier, suggesting wider dissemination of current educational materials is needed.[78]

Beyond the education of physicians and nurses within geriatric emergency care, the successful care of older adults in the ED requires a multidisciplinary approach including the active engagement of social workers, case managers, physical and occupational teams, and coordination with outpatient clinicians. This multidisciplinary approach is not only required for GED accreditation and recommended within the GED guidelines, but is also associated with meaningful patient-centered outcomes.[23,25,79]

ANTICIPATED CHALLENGES AND FUTURE OPPORTUNITIES

GEDs confront an array of counterarguments. One critique concerns continued partitioning of emergency care into cardiac, neurologic, trauma, pediatric, and geriatric care, which seems to deviate from emergency medicine's founding vision of a single site capable of delivering care to anyone, anytime, for anything.[80] Another argument is the lack of proof that GED-recommended protocols improve patient-centric outcomes. In fact, some early studies have been disappointing.[81–83] Lack of effectiveness is also problematic for health care system leaders seeking cost-effectiveness before investing in GEDs.[9,84] However, early studies demonstrating lack of effectiveness provide the intellectual foundations to formulate interventions that are more effective and targeted subsets that may benefit. In doing so, the "failed" studies provide valuable lessons about patient recruitment, measures of geriatric vulnerability, and outcomes to assess. Some of the studies have shown measurable benefit.[22,84–86] Some GED studies also demonstrate previously unrecognized scientific barriers between emergency medicine and other specialties, and physician and nurse research methods.[87] Another positive consequence of the increasing pace of GED research and funding opportunities is that the next generation of clinical investigators is developing, so current knowledge gaps will soon close.[88]

SUMMARY

As more older adults present to the nation's EDs for care, emergency medicine has witnessed a concurrent increase in the recognition of the importance of geriatric emergency medicine as a field. Although higher quality research continues to emerge in this field, some of which has led to the establishment of GED best practice guidelines and accreditation standards, many EDs around the country are likely underprepared for this resource-intense population. This article seeks to educate EMPs and highlight high-value care practice trends to inform and prioritize decision-making for this unique patient population.

CLINICS CARE POINTS

- The number of geriatric patients visiting the ED has outpaced the educational emphasis in training programs and clinical resources available in the nation's EDs dedicated to caring for this population.
- The Geriatric Emergency Department Guidelines, published in 2014, should be consulted when implementing new clinical practices aimed at improving the care of older adults.
- Geriatric screening tools, studied specifically in the ED, are available within the domains of falls, delirium, elder abuse, functional capacity, vulnerability, frailty, and dementia.
- Further research in geriatric emergency care aimed at identifying high-value, cost-effective strategies is warranted.

DISCLOSURE

P.D. Magidson: None. C.R. Carpenter: Paid consultant for the Geriatric Emergency Department Collaborative with funding from the John A. Hartford Foundation and Gary and Mary West Foundation. Paid consultant on the Steering Committee for the Clinical-Scientists Transdisciplinary Aging Research (Clin-STAR) Coordinating Center. Serves on American College of Emergency Physician's (ACEP) Geriatric Emergency Department Accreditation Board of Governors, and ACEP's Clinical Policy Committee. Serves on Society for Academic Emergency Medicine Board of Directors. Deputy Editor-in-Chief of *Academic Emergency Medicine* and Associate Editor of the *Journal of the American Geriatrics Society*. He is Chair of the Schwartz-Reisman Emergency Medicine Institute International Advisory Board.

REFERENCES

1. Reuben D, Bradley T, Zsanziger J, et al. The critical shortage of geriatrics faculty. J Am Geriatr Soc 1993;41(5):560–9.
2. Hwang U, Morrison RS. The geriatric emergency department. J Am Geriatr Soc 2007;55(11):1873–6.
3. Terrell KM, Hustey FM, Hwang U, et al. Quality indicators for geriatric emergency care. Acad Emerg Med 2009;16(5):441–9.
4. Hogan TM, Losman ED, Carpenter CR, et al. Development of geriatric competencies for emergency medicine residents using an expert consensus process. Acad Emerg 2010;17(3):316–24.
5. Carpenter CR, Heard K, Wilber S, et al. Research priorities for high-quality geriatric emergency care: medication management, screening, and prevention and functional assessment. Acad Emerg Med 2011;18(6):644–54.
6. Carpenter CR, Shah MN, Hustey FM, et al. High yield research opportunities in geriatric emergency medicine: prehospital care, delirium, adverse drug events, and falls. J Gerontol A Biol Sci Med Sci 2011;66 A(7):775–83.

7. Hogan TM, Olade TO, Carpenter CR. A profile of acute care in an aging America: snowball sample identification and characterization of United States geriatric emergency departments in 2013. Acad Emerg Med 2014;21(3):337–46.

8. Hwang U, Shah MN, Han JH, et al. Transforming emergency care for older adults. Health Aff (Millwood) 2013;32(12):2116–21.

9. Lo AX, Carpenter CR. Balancing evidence and economics while adapting emergency medicine to the 21st century's geriatric demographic imperative. Acad Emerg Med 2020;27(10):1070–3.

10. Pines JM, Edginton S, Aldeen AZ. What we can do to justify hospital investment in geriatric emergency departments. Acad Emerg Med 2020;27(10):1074–6.

11. Hwang U, Carpenter CR. The geriatric emergency department. In: Wiler J, Pines J, Ward M, editors. Value and quality innovations in acute and emergency care. Cambridge, UK: Cambridge; 2017. p. 82–90.

12. United States Census Bureau. An aging nation: projected number of children and older adults 2017. Available at: https://www.census.gov/library/visualizations/2018/comm/historic-first.html. Accessed March 2, 2020.

13. United States Census Bureau. 2017 national population projections tables: main series 2017. Available at: https://www.census.gov/data/tables/2017/demo/popproj/2017-summary-tables.html. Accessed March 2, 2020.

14. Rui P, Kang K. National hospital ambulatory medical care survey: 2017 emergency department summary tables. National Center for Health Statistics. 2017. Available at: file:///C:/Users/pmagids1/Desktop/2017_ed_web_tables-508.pdf. Accessed March 2, 2020.

15. Niska R, Bhuiya F, Xu J. National hospital ambulatory medical care survey: 2007 emergency department summary. Natl Health Stat Rep 2010;(26):1–32.

16. Strange GR, Chen EH. Use of emergency departments by elder patients: a five-year follow-up study. Acad Emerg Med 1998;5(12):1157–63.

17. Pines JM, Mullins PM, Cooper JK, et al. National trends in emergency department use, care patterns, and quality of care of older adults in the United States. J Am Geriatr Soc 2013;61(1):12–7.

18. Aminzadeh F, Dalziel WB. Older adults in the emergency department: a systematic review of patterns of use, adverse outcomes, and effectiveness of interventions. Ann Emerg Med 2002;39(3):238–47.

19. Singal BM, Hedges JR, Rousseau EW, et al. Geriatric patient emergency visits. Part I: comparison of visits by geriatric and younger patients. Ann Emerg Med 1992;21(7):802–7.

20. Lowenstein SR, Crescenzi CA, Kern DC, et al. Care of the elderly in the emergency department. Ann Emerg Med 1986;15(5):528–35.

21. Wilber ST, Blanda M, Gerson LW. Does functional decline prompt emergency department visits and admission in older patients? Acad Emerg Med 2006; 13(6):680–2.

22. Carpenter CR, Platts-Mills TF. Evolving prehospital, emergency department, and "inpatient" management models for geriatric emergencies. Clin Geriatr Med 2013;29(1):31–47.

23. ACEP, AGS, ENA, SAEM. Geriatric emergency department guidelines. Ann Emerg Med 2014;63(5):e7–25.

24. Schumacher JG, Hirshon JM, Magidson P, et al. Tracking the rise of geriatric emergency departments in the United States. J Appl Gerontol 2020;39(8):871–9.

25. ACEP. Criteria for Levels 1,2 & 3. ACEP Geriatric Emergency Department Accreditation. Available at: https://www.acep.org/globalassets/sites/geda/documnets/geda-criteria-final_1.17.2019.pdf. Accessed March 3, 2020.

26. Southerland LT, Lo AX, Biese K, et al. Concepts in practice: geriatric emergency departments. Ann Emerg Med 2020;75(2):162–70.

27. ACEP. Geriatric Emergency Department Accreditation List. 2020. Available at: https://www.acep.org/globalassets/sites/geda/documnets/geda-accreditation-list.xlsx. Accessed June 15, 2020.

28. Carpenter CR, Despain B, Keeling TN, et al. The six-item screener and AD8 for the detection of cognitive impairment in geriatric emergency department patients. Ann Emerg Med 2011;57(6):653–61.

29. Han JH, Zimmerman EE, Cutler N, et al. Delirium in older emergency department patients: recognition, risk factors, and psychomotor subtypes. Acad Emerg Med 2009;16(3):193–200.

30. Tirrell G, Sri-on J, Lipsitz LA, et al. Evaluation of older adult patients with falls in the emergency department: discordance with national guidelines. Acad Emerg Med 2015;22(4):461–7.

31. Pereira G, Bulik CM, Weaver MA, et al. Malnutrition among cognitively intact, non-critically ill older adults in ED. Ann Emerg Med 2015;65(1):85–91.

32. Hustey FM. The use of a brief depression screen in older emergency department patients. Acad Emerg Med 2005;12(9):905–8.

33. Carpenter CR, Griffey RT, Stark S, et al. Physician and nurse acceptance of technicians to screen for geriatric syndromes in the emergency department. West J Emerg Med 2011;12(4):489–95.

34. Hayden SR, Brown MD. Likelihood ratio: a powerful tool for incorporating the results of a diagnostic test into clinical decisionmaking. Ann Emerg Med 1999; 33(5):575–80.

35. Carpenter CR, Meisel ZF. Overcoming the tower of Babel in medical science by finding the "EQUATOR": research reporting guidelines. Acad Emerg Med 2017; 24(8):1030–3.

36. Carpenter CR, Émond M. Pragmatic barriers to assessing post-emergency department vulnerability for poor outcomes in an ageing society. Neth J Med 2016;74(8):327–9.

37. Carpenter CR, Mooijaart SP. Geriatric screeners 2.0: time for a paradigm shift in emergency department vulnerability research. J Am Geriatr Soc 2020;68(7): 1402–5.

38. Caterino JM, Karaman R, Arora V, et al. Comparison of balance assessment modalities in emergency department elders: a pilot cross-sectional observational study. BMC Emerg Med 2009;9:19.

39. Chow RB, Lee A, Kane BG, et al. Effectiveness of the "Timed Up and Go" (TUG) and the chair test as screening tools for geriatric fall risk assessment in the ED. Am J Emerg Med 2019;37(3):457–60.

40. Hendrich AL, Bender PS, Nyhuis A. Validation of the Hendrich II fall risk model: a large concurrent case/control study of hospitalized patients. Appl Nurs Res 2003; 16(1):9–21.

41. Patterson BW, Repplinger MD, Pulia MS, et al. Using the Hendrich II inpatient fall risk screen to predict outpatient falls after ED visits. J Am Geriatr Soc 2018;66(4): 760–5.

42. Carpenter CR, Scheatzle MD, D'Antonio JA, et al. Identification of fall risk factors in older adult emergency department patients. Acad Emerg Med 2009;16(3): 211–9.

43. Carpenter CR, Avidan MS, Wildes T, et al. Predicting geriatric falls following an episode of emergency department care: a systematic review. Acad Emerg Med 2014;21(10):1069–82.

44. Han JH, Wilson A, Graves AJ, et al. A quick and easy delirium assessment for non-physician research personnel. Am J Emerg Med 2016;34(6):1031–6.
45. Baten V, Busch HJ, Busche C, et al. Validation of the brief confusion assessment method for screening delirium in elderly medical patients in a German emergency department. Acad Emerg Med 2018;25(11):1251–62.
46. Han JH, Wilson A, Vasilevskis EE, et al. Diagnosing delirium in older emergency department patients: validity and reliability of the delirium triage screen and the brief confusion assessment method. Ann Emerg Med 2013;62(5):457–65.
47. Mariz J, Castanho TC, Teixeira J, et al. Delirium diagnostic and screening instruments in the emergency department: an up-to-date systematic review. Geriatr 2016;1(3):22.
48. Bellelli G, Morandi A, Davis DHJ, et al. Validation of the 4AT, a new instrument for rapid delirium screening: a study in 234 hospitalised older people. Age Ageing 2014;43(4):496–502.
49. Gagné AJ, Voyer P, Boucher V, et al. Performance of the French version of the 4AT for screening the elderly for delirium in the emergency department. Can J Emerg Med 2018;20(6):903–10.
50. Yaffe MJ, Wolfson C, Lithwick M, et al. Development and validation of a tool to improve physician identification of elder abuse: the Elder Abuse Suspicion Index (EASI)©. J Elder Abuse Negl 2008;20(3):276–300.
51. Neale AV, Scott RO, Sengstock MC, et al. Validation of the Hwalek-Sengstock elder abuse screening test. J Appl Gerontol 1991;10(4):406–18.
52. Strasser SM, Smith M, Weaver S, et al. Screening for elder mistreatment among older adults seeking legal assistance services. West J Emerg Med 2013;14(4):309–15.
53. Fulmer T, Paveza G, Abraham I, et al. Elder neglect assessment in the emergency department. J Emerg Nurs 2000;26(5):436–43.
54. Fulmer T. Elder abuse and neglect assessment. J Gerontol Nurs 2003;29(6):4–5.
55. Katz S, Down T, Cash H, et al. Progress in the development of the index of ADL. Gerontologist 1970;10(1):20–30.
56. Carpenter CR, Shelton E, Fowler S, et al. Risk factors and screening instruments to predict adverse outcomes for undifferentiated older emergency department patients: a systematic review and meta-analysis. Acad Emerg Med 2015;22(1):1–21.
57. McCusker J, Bellavance F, Cardin S, et al. Detection of older people at increased risk of adverse health outcomes after an emergency visit: the ISAR screening tool. J Am Geriatr Soc 1999;47(10):1229–37.
58. O'Caoimh R, Costello M, Small C, et al. Comparison of frailty screening instruments in the emergency department. Int J Environ Res Public Health 2019;16(19):1–13.
59. Lewis ET, Dent E, Alkhouri H, et al. Which frailty scale for patients admitted via emergency department? A cohort study. Arch Gerontol Geriatr 2019;80:104–14.
60. Rockwood K, Song X, MacKnight C, et al. A global clinical measure of fitness and frailty in elderly people. CMAJ 2005;173(5):489–95.
61. Kaeppeli T, Rueegg M, Dreher-Hummel T, et al. Validation of the Clinical Frailty Scale for prediction of thirty-day mortality in the emergency department. Ann Emerg Med 2020;76(3):291–300.
62. Lo AX, Heinemann AW, Gray E, et al. Inter-rater reliability of clinical frailty scores for older patients in the emergency department. Acad Emerg Med 2020. https://doi.org/10.1111/acem.13953.

63. Rolfson DB, Majumdar SR, Tsuyuki R, et al. Validity and reliability of the Edmonton Frail Scale. Age Ageing 2008;35(5):526–9.

64. Morley J, Malmstrom T, Miller D. A simple frailty questionnaire (FRAIL) predicts outcomes in middle aged African Americans. J Nutr Health Aging 2012;16(7): 601–8.

65. Carpenter CR, Banerjee J, Keyes D, et al. Accuracy of dementia screening instruments in emergency medicine: a diagnostic meta-analysis. Acad Emerg Med 2019;26(2):226–45.

66. Costa AP, Hirdes JP, Heckman GA, et al. Geriatric syndromes predict postdischarge outcomes among older emergency department patients: findings from the interRAI multinational emergency department study. Acad Emerg Med 2014;21(4):422–33.

67. Theou O, Campbell S, Malone ML, et al. Older adults in the emergency department with frailty. Clin Geriatr Med 2018;34(3):369–86.

68. Schnitker L, Martin-Khan M, Beattie E, et al. Negative health outcomes and adverse events in older people attending emergency departments: a systematic review. Australas Emerg Nurs J 2011;14(3):141–62.

69. Jones J, Dougherty J, Cannon L, et al. A geriatrics curriculum for emergency medicine training programs. Ann Emerg Med 1986;15(11):1275–81.

70. Jones JS, Rousseau EW, Schropp MA, et al. Geriatric training in emergency medicine residency programs. Ann Emerg Med 1992;21(7):825–9.

71. Snider T, Melady D, Costa AP. A national survey of Canadian emergency medicine residents' comfort with geriatric emergency medicine. Can J Emerg Med 2017;19(1):9–17.

72. Prendergast HM, Jurivich D, Edison M, et al. Preparing the front line for the increase in the aging population: geriatric curriculum development for an emergency medicine residency program. J Emerg Med 2010;38(3):386–92.

73. Biese KJ, Roberts E, Lamantia M, et al. Effect of a geriatric curriculum on emergency medicine resident attitudes, knowledge, and decision-making. Acad Emerg Med 2011;18(10 Suppl 2):92–6.

74. Rosen T, Liu SW, Cameron-Comasco L, et al. Geriatric emergency medicine fellowships: current state of specialized training for emergency physicians in optimizing care for older adults. AEM Educ Train 2020;4(Suppl 1):S122–9.

75. Désy PM, Prohaska TR. The Geriatric Emergency Nursing Education (GENE) course: an evaluation. J Emerg Nurs 2008;34(5):396–402.

76. Somes J. Geriatric Emergency Nurse Education (GENE) course premieres in September. J Emerg Nurs 2004;30(3):200–1.

77. Donatelli NS, Somes J. The geriatric bookworm: resources for those interested in the geriatric population. J Emerg Nurs 2014;40(4):390–3.

78. Wolf LA, Delao AM, Malsch AJ, et al. Emergency nurses' perception of geriatric readiness in the ED setting: a mixed-methods study. J Emerg Nurs 2019;45(4): 374–85.

79. Southerland LT, Stephens JA, Carpenter CR, et al. Study protocol for IMAGE: implementing multidisciplinary assessments for geriatric patients in an emergency department observation unit, a hybrid effectiveness/implementation study using the Consolidated Framework for Implementation Research. Implement Sci Commun 2020;1(1):1–12.

80. Zink BJ. Anyone, anything, anytime: a history of emergency medicine. 2nd edition. Dallas (TX): American College of Emergency Physicians; 2018.

81. Biese KJ, Busby-Whitehead J, Cai J, et al. Telephone follow-up for older adults discharged to home from the emergency department: a pragmatic randomized controlled trial. J Am Geriatr Soc 2018;66(3):452–8.
82. Arendts G, Love J, Nagree Y, et al. Rates of delirium diagnosis do not improve with emergency risk screening: results of the emergency department delirium initiative trial. J Am Geriatr Soc 2017;65(8):1810–5.
83. Morello RT, Soh SE, Behm K, et al. Multifactorial falls prevention programmes for older adults presenting to the emergency department with a fall: systematic review and meta-analysis. Inj Prev 2019;25(6):557–64.
84. Aldeen AZ, Courtney D, Lindquist LA, et al. Geriatric emergency department innovations: preliminary data for the geriatric nurse liaison model. J Am Geriatr Soc 2014;62(9):1781–5.
85. Prusaczyk B, Cherney SM, Carpenter CR, et al. Informed consent to research with cognitively impaired adults: transdisciplinary challenges and opportunities. Clin Gerontol 2017;40(1):63–73.
86. Hwang U, Carpenter C. Assessing geriatric vulnerability for post emergency department adverse outcomes: challenges abound while progress is slow. Emerg Med J 2016;33(1):2–3.
87. Kennedy M, Hwang U, Han JH. Delirium in the emergency department: moving from tool-based research to system-wide change. J Am Geriatr Soc 2020; 68(5):956–8.
88. Rosen T, Shah M, Lundebjerg NE, et al. Impact of Jahnigen/GEMSSTAR scholarships on careers of recipients in emergency medicine and on development of geriatric emergency medicine. Acad Emerg Med 2018;25(8):911–20.

Geriatric Trauma

Drew Clare, MD[a],*, Korie L. Zink, MD, MS[b]

KEYWORDS

- Geriatric patient • Older adult • Trauma • Fall • Head injury • Hip fracture

KEY POINTS

- Geriatric trauma is an increasingly prevalent and historically under-triaged presentation in emergency medicine.
- Geriatric trauma patients deserve special consideration due to baseline physiologic differences and unique injury patterns.
- Geriatric trauma patients should have comprehensive evaluations, including assessment of baseline function, medications, and access to care.

INTRODUCTION/EPIDEMIOLOGY

Geriatric trauma is a rapidly evolving area of interest in emergency medicine (EM). As the population ages, emergency physicians (EPs) can expect to see a surge in geriatric patients presenting with all common chief complaints, in particular trauma.[1] Geriatric patients are defined as any patients 65 years of age or older.[2] The geriatric population continues to grow, with 69 million Americans anticipated to be older than 65 by 2030. The incidence of geriatric trauma will rise with this growth.[3,4] More than 1 million geriatric patients experience trauma annually, and this number will continue to increase.[5]

As of 2011, the average age of a trauma patient discharged from the hospital in the United States is 59, up from 54 in 2000.[6] The latest data suggest geriatric patients represent 30.75% of all trauma patients.[7] Older adults who experience trauma have worse clinical outcomes compared with younger patients.[8] The traumatic case fatality rate increases significantly after age 65; trauma patients between ages 35 and 44 have an expected case fatality rate of 3.35, whereas those ages 75 to 84 have a rate of 6.66. Even if a traumatic injury does not cause immediate death or serious injury, geriatric patients who experience traumatic injuries have an increased mortality within the next 12 months.[9]

[a] Department of Emergency Medicine, University of Florida, 655 W 8th st, Jacksonville, FL 32209, USA; [b] Johns Hopkins University, 1830 E. Monument St, St 6-100, Baltimore, MD 21224, USA
* Corresponding author. ;
E-mail address: Drew.clare@jax.ufl.edu
Twitter: @koriezinkmd (K.L.Z.)

Emerg Med Clin N Am 39 (2021) 257–271
https://doi.org/10.1016/j.emc.2021.01.002
0733-8627/21/© 2021 Elsevier Inc. All rights reserved.

The most common mechanism for trauma in older patients is falls.[7] Ground-level falls account for approximately 2.1 million emergency department (ED) visits per year. Geriatric patients have a mortality of 7% to 11% after falls and have increased incidence of hospital and intensive care unit (ICU) admission compared with younger patients. The case fatality rate for geriatric patients who fall ranges from 4.04 (ages 65–74) to 8.11 (ages >84). Although ground-level falls are much more prevalent than other mechanisms of trauma in geriatric patients, other mechanisms typically seen include motor vehicle accidents, pedestrians struck by a vehicle, injuries related to other forms of transport, firearm injuries, and lacerations/penetrating injuries.

This article outlines common presentations for trauma in older adults, management strategies, and special circumstances that should be considered.

AGE-RELATED CHANGES IN OLDER ADULTS
Vital Signs

The geriatric population has more comorbidities than younger populations. Special consideration should be taken when determining normal vital signs in the setting of trauma, given physiologic changes of aging as well as increase in comorbidities. Many geriatric patients are on medications for cardiac conditions, such as β-blockers, which may slow their heart rate artificially or blunt a physiologic tachycardic response to stress or hemorrhage. Additionally, many patients have chronic hypertension that may or may not be controlled with medications. It is crucial to obtain an accurate medication list for these patients as well as to determine when they last took each medication. Physicians who remain cognizant of these vital sign nuances can avoid the pitfalls of being falsely reassured by the lack of tachycardia or a normal blood pressure (for example, a systolic blood pressure of 110 mm Hg when a patient's baseline is 160 mm Hg). Further information can be found in **Table 1**.[2]

Frailty

Geriatric trauma patients present a challenge from a physiologic perspective. Generally, geriatric patients with preexisting conditions have higher morbidity and are more likely to die within 5 years of a traumatic injury.[10] EPs must consider comorbidities, medications, and baseline functional status (eg, ambulatory ability and cognitive deficits) carefully when evaluating geriatric patients.

Generally, geriatric patients are more likely to be considered frail than their younger counterparts. Frailty, defined as the age-associated decline in physiologic function across multiple organ systems, makes patients both more likely to experience trauma (in particular falls) and to have poor outcomes after a trauma.[11,12]

Neurologic Considerations

From a neurologic perspective, geriatric patients are more likely to have neurocognitive impairments, such as dementia, which could influence the accuracy of a medical history.[13] They are more likely to have had prior cerebrovascular accidents, often with residual neurologic deficits. This can make it challenging to accurately assess for new deficits from a traumatic injury. Geriatric patients are more likely to be on anticoagulants or antiplatelets and also have decreased brain volume, making intracranial bleeds more prevalent and often more difficult to manage.[14]

Cardiopulmonary Considerations

From a cardiopulmonary perspective, geriatric patients are much more likely to be on medications that alter hemodynamics. Additionally, they have a higher incidence of baseline cardiovascular disease. Blunt cardiac injury has a higher mortality in patients

Table 1
Vital sign considerations in geriatric trauma patients[2]

Vital Sign	Special Considerations in Geriatric Population	Concerning Values in Geriatric Patient	Traditional Trauma Activation Vitals
Blood pressure	• Frequent use of antihypertensive medications	• SBP <110 mm Hg • SBP 40 mm Hg less than baseline	• SBP <90 mm Hg
Heart rate	• β-blocker, calcium channel blocker usage may blunt hemodynamic response to stress - comorbidities, such as heart failure and ACS	• Heart rate >90 bpm	• Heart rate >120 bpm
Respiratory rate	• Decreased ability to compensate for pulmonary injuries; less pulmonary reserve; may fatigue/need intervention earlier	• Rate may be normal, while still experiencing hypoxia/hypercarbia • RR <10 is particularly worrisome.	• RR <10 or >30
Oxygen saturation	• Challenge to recognize hypoxia/hypercarbia in patients with an atypical baseline	• Baseline may be 88%–92% rather than 100%.	• Oxygen saturation <93%

Abbreviations: ACS, acute coronary syndrome; RR, respiratory rate; SBP, systolic blood pressure.

with existing cardiac conditions.[15] Physiologically, older adults have a decline in overall respiratory function, including decreased functional residual capacity, and a higher incidence of pulmonary comorbidities, such as chronic obstructive pulmonary disease, with associated decrease in lung compliance.[13] As a result, injuries that may not have significant implications in younger patients, such as rib fractures and pulmonary contusions, have a larger impact on geriatric patients. The most common posttraumatic hospital complication is pneumonia, which can have delayed resolution in patients with poor baseline pulmonary function.[16]

Musculoskeletal Considerations

Geriatric patients are more prone to musculoskeletal injuries compared with younger patients because they are more likely to be deconditioned and also have bone pathology, such as osteoporosis. They are more likely to suffer fractures and dislocations from minor trauma.[17] Orthopedic injuries that may have minimal impact on the lives of younger patients can have a profound impact on functional independence, and even mortality, of geriatric patients.[17]

COMMON INJURIES
Head Injuries

Outcomes for geriatric patients who experience head injuries unequivocally are worse than in younger patients.[18] Traumatic brain injuries (TBIs) predominantly are caused by ground-level falls and are a leading cause of mortality in geriatric patients.[19] Studies show a mortality of up to 74% in patients older than 65.[18] Mortality for geriatric head injury patients with a Glasgow Coma Scale score less than 8 is extremely high, and in some studies a low Glasgow Coma Scale score is thought to be predictive of death.[18,20] Recovery from serious head injuries often is delayed and results in worse cognitive and psychosocial function in older adults compared with their younger counterparts.[21]

As patients age, the incidence of subdural hematoma after a head injury increases significantly. This is due partly to the inherent changes in vasculature and white matter in geriatric patients and exacerbated by the increased prevalence of antiplatelet and anticoagulant therapy in this population.[22] Geriatric patients on anticoagulation may have a delayed presentation of intracranial hemorrhage, necessitating a longer period of observation after their injury.[23] Historically, there has been controversy surrounding observation, repeat neurologic examinations, and repeat head imaging. Current data suggest head computed tomography (CT) at the time of presentation is sufficient for patients with a normal neurologic examination, patients with therapeutic/subtherapeutic international normalized ratio (INR) (if on warfarin), and for those taking novel oral anticoagulants.[24] For those patients with a supratherapeutic INR, further observation likely is necessary; however, there remains no consensus on whether serial neurologic examinations are sufficient or if repeat imaging is warranted.

If there is an acute intracranial hemorrhage, the patient should be resuscitated as needed and evaluated by a neurosurgeon, and reversal of anticoagulation (if present) should be initiated. If the head CT is unremarkable and the patient otherwise is safe for discharge, the EP frequently is tasked with the decision on whether to continue or hold anticoagulation, particularly in patients with frequent falls. There are studies suggesting that patients with frequent falls do not have an increased risk of major bleeding, thus making it safe to continue anticoagulation.[25] Other studies show that there are increased rates of intracranial hemorrhage in patients with frequent falls; however, there are no differences between patients on warfarin and those on aspirin only. Additionally, within this study those in the warfarin group showed that the drug was protective against stroke, intracranial hemorrhage, myocardial infarction (MI), and death.[26] Finally, there are data to suggest that patients on warfarin would need to fall 295 times in a year for the risk of fall-related intracranial hemorrhage would outweigh the benefit of the warfarin itself.[27]

Although these data suggest that continuing anticoagulation is safe for patients, in particular those with multiple stroke risk factors, it is prudent for EPs to evaluate each patient individually. This can be done by considering the underlying pathology being addressed with warfarin and making a calculated risk-benefit assessment using previously validated clinical decision rules when possible. The CHA_2DS_2-VASc score assesses the risk of stroke for patients with atrial fibrillation, a common reason for anticoagulation in the geriatric population.[27] The risk of stroke given by this score can be weighed against the risk of major bleeding while taking anticoagulation, which can be calculated by the HAS-BLED score.[28] If the risk of stroke exceeds the risk of major bleeding, then anticoagulation may be favored, even in light of fall risk.

Spinal Injuries

Geriatric patients are more likely to have baseline spinal pathology, such as arthritis, osteoporosis, stenosis, or disk disease, than younger patients. These comorbidities predispose patients to more severe cervical (C)-spine injuries from lesser impact trauma. Although young patients have the highest risk of C-spine injury at C4-7 (the most mobile portion of the C-spine), geriatric patients have increased spinal rigidity and are more likely to suffer from injuries to odontoid and C2.[29] Therefore, C-spine imaging often is warranted in geriatric patients with blunt trauma that may have affected the C-spine.[2] Notably, 50% of C-spine injuries in geriatric patients are unstable, so the risk of missing this diagnosis, particularly after a low-impact trauma, is very high. Many radiologists recommend that any geriatric trauma patient who has a mechanism or findings severe enough to consider a head CT also should undergo cervical spine imaging.[29]

Evaluation of C-spine injuries in geriatric patients generally should be done with cross-sectional imaging as opposed to plain films. When using clinical decision-making tools to determine whether these patients need a C-spine CT, EPs often look to Canadian C-spine and National Emergency X-Radiography Utilization Study (NEXUS) rules (**Box 1**). Based on the Canadian C-spine rule, patients 65 and older are not considered low risk enough to forego imaging; therefore, limiting the utility of this tool in geriatric patients. On the other hand, the NEXUS criteria do not include age as a risk-stratifying factor, allowing its usage in older adults.[30] A subgroup analysis of approximately 3000 older adults included in the original NEXUS study reveals a sensitivity of 100% (CI, 97.1%–100%) in older adults for clinically significant C-spine injury.[31] Given the lack of a robust external validation of NEXUS, however, specifically in geriatric patients, some clinicians are hesitant to utilize this tool in older adults and prefer liberal imaging. For those patients who do receive a CT scan, EPs may be challenged with having to "clear the C-spine" after the negative imaging in patients with cognitive impairment. There is literature suggesting that magnetic resonance imaging (MRI) to evaluate for occult C-spine injury in blunt trauma can change management up to 6% of the time[32]; however, other data suggest that the incidence of occult C-spine injuries in this setting is as low as 0.12%, even in obtunded patients.[33] This likely is due to the high quality of modern CT scanners. Furthermore, another systematic review recommends removing the C-collar after negative high-quality CT scan alone (a guideline put forth by the Eastern Association for the Surgery of Trauma).[34] None of these studies addresses older adults in particular, which may make this information unclear, and the decision to remove a C-collar without confirmatory MRI a difficult one. Further issues surround the use of C-collars, which have been shown to cause discomfort, tissue breakdown, increased aspiration risk, and worsened delirium.[35] It is helpful to involve the family in the discussion around the removal of the C-collar after CT scan alone versus obtaining an MRI as well as to consider the patient's wishes, underlying functional status, and goals of care. Finally, if a patient must be sedated for MRI, the EP needs to consider the risks of sedative administration versus the likelihood of advanced imaging changing management.

Box 1
National Emergency X-Radiography Utilization Study criteria: cervical spine imaging recommended unless all criteria met

C-spine imaging is recommended unless all the following criteria are met:

No posterior midline C-spine tenderness

No evidence of intoxication

Normal level of alertness

No focal neurologic deficit

No painful distracting injuries

Data from Hoffman JR, Mower WR, Wolfson AB, et al. Validity of a set of clinical criteria to rule out injury to the cervical spine in patients with blunt trauma. National emergency X-radiography utilization study group. N Engl J Med 2000;343(2):94–9.

Vertebral fractures are some of the most common osteoporotic fractures in geriatric patients. They are most common from T10 down into the lumbar spine. Recent studies suggest that most of the fractures are nonoperative and that spine immobilization can lead to worse outcomes. Therefore, early ambulation with a supportive brace often is indicated for vertebral fractures without neurologic compromise in geriatric patients.[36,37]

Thoracic Injuries

Geriatric patients who suffer from blunt trauma often sustain rib fractures. Age is one of the strongest predictors of mortality after rib fractures.[38] Rib fractures are a surrogate for major trauma, because 90% of patients with rib fractures have other traumatic injuries.[39] Geriatric patients with rib fractures have double the mortality rates of young patients with rib fractures and this number increases proportionally with each additional rib fracture.[40] Additionally, the risk of pneumonia, hypoventilation, pneumothorax, and respiratory failure increases with the number of fractured ribs in geriatric patients.[39] In older patients who suffer from rib fractures, up to 34% subsequently develop pneumonia, which significantly increases risk of mortality.[16] As a result of this, geriatric patients with multiple rib fractures usually benefit from inpatient management.

Multiple studies have demonstrated that appropriate analgesia lowers the risk of poor outcomes in geriatric patients with rib fractures, and many trauma centers have specific "rib fracture protocols" to manage pain (**Table 2**).[13] These protocols include multimodal analgesia in addition to pulmonary therapy, such as incentive spirometer. One study in 2005 found that epidural analgesia reduces mortality in patients with multiple rib fractures.[41] Although rib fractures in geriatric patients historically have been managed conservatively, there has been recent advocacy for operative management, particularly for rib plating. Studies on rib plating and fracture fixation thus far have demonstrated lower mortality, decreased posttraumatic complications, and shorter rehabilitation periods than patients managed conservatively.[42]

Abdominal Injury

Geriatric patients who suffer from abdominal trauma have a lower likelihood of operative management, but those who undergo surgery have worse outcomes than younger patients. Identifying intraabdominal injuries early can allow for maximal medical management and many clinicians have a lower threshold to image geriatric patients than younger patients. For patients who suffer from splenic injury, age predicts overall mortality rates.[43] Geriatric patients are more likely to have underlying

Table 2 Sample rib fracture protocol[13]	
Intervention	**Dosing**
Nonopiates	Acetaminophen scheduled dosing Ibuprofen scheduled dosing Lidocaine patch 5%
Regional	Nerve blocks (serratus anterior plane) Consider catheter placement by anesthesiology for continuous administration
Opiates	Morphine or hydromorphone, as needed Consider patient-controlled analgesia for severe refractory pain
Nursing	Frequent incentive spirometer use Pulmonary toilet

liver and kidney disease, which can make obtaining certain diagnostics more challenging. Previously it was thought that patients with poor baseline renal function could sustain acute kidney injuries from intravenous contrast administration; however, there is a growing body of literature suggesting that this is untrue.[44,45] Considering the recent literature, trauma patients undergoing abdominal imaging with high suspicion for injury should receive intravenous contrast for better results, because the risk profile is lower than previously thought.

Orthopedic Injuries

As discussed previously, geriatric patients have higher incidence of osteoporosis and sarcopenia (loss of muscle mass), increasing the likelihood of bony injury after trauma. The most common orthopedic injury in this population is forearm fractures, followed by hip fractures. Sarcopenia, in general, increases the likelihood that geriatric patients need rehabilitation and possible prolonged hospitalization after injuries.[13,46]

There are several common types of fractures sustained at the hip or proximal femur, and older adults are particularly susceptible to these injuries. Fractures of the femoral neck are intracapsular injuries in which the 1-year mortality increases with associated medical comorbidities, such as chronic renal failure and congestive heart failure.[47] Intertrochanteric fractures occur between the greater and lesser trochanter and typically occur in an older age group than those with femoral neck fractures. Clinically, a patient's leg usually is shortened and externally rotated. Finally, subtrochanteric femur fractures occur in the region 5 cm distal to the lesser trochanter. Low-energy mechanisms should increase suspicion for pathologic fractures and further work-up.

Despite the frequency of hip fractures in older adults, the true emergent nature of a hip fracture in a geriatric patient often is underappreciated. The overall 1-year mortality of an older adult after a hip fracture is 21.2%, on par with the mortality of 24% in adults over age 65 with acute MI.[48,49] Surgical intervention is recommended in most geriatric hip fractures, except in patients who are nonambulatory or have multiple medical comorbidities that preclude surgery. The urgency in which the fracture should be repaired is underappreciated as well. In geriatric patients undergoing operative repair of a hip fracture, pulmonary complications were decreased if the surgery was performed within less than 24 hours.[50] Other studies suggest that repair within 12 hours has improvement in 30-day mortality compared with those repaired after 12 hours.[51] Delays to surgery are associated with increased 30-day mortality, 1-year mortality, and incidences of pulmonary embolisms, MI, and pneumonia. Delays in operative interventions were more likely seen in those that presented to academic institutions and during nights and weekends.[52]

Similar to those with hip fractures, geriatric patients with pelvic fractures also have a higher likelihood of developing complications and have higher overall mortality rates than younger patients. Older patients more frequently sustain lateral compression fractures, which can have associated vascular injury necessitating invasive procedures.[53] Missed pelvic and hip fractures may lead to increased nonunion, avascular necrosis, and morbidity.[54] It is important to maintain a high level of suspicion for pelvic and hip fractures and to obtain further imaging studies, such as CT or MRI, in patients who have significant pain or difficulty ambulating in the setting of a nondiagnostic radiograph. MRI has been shown to have greater sensitivity for fractures of the pelvis and proximal femur compared with CT; however, CT available is more widely.[55]

Polytrauma

Overall, polytrauma carries a mortality rate of 36% for geriatric patients. Polytrauma patients often have complicated hospital courses. One study found that the most common complications were delirium, pneumonia, and electrolyte abnormalities.[56] Fatalities directly from trauma in geriatric patients most likely are related to neurologic damage from TBIs and exsanguination.[56]

MANAGEMENT
Trauma Activation and Consulting Services

There is evidence suggesting geriatric patients who experience trauma have better outcomes if they present to a trauma center that serves a higher proportion of older trauma patients. One study shows such patients were 34% less likely to die if cared for at a higher-volume trauma center.[5] Access to a trauma team plays a large role in the outcomes of trauma patients. Trauma team activation at trauma centers often is a crucial component of adequate trauma care, yet geriatric trauma patients are more likely to be under-triaged and not have all trauma resources utilized in their care.[57] Geriatric trauma patients who have comprehensive trauma evaluations by a trained trauma team on arrival ultimately have fewer complications and stay in the ED and hospital for less time.[58] Not every geriatric patient who falls can be seen at a trauma center, so this patient population likely is encountered in all practice environments. The EP can mitigate the lack of a trauma team with early recognition of traumatic injuries and aiming for early, thorough evaluation of all geriatric trauma patients. This includes timely radiographic diagnostics and involving consulting services to improve outcomes and decrease patient length of stay (LOS).[59] One level 1 trauma center opted to activate the trauma team for any trauma patient greater than age 70 and found that doing this resulted in both a decreased ED LOS and overall improvement in mortality.[60]

Because it is important to have access to an equipped trauma team for geriatric trauma evaluations, it is also important to have resources for a comprehensive assessment of geriatric patients overall. Having a geriatrician available for consulting on trauma patients has been shown to improve outcomes in these patients and decrease hospital LOS.[8] Specifically, geriatricians help reduce hospital-acquired complications, such as falls, functional decline, and delirium, while also evaluating new and existing medical conditions.[61] A formal comprehensive geriatric assessment improves outcomes for medical and surgical geriatric patients alike and is strongly recommended for trauma patients. Additionally, the early involvement of a palliative care team can strongly benefit patients with a high chance of accelerated death (such as those over age 80 suffering a hip fracture and geriatric patients with multiple rib fractures, TBI, or polytrauma), in addition to benefiting their families and the hospital system as a whole.[62,63] Early palliative care consultation, even initiated from the ED, can decrease patient pain and suffering, decrease family anxiety, improve patient/family understanding of goals of care, decrease hospital LOS, decrease ICU admissions, and decrease hospital system costs.[13,64]

Pain Management

Pain control can be difficult in geriatric patients. Physiologic changes that occur with aging can influence the effects and metabolism of pain medication. For example, having a lower overall plasma volume, decreased muscle mass, and increased body fat can give lipid-soluble medications, such as fentanyl, a longer duration of action. Medications with lower lipid-solubility, such as morphine, can have a much more potent effect than desired.[65] Additionally, many geriatric patients are on multiple home medications, and polypharmacy can present a risk when prescribing acute doses of opioid pain medications. Many well-intended physicians prioritize the risks of acute pain management while dosing geriatric trauma patients, which can lead to the undertreatment of pain in these patients.[66,67] Undertreating pain is a frequent cause of delirium, but over-medication, particularly with opioids, also can contribute to delirium, exacerbation of dementia, or sedation.

There are several options for acute pain management in geriatric patients. Acetaminophen has relatively few side effects and contraindications.[68] Nonsteroidal anti-inflammatory drugs (NSAIDs) have a higher risk profile and can cause renal dysfunction and gastrointestinal bleeds. In the acute setting, however, topical NSAIDs have similar effectiveness to oral ones and have lower systemic effects.[69] Ketamine can be considered for acute management if trying to avoid opioid analgesia; however, the data for ketamine safety in older adults are sparse. Ketamine also is noted to cause psychogenic side effects that may be difficult to mediate; thus, it is recommended to use a low-dose ketamine infusion if necessary.[70] If using opioids, it is recommended to use a low dose (25%–50% less) for a short duration, primarily in the setting of failure of other pain management techniques.[71,72]

Regional anesthesia, including local or epidural blocks, also can provide pain relief to patients and is considered superior to opioid analgesia. Epidural analgesia has been associated with a reduction in mortality for patients with multiple rib fractures.[41] Peripheral nerve blocks act faster and last longer in geriatric patients, with fewer systemic side effects than oral or parenteral pain management options.[73] It is increasingly common to see a variety of ultrasound-guided nerve blocks performed in the ED. Overall, considering a multimodal approach to pain management can help minimize risks of use of any 1 method, while increasing pain control for patients.

DISPOSITION CONSIDERATIONS

Geriatric patients with traumatic injuries have a high likelihood of being admitted to the hospital. Ideally, they are admitted to a trauma service with a geriatrics consult, so that their specific injuries can be addressed while also receiving a holistic evaluation of their medical condition. In many academic hospitals, patients with isolated orthopedic injuries and multiple comorbidities are admitted to the internal medicine service for management. Admitting these patients to internal medicine can increase their LOS significantly, particularly for those with hip fractures.[74] Hip fracture patients have a similar number of postoperative complications, whether admitted to medicine or orthopedic services.[75] Regardless of the arrangement, it is helpful to draft interdepartmental protocols for common injuries, such as hip fractures.

When discharging older adults, there are several barriers that should be considered (**Box 2**). Whether the patient is coming from home or a nursing facility, it is important to consider elder abuse or neglect. If the patient lives alone, assessment is needed to see if they can care for themselves or if they have family support. This is important particularly in terms of medication administration, activities of daily living (ADLs), and ambulatory function. Finally, and importantly, employing rehabilitation services in the ED to ensure safe disposition is gaining acceptance.

Medications often are prescribed after ED visits; however, this is a major opportunity for improvement in the care of older adults. Careful review of a patient's medication list is prudent, and avoidance of polypharmacy has important safety implications. Many older adults have several prescribers, and as a result it becomes easier to unintentionally create unsafe medication interactions. Polypharmacy is a major cause for falls in older adults, and it has been documented that up to 37% of geriatric patients are on anticholinergic medication.[76] To ensure safety in prescribing medications to the geriatric population, a list of dangerous medications (Beers Criteria) has

---

Box 2
Disposition considerations in geriatric patients

Safe discharge plan
- Ability to perform/has assistance with ADLs
- Discussion with caretaker regarding plan of care, new medications, follow-up plan

Screen for elder abuse for example, Elder Abuse Suspicion Index[82]

Occupational therapy evaluation or ability to perform ADLs

Vision/ability to safely take appropriate medications

Physical therapy evaluation or ambulatory assessment

Cognitive assessment

Medication reconciliation/review of Beers Criteria

---

been compiled by the American Geriatrics Society (AGS).[77] Some institutions have incorporated clinical support tools, such as medication order sets, which have shown substantial reduction in inappropriate prescribing.[78] ED-based pharmacists also can be a valuable resource.

Regarding falls, the AGS has recommended that all older adults who fall get a risk assessment. This includes, but is not limited to, medication review, visual acuity, ambulatory/gait evaluation, and assessment for postural hypotension.[3] This does not necessarily need to occur on the index ED visit. A patient's caregiver or primary care physician should be notified to ensure expeditious follow-up because up to 30% of patients fall again in 1 year, and up to 12% fall multiple times.[79] Although not possible in all EDs, a physical therapy evaluation when available can reduce ED revisits significantly.[79,80] Recently, a randomized controlled trial centered around a fall prevention program showed a number needed to treat of 3 to prevent revisits, 6 to prevent recurrent falls, and 9 to prevent a hospitalization. This program was centered around EP, pharmacist, and physical therapist evaluation.[81]

SUMMARY

In summary, there are several considerations in the care of the geriatric trauma population. Recognition of physiologic and vital sign differences, prompt evaluation and diagnostic imaging, and timely consultations for definitive management decrease the mortality of the geriatric trauma patient. Finally, a comprehensive evaluation of medication safety, ambulatory function, and appropriate follow-up all are imperative and improve clinical outcomes.

CLINICS CARE POINTS

- EPs should familiarize themselves with the age-related physiologic changes common among older adults. Special consideration should be given to vital signs and medications that affect them.
- Early evaluation of the geriatric trauma patient, even with seemingly benign mechanisms, can save lives.
- Discharge after normal noncontrast head CT is sufficient for anticoagulated patients who are neurologically intact, have a therapeutic INR, or are on direct oral anticoagulants. Those with a supratherapeutic INR require at minimum further observation.
- Cessation of anticoagulation likely is unnecessary following an ED visit for head injury. Consideration should be given to the reason for the patient being anticoagulated and the risk/benefits of cessation versus bleeding from future trauma.

- C-collars should be removed after negative C-spine CT in the alert, neurologically intact patient. For patients with dementia, or other mental status changes, the data are less clear. The authors recommend discussion with the family regarding patient's wishes and risks/benefits of sedation for MRI versus diagnostic yield, if necessary.
- EPs should familiarize themselves with the list of medications to avoid in the elderly (Beers Criteria).
- Physical therapy evaluation of the geriatric patient after a fall, whether in the ED or on follow-up, is vital for the prevention of further injury.

DISCLOSURE

The authors have nothing to disclose.

REFERENCES

1. MacKenzie EJ, Morris JAJ, Smith GS, et al. Acute hospital costs of trauma in the united states: implications for regionalized systems of care. J Trauma Acute Care Surg 1990;30(9):1096–103.
2. Bonne S, Schuerer DJE. Trauma in the older adult: epidemiology and evolving geriatric trauma principles. Clin Geriatr Med 2013;29(1):137–50.
3. Huntzinger A. AGS releases guideline for prevention of falls in older persons - practice guidelines. Am Fam Physician 2010;82(1):81–2.
4. Trauma Facts - The American association for the surgery of trauma. Available at: https://www.aast.org/trauma-facts. Accessed June 23, 2020.
5. Zafar SN, Obirieze A, Schneider EB, et al. Outcomes of trauma care at centers treating a higher proportion of older patients: the case for geriatric trauma centers. J Trauma Acute Care Surg 2015;78(4):852–9.
6. DiMaggio C, Ayoung-Chee P, Shinseki M, et al. Traumatic injury in the United States: In-patient epidemiology 2000-2011. Injury 2016;47(7):1393–403.
7. Chang MC. National trauma data bank annual report. Chicago, IL: American College of Surgeons; 2016.
8. Eagles D, Godwin B, Cheng W, et al. A systematic review and meta-analysis evaluating geriatric consultation on older trauma patients. J Trauma Acute Care Surg 2020;88(3):446–53.
9. Friesendorff M, von McGuigan FE, Wizert A, et al. Hip fracture, mortality risk, and cause of death over two decades. Osteoporos Int 2016;10(7):2945–53.
10. Gubler KD, Davis R, Koepsell T, et al. Long-term survival of elderly trauma patients. Arch Surg 1997;132(9):1010–4.
11. Chen X, Mao G, Leng SX. Frailty syndrome: an overview. Clin Interv Aging 2014; 9:433–41.
12. Joseph B, Pandit V, Zangbar B, et al. Superiority of frailty over age in predicting outcomes among geriatric trauma patients: a prospective analysis. JAMA Surg 2014;149(8):766–72.
13. Llompart-Pou JA, Pérez-Bárcena J, Chico-Fernández M, et al. Severe trauma in the geriatric population. World J Crit Care Med 2017;6(2):99–106.
14. Thompson HJ, McCormick WC, Kagan SH. Traumatic brain injury in older adults: epidemiology, outcomes, and future implications. J Am Geriatr Soc 2006;54(10): 1590–5.
15. Singh S, Angus LD. Blunt cardiac injury. In: StatPearls. StatPearls Publishing; 2020. Available at: https://www.ncbi.nlm.nih.gov/books/NBK532267/. Accessed June 24, 2020.

16. Bergeron E, Lavoie A, Clas D, et al. Elderly trauma patients with rib fractures are at greater risk of death and pneumonia. J Trauma 2003;54(3):478–85.
17. Reske-Nielsen C, Medzon R. Geriatric trauma. Emerg Med Clin North Am 2016; 34(3):483–500.
18. Jacobs DG, Plaisier BR, Barie PS, et al. Practice management guidelines for geriatric trauma: the EAST practice management guidelines work group. J Trauma 2003;54(2):391–416.
19. Dams-O'Connor K, Cuthbert JP, Whyte J, et al. Traumatic brain injury among older adults at level I and II trauma centers. J Neurotrauma 2013;30(24):2001–13.
20. Rozzelle CJ, Wofford JL, Branch CL. Predictors of hospital mortality in older patients with subdural hematoma. J Am Geriatr Soc 1995;43:240–4.
21. Gardner RC, Dams-O'Connor K, Morrissey MR, et al. Geriatric traumatic brain injury: epidemiology, outcomes, knowledge gaps, and future directions. J Neurotrauma 2018;35(7):889–906.
22. O'Neill KM, Jean RA, Savetamal A, et al. When to admit to observation: predicting length of stay for anticoagulated elderly fall victims. J Surg Res 2020;250:156–60.
23. Donzé J, Clair C, Hug B, et al. Risk of falls and major bleeds in patients on oral anticoagulation therapy. Am J Med 2012;125(8):773–8.
24. Battle B, Sexton KW, Fitzgerald RT. Understanding the value of repeat head CT in elderly trauma patients on anticoagulant or antiplatelet therapy. J Am Coll Radiol 2018;15(2):319–21.
25. Gage BF, Birman-Deych E, Kerzner R, et al. Incidence of intracranial hemorrhage in patients with atrial fibrillation who are prone to fall. Am J Med 2005;118(6): 612–7.
26. Man-Son-Hing M, Nichol G, Lau A, et al. Choosing antithrombotic therapy for elderly patients with atrial fibrillation who are at risk for falls. Arch Intern Med 1999;159(7):677–85.
27. Ntaios G, Lip GYH, Makaritsis K, et al. CHADS$_2$, CHA$_2$S$_2$DS$_2$-VASc, and long-term stroke outcome in patients without atrial fibrillation. Neurology 2013;80(11): 1009–17.
28. Pisters R, Lane DA, Nieuwlaat R, et al. A novel user-friendly score (HAS-BLED) to assess 1-year risk of major bleeding in patients with atrial fibrillation: the euro heart survey. Chest 2010;138(5):1093–100.
29. Sadro CT, Sandstrom CK, Verma N, et al. Geriatric trauma: a radiologist's guide to imaging trauma patients aged 65 years and older. Radiographics 2015;35(4): 1263–85.
30. Hoffman JR, Mower WR, Wolfson AB, et al. Validity of a set of clinical criteria to rule out injury to the cervical spine in patients with blunt trauma. National emergency X-radiography utilization study group. N Engl J Med 2000;343(2):94–9.
31. Touger M, Gennis P, Nathanson N, et al. Validity of a decision rule to reduce cervical spine radiography in elderly patients with blunt trauma. Ann Emerg Med 2002;40(3):287–93.
32. Schoenfeld AJ, Bono CM, McGuire KJ, et al. Computed tomography alone versus computed tomography and magnetic resonance imaging in the identification of occult injuries to the cervical spine: a meta-analysis. J Trauma 2010;68(1): 109–14.
33. Malhotra A, Wu X, Kalra VB, et al. Utility of MRI for cervical spine clearance after blunt traumatic injury: a meta-analysis. Eur Radiol 2017;27(3):1148–60.
34. Patel MB, Humble SS, Cullinane DC, et al. Cervical spine collar clearance in the obtunded adult blunt trauma patient: a systematic review and practice

management guideline from the Eastern association for the surgery of trauma. J Trauma Acute Care Surg 2015;78(2):430–41.

35. Dehner C, Hartwig E, Strobel P, et al. Comparison of the relative benefits of 2 versus 10 days of soft collar cervical immobilization after acute whiplash injury. Arch Phys Med Rehabil 2006;87(11):1423–7.

36. Cantor JB, Lebwohl NH, Garvey T, et al. Nonoperative management of stable thoracolumbar burst fractures with early ambulation and bracing. Spine 1993; 18(8):971–6.

37. Weerink LBM, Folbert EC, Kraai M, et al. Thoracolumbar spine fractures in the geriatric fracture center: early ambulation leads to good results on short term and is a successful and safe alternative compared to immobilization in elderly patients with two-column vertebral fractures. Geriatr Orthop Surg Rehabil 2014; 5(2):43–9.

38. Brasel KJ, Guse CE, Layde P, et al. Rib fractures: relationship with pneumonia and mortality. Crit Care Med 2006;34(6):1642–6.

39. Coary R, Skerritt C, Carey A, et al. New horizons in rib fracture management in the older adult. Age Ageing 2020;49(2):161–7.

40. Bulger EM, Arneson MA, Mock CN, et al. Rib fractures in the elderly. J Trauma 2000;48(6):1040–7.

41. Flagel BT, Luchette FA, Reed RL, et al. Half-a-dozen ribs: the breakpoint for mortality. Surgery 2005;138(4):717–25.

42. Fitzgerald MT, Ashley DW, Abukhdeir H, et al. Rib fracture fixation in the 65 years and older population: a paradigm shift in management strategy at a Level I trauma center. J Trauma Acute Care Surg 2017;82(3):524–7.

43. Da Costa J-P, Laing J, Kong VY, et al. A review of geriatric injuries at a major trauma centre in South Africa. S Afr Med J 2020;110(1):44–8.

44. McGillicuddy EA, Schuster KM, Kaplan LJ, et al. Contrast-induced nephropathy in elderly trauma patients. J Trauma 2010;68(2):294–7.

45. Hinson JS, Ehmann MR, Fine DM, et al. Risk of acute kidney injury after intravenous contrast media administration. Ann Emerg Med 2017;69(5):577–86.e4.

46. Kozar RA, Arbabi S, Stein DM, et al. Injury in the aged: geriatric trauma care at the crossroads. J Trauma Acute Care Surg 2015;78(6):1197–209.

47. Brox WT, Roberts KC, Taksali S, et al. The American academy of orthopaedic surgeons evidence-based guideline on management of hip fractures in the elderly. J Bone Joint Surg Am 2015;97:1196.

48. Schnell S, Friedman SM, Mendelson DA, et al. The 1-year mortality of patients treated in a hip fracture program for elders. Geriatr Orthop Surg Rehabil 2010; 1(1):6–14.

49. Kochar A, Chen AY, Sharma PP, et al. Long-term mortality of older patients with acute myocardial infarction treated in US clinical practice. J Am Heart Assoc 2018;7(13):e007230.

50. Fu MC, Boddapati V, Gausden EB, et al. Surgery for a fracture of the hip within 24 hours of admission is independently associated with reduced short-term postoperative complications. Bone Joint J 2017;99-B(9):1216–22.

51. Bretherton CP, Parker MJ. Early surgery for patients with a fracture of the hip decreases 30-day mortality. Bone Joint J 2015;97-B(1):104–8.

52. Pincus D, Ravi B, Wasserstein D, et al. Association between wait time and 30-day mortality in adults undergoing hip fracture surgery. JAMA 2017;318(20): 1994–2003.

53. Henry SM, Pollak AN, Jones AL, et al. Pelvic fracture in geriatric patients: a distinct clinical entity. J Trauma 2002;53(1):15–20.

54. Parker MJ. Missed hip fractures. Arch Emerg Med 1992;9(1):23–7.
55. Cabarrus MC, Ambekar A, Lu Y, et al. MRI and CT of insufficiency fractures of the pelvis and the proximal femur. Am J Roentgenol 2008;191(4):995–1001.
56. de Vries R, Reininga IHF, Pieske O, et al. Injury mechanisms, patterns and outcomes of older polytrauma patients-An analysis of the dutch trauma registry. PLoS One 2018;13(1):e0190587.
57. Hung KK, Yeung JHH, Cheung CSK, et al. Trauma team activation criteria and outcomes of geriatric trauma: 10 year single centre cohort study. Am J Emerg Med 2019;37(3):450–6.
58. Wiles LL, Day MD. Delta alert: expanding gerotrauma criteria to improve patient outcomes. J Trauma Nurs 2018;25(3):159–64.
59. Fernandez FB, Ong A, Martin AP, et al. Success of an expedited emergency department triage evaluation system for geriatric trauma patients not meeting trauma activation criteria. Open Access Emerg Med 2019;11:241–7.
60. Hammer PM, Storey AC, Bell T, et al. Improving geriatric trauma outcomes: a small step toward a big problem. J Trauma Acute Care Surg 2016;81(1):162–7.
61. Fallon WFJ, Rader E, Zyzanski S, et al. Geriatric outcomes are improved by a geriatric trauma consultation service. J Trauma Acute Care Surg 2006;61(5):1040–6.
62. Bowman J, George N, Barrett N, et al. Acceptability and reliability of a novel palliative care screening tool among emergency department providers. Acad Emerg Med 2016;23(6):694–702.
63. George N, Barrett N, McPeake L, et al. Content validation of a novel screening tool to identify emergency department patients with significant palliative care needs. Acad Emerg Med 2015;22(7):823–37.
64. Wu FM, Newman JM, Lasher A, et al. Effects of initiating palliative care consultation in the emergency department on inpatient length of stay. J Palliat Med 2013;16(11):1362–7.
65. Turnheim K. When drug therapy gets old: pharmacokinetics and pharmacodynamics in the elderly. Exp Gerontol 2003;38(8):843–53.
66. Weiner DK, Rudy TE. Attitudinal barriers to effective treatment of persistent pain in nursing home residents. J Am Geriatr Soc 2002;50(12):2035–40.
67. Rajan J, Behrends M. Acute pain in older adults: recommendations for assessment and treatment. Anesthesiol Clin 2019;37(3):507–20.
68. Mian P, Allegaert K, Spriet I, et al. Paracetamol in older people: towards evidence-based dosing? Drugs Aging 2018;35(7):603–24.
69. Rannou F, Pelletier J-P, Martel-Pelletier J. Efficacy and safety of topical NSAIDs in the management of osteoarthritis: evidence from real-life setting trials and surveys. Semin Arthritis Rheum 2016;45(4 Suppl):S18–21.
70. Motov S, Mann S, Drapkin J, et al. Intravenous subdissociative-dose ketamine versus morphine for acute geriatric pain in the Emergency department: a randomized controlled trial. Am J Emerg Med 2019;37(2):220–7.
71. Shah A, Hayes CJ, Martin BC. Factors influencing long-term opioid use among opioid naive patients: an examination of initial prescription characteristics and pain etiologies. J Pain 2017;18(11):1374–83.
72. Mann C, Pouzeratte Y, Eledjam J-J. Postoperative patient-controlled analgesia in the elderly: risks and benefits of epidural versus intravenous administration. Drugs Aging 2003;20(5):337–45.
73. Hanks RK, Pietrobon R, Nielsen KC, et al. The effect of age on sciatic nerve block duration. Anesth Analg 2006;102(2):588–92.

74. Greenberg SE, VanHouten JP, Lakomkin N, et al. Does admission to medicine or orthopaedics impact a geriatric hip patient's hospital length of stay? J Orthop Trauma 2016;30(2):95–9.
75. Chuang CH, Pinkowsky GJ, Hollenbeak CS, et al. Medicine versus orthopaedic service for hospital management of hip fractures. Clin Orthop Relat Res 2010; 468(8):2218–23.
76. Britt DMI, Day GS. Over-prescribed medications, under-appreciated risks: a review of the cognitive effects of anticholinergic medications in older adults. Mo Med 2016;113(3):207–14.
77. Croke L. Beers criteria for inappropriate medication use in older patients: an update from the AGS. Am Fam Physician 2020;101(1):56–7.
78. Stevens M, Hastings SN, Markland AD, et al. Enhancing quality of provider practices for older adults in the emergency department (EQUiPPED). J Am Geriatr Soc 2017;65(7):1609–14.
79. O'Loughlin JL, Robitaille Y, Boivin JF, et al. Incidence of and risk factors for falls and injurious falls among the community-dwelling elderly. Am J Epidemiol 1993; 137(3):342–54.
80. Lesser A, Israni J, Kent T, et al. Association between physical therapy in the emergency department and emergency department revisits for older adult fallers: a nationally representative analysis. J Am Geriatr Soc 2018;66(11):2205–12.
81. Goldberg EM, Resnik L, Marks SJ, et al. GAPcare: the geriatric acute and post-acute fall prevention intervention-a pilot investigation of an emergency department-based fall prevention program for community-dwelling older adults. Pilot Feasibility Stud 2019;5:106.
82. Yaffe MJ, Wolfson C, Lithwick M, et al. Development and validation of a tool to improve physician identification of elder abuse: the elder abuse suspicion index (EASI). J Elder Abuse Negl 2008;20(3):276–300.

Resuscitation of the Critically Ill Older Adult

Kami M. Hu, MD[a,b,]*, Robert M. Brown, MD[c]

KEYWORDS

- Geriatrics • Shock • Resuscitation • Critical care • Goals of care

KEY POINTS

- Adults older than 65 years represent an increasing proportion of the population that is at increased risk of critical illness and death.
- Due to the physiologic changes of aging, the presentation of critical illness varies in the older population, as do the goal metrics of successful resuscitation.
- Although age does not limit clinical outcomes, comorbidities and poor functional status can. The most appropriate management provides the care that best incorporates prognosis with the patient's personal goals of care.

EPIDEMIOLOGY OF CRITICAL ILLNESS IN OLDER ADULTS

There is no agreement as to when old age begins, but the widely accepted age for the purposes of research and epidemiologic tracking is 65 years. It is predicted that 83.7 million Americans, one-fifth of the population, will be older than 65 in 2050.[1] The mortality and complexity of disease in this cohort is significant. Intensive care unit (ICU) utilization in the United States by patients 65 and older has increased in the past 20 years,[2] with an increasing proportion of admissions in patients 85 and older.[3] In Europe, the overall median age of ICU patients is already 65 years[4] and even older in surgical ICUs.[5] The number of medical comorbidities increases from an average 2.6 (SD 2.09) in the 65-year to 84-year age range to 3.62 (SD 2.30) in the 85 years and older cohort.[6] Comorbidities combined with age, sex, and type of admission are predictive of mortality,[7] and mortality increases with age in the ICU independent of illness severity and treatment intensity.[8]

[a] Department of Emergency Medicine, University of Maryland School of Medicine, 110 South Paca Street, 6th Floor, Suite 200, Baltimore, MD 21201, USA; [b] Department of Internal Medicine, University of Maryland School of Medicine, 110 South Paca Street, 6th Floor, Suite 200, Baltimore, MD 21201, USA; [c] Department of Emergency Medicine, Virginia Tech Carilion School of Medicine, Carilion Roanoke Memorial Hospital, 1906 Belleview Ave SE, Roanoke, VA 24014, USA
* Corresponding author. Department of Emergency Medicine, University of Maryland School of Medicine, 110 South Paca Street, 6th Floor, Suite 200, Baltimore, MD 21201.
E-mail address: khu@som.umaryland.edu
Twitter: @kwhomd (K.M.H.)

Emerg Med Clin N Am 39 (2021) 273–286
https://doi.org/10.1016/j.emc.2020.12.001
0733-8627/21/© 2020 Elsevier Inc. All rights reserved.

PHYSIOLOGY OF AGING AND CRITICAL ILLNESS

The natural changes that occur during the normal aging process put the older patient at risk for higher severity of illness due to a decreased ability to tolerate and respond to said illness. The exact mechanism for these changes and the reasons for the variation in age at which different patients experience them is unclear, but leading theories involve an interplay between genetic predisposition and free radical damage.[9]

Cardiovascular

The cardiovascular system undergoes a great deal of change that, unsurprisingly, has downstream effects in the response to critical illness as well as to the resuscitation delivered. Advancing age is an inherent risk factor for the development of cardiovascular disease; arteriosclerosis contributes to hypertension and secondary decreases in left ventricular compliance due to hypertrophy.[10] Conduction abnormalities increase as myocytes decrease and undergo fibrotic changes, and the heart becomes less responsive to sympathetic drive, becoming inherently less able to mount compensatory heart rate increases to improve cardiac output. Myocyte hypertrophy and fibrosis lead to impaired relaxation and diastolic dysfunction, so although the older heart is more reliant on preload, it is also less tolerant of overaggressive fluid resuscitation and is at higher risk for development of pulmonary edema.[10,11] Older patients have higher incidences of cardiac arrhythmia[12] and coronary artery disease,[13] placing them at risk for secondary decompensation even if their primary disease process is not cardiac in nature, and contributing to an overall decreased cardiac reserve.

Pulmonary

The aging body seems primed for respiratory failure, with various components of the pulmonary system degrading with age. Increasing kyphosis causes decreased chest wall compliance while respiratory muscles weaken. Changes to the lung parenchyma (loss of elasticity, alveolar dilatation, and small airway collapse) decrease surface area for gas exchange and complete the trifecta responsible for decreased maximal inspiratory and expiratory flows, decreased oxygen tension, and ventilation-perfusion mismatch.[14] Older adults have decreased chemoreceptor sensitivity to hypoxia and hypercapnia, and with their decreased reserve can decompensate rapidly.[14] Immunosenescence and decreased mucociliary clearance, often accompanied by impaired swallowing, increases risk and incidence of aspiration in this population.[15]

Renal

The renal system also undergoes age-related decline, with the onset and extent of said decline depending on genetics, gender, and medical comorbidity.[16] With aging, there is a decrease in glomerular filtration rate (GFR) due loss of functioning nephrons secondary to glomerular sclerosis, as well as alterations in glomerular pressure and renal blood flow due to increased vascular resistance. This decrease in GFR may not be readily evident, as a decreased overall muscle mass results in a lower serum creatinine. Decreased renal tubular function and decreased renin-angiotensin-aldosterone system activity lead to a decreased ability to regulate fluid, electrolytes, and acid-base balance. Older, relatively healthy individuals may, despite decreases in GFR, still have relatively intact renal function at baseline, but functional reserve is markedly reduced[16] and results of dysfunction in critical illness can be life-limiting.

Hepatic, Endocrine, Neurologic, Immunologic

Other organ systems undergo changes with advancing age as well. Although the cellular function of the liver is generally well-preserved, there is decreased activity of the cytochrome P450 system and decreased drug clearance.[17,18] Due to decreased hepatic flow, the liver has a lower tolerance for ischemia,[17] such as that experienced in shock. There is an overall decreased basal metabolic rate, and older patients are at higher risk for development of hypothyroidism and diabetes.[19] The brain's autoregulation of cerebral perfusion is diminished,[20] leading to increased sensitivity to acute changes and extremes of blood pressure. There is inherent neurocognitive degeneration with aging,[21] and older patients have a higher risk of delirium, which is associated with increased mortality.[22] The immunosenescence of aging leads to an impaired antibody and cellular response to infections, and poor nutrition status worsens immune function and otherwise hinders the aging body's ability to recuperate from severe illness, leading to increased mortality.[23]

MANAGEMENT OF SHOCK IN THE OLDER ADULT
Shock Assessment

Frank hypotension is an obvious clue to the presence of a potential shock state, but critical illness can be present without marked vital sign abnormalities. Clinicians should be aware of alterations in potential presenting features of critical illness and decreased perfusion in older adult so as not to miss occult shock or impending decompensation (**Table 1**).

Initial Steps

Although critically ill patients usually receive simultaneous interventions, initial steps should follow the standard "C-A-B" algorithm, actively working to stabilize hypotensive patients to optimize hemodynamics and avoid peri-intubation cardiac arrest should an emergent intubation be indicated. Large-bore intravenous (IV) access is ideal for resuscitation, both for rapidity of fluid infusion and for peripheral vasopressor use. Multiple IVs are usually necessary for infusion of all the medications and therapies needed.

A full set of laboratory tests should be obtained, including venous blood gas, lactate, complete blood count with differential, comprehensive metabolic panel, prothrombin time/international normalized ratio, and partial thromboplastin time, with consideration for troponin if an electrocardiogram indicates potential ischemia and fibrinogen if there is concern for disseminated intravascular coagulation. Blood cultures should be obtained for patients with unexplained hypotension or with apparent infection. Further investigation for the source of possible infection should be pursued via urinalysis and urine culture (via catheterized sample if the patient is altered) as well as chest radiograph and sputum culture if the patient is able to provide one. An endotracheal aspirate should be obtained in patients who are intubated. Additional diagnostics depend on patient presentation and etiology of shock. Emergency physicians should have a low threshold to obtain computed tomography imaging of the brain in patients with depressed mental status and should pursue more expansive imaging of additional organ systems if the patient is unable to provide history or react to examination.

Point-of-Care Ultrasound

In undifferentiated shock, bedside ultrasound or POCUS (point-of-care ultrasound) is a key diagnostic tool. Evaluation of the heart identifies ventricular dysfunction, right

Table 1
Shock assessment in the critically ill older adult

	Vital Signs		Physical Examination
Heart rate	• Compensatory tachycardia may be absent due to meds, heart disease	Mental status	• Altered mentation an underrecognized sign of shock[31,32] • CAM-ICU improves delirium detection in the ED[32] (100% Sn, 98% Sp)
Blood pressure	• Chronic hypertension[24] may obscure relative hypotension • Shock index is a good early indicator of acuity[25] and mortality risk[26,27]	Capillary refill time	• Detects hypoperfusion (>3 s) and can guide resuscitation • Predicts mortality[33,34]
Respiratory rate	• Baseline respiratory rate higher than average adult[28] • Further tachypnea indicative of illness[28]	Skin	• Higher skin mottling scores a strong predictor of mortality[35,36] • Improvement in mottling with resuscitation linked to better outcomes[35,36]
Temperature	• Lower baseline temperatures[29] • 1/3 of patients afebrile despite infection[30]	Urine output	• Decrease in urine output a sign of renal injury and marker of mortality[37]

Abbreviations: CAM-ICU, confusion assessment method for the intensive care unit; ED, emergency department; Sn, sensitivity; Sp, specificity.

heart strain from massive pulmonary embolism (PE), valvular insufficiency, tamponade, or hypovolemia. The remainder of the RUSH (Rapid Ultrasound in Shock and Hypotension) examination can identify tension pneumothorax, intraperitoneal hemorrhage, or aortic pathology.[38]

Ultrasound can and should be used to guide resuscitation.[39] Although there are many methods to assess volume responsiveness, one of the best validated is stroke volume and cardiac output calculated via the velocity time integral (VTI) of the left ventricular outflow tract (LVOT). The accuracy of LVOT-VTI has been confirmed by correlation with invasive monitoring by pulmonary artery catheter intermittent thermodilution,[40] and measurements of pre-passive and post-passive leg raise LVOT-VTI is a quick, validated way to assess for IV fluid responsiveness.[41] In cases in which the LVOT cannot be visualized, carotid VTI measurement for carotid blood flow has also been validated.[42] It should be noted that there are currently no studies specifically investigating resuscitative ultrasound in older patients, and most studies have an average age range from 53 to 69 years.[41]

Dynamic assessments should be chosen over static assessments of volume responsiveness. Volume tolerance assessed via pulse wave Doppler of the hepatic,[43] portal,[44] or internal jugular[45] circulation is possible but interpretability depends on the experience of the sonographer.

Hypovolemic Shock

Older patients with hypovolemic shock should be resuscitated with crystalloid or blood products as appropriate. Given the greater difficulty in maintaining appropriate acid-base balance in older adults,[16] balanced solutions such as plasmalyte or lactated Ringer's, rather than normal saline, should be used when able to avoid contribution to or development of hyperchloremic metabolic acidosis and further renal dysfunction.[46] The emergency physician should use cardiac POCUS or prior echocardiographic documentation to determine if right heart strain, diastolic dysfunction, or reduced ejection fraction necessitate a slower infusion to prevent exacerbating heart failure or precipitating pulmonary edema.

Patients with hemorrhagic shock should be transfused with whole blood (packed red blood cells, plasma, platelets) in 1:1:1 fashion,[47] preferably by activating a prearranged massive transfusion protocol, while working toward emergent, definitive hemorrhage control.[47–49] Crystalloid infusions should be strongly avoided, if possible, to prevent hemodilution and hypothermia, both of which worsen coagulopathy.[50] Reversing therapeutic anticoagulation using the appropriate reversal agents is necessary; in immediately life-threatening hemorrhage associated with anticoagulation, prothrombin complex concentrate should be given emergently.

Depending on the etiology, permissive hypotension should be allowed to avoid disrupting fragile clots only until definitive source control can be obtained. Data extrapolated from trauma research demonstrate benefits to targeting lower systolic (>70–80 mm Hg) and mean arterial pressures (>50 mm Hg) in cases of hemorrhagic shock,[51] and the Society for Vascular Surgery recommends targeting systolic pressures of 70 to 90 mm Hg in cases of ruptured abdominal aortic aneurysm.[52] Although analyses using data from the National Trauma Data Bank National Sample Program indicate that presenting systolic blood pressures less than 110 mm Hg are associated with increased mortality rates in patients older than 60 years,[53] a later study did not find evidence of interaction between age and initial blood pressure on mortality.[54] Prompt, definitive hemostasis remains key to prevent prolonged hypoperfusion to organ systems and to improve outcomes regardless of age.

The appropriate hemoglobin transfusion goals in nonbleeding older patients is debated. The current recommendation remains to target a goal hemoglobin level greater than 7 g/dL based on critical care literature supporting this practice,[55,56] but it is worth noting that a more recent meta-analysis examining non–critically ill, mostly postsurgical patients older than 65 years found a mortality benefit with a more liberal transfusion strategy[57] and further investigation is needed.

Cardiogenic Shock

There are much higher incidences of primary cardiac illness, such as heart block or myocardial infarction (MI) in older adults. Roughly 6.5 million US adults have heart failure,[58] an increasing proportion of which have preserved ejection fraction.[59] When heart function is worsened or there is development of new heart failure secondary to an acute insult such as MI or PE, treatment of the underlying pathology with support of cardiac function is key and may require pharmacologic, electrical, or mechanical support. A cardiogenic component to shock can accompany other types of shock as well, as in stress cardiomyopathy.

Determining mixed shock states without ultrasound can be difficult. Mixed venous oxygen ($ScvO_2$) less than 70% from a superior vena cava central line or peripheral intravenous central catheter could be indicative of cardiogenic shock,[60] but may fail to detect the cardiac component in states of decreased oxygen requirement, such as neuromuscular blockade,[61] or high blood flow with decreased extraction, such as sepsis.[62] Likewise, it would be incorrect to assume cardiogenic shock in high-demand states such as after a seizure, in hypoxemic states such as acute respiratory distress syndrome (ARDS), or in the setting of severe anemia.[63]

Epinephrine at inotropic doses (0.01–0.05 μg/kg per hour) is generally recommended in the emergency department due to the easy titratability and vasoconstrictive effects of epinephrine, which can obviate the need for other vasopressors. Dobutamine and milrinone, while providing good inotropic effect, usually cause peripheral vasodilation that often requires the addition of norepinephrine. In the case of cardiogenic shock secondary to acute MI, norepinephrine is recommended over epinephrine due to higher incidence of refractory shock with epinephrine use.[64] Emergency physicians should be prepared for secondary arrhythmias arising from use of inotropic medications given their arrhythmogenicity[65] and the increased propensity of the older and critically ill populations to develop arrhythmias such as rapid atrial fibrillation or ventricular tachycardia.[12,66,67] In borderline hypotensive patients or those on vasopressors, the options to manage these rhythms are limited to relatively hemodynamically stable medications such as digoxin (for atrial fibrillation) or slow amiodarone bolus, or even electric cardioversion if hemodynamics are worsened.

Distributive Shock

In patients with distributive or septic shock, existing evidence supports the avoidance of overaggressive IV fluid resuscitation[68,69] and points to potential benefits with early administration of vasopressors.[70] Although the Surviving Sepsis Campaign guidelines make a general recommendation for a mean arterial pressure goal of 65 mm Hg or greater in septic shock,[71] the recent 65 Trial indicates that a lower goal of 60 mm Hg may be a safe alternative in patients older than 65 years.[72]

Additional IV fluid administration after an initial bolus should ideally be given only if patients demonstrate fluid responsiveness by passive leg raise and ultrasound[41] or by pulse pressure variability.[73] Although the Surviving Sepsis Guidelines suggest following the lactate levels to determine additional need for crystalloid,[71] a large, multicenter, randomized controlled trial found that lactate was no better than capillary refill to gauge resuscitation, and the cohort relying on lactate clearance demonstrated a trend toward worsened mortality.[34] Lactate-based fluid resuscitation often leads to excessive IV fluid administration, a practice increasingly linked to either no improvement[74] or harm.[75] Elevated lactate is associated with greater mortality, but because it rises with beta-adrenergic stimulation,[76] its failure to clear is an indicator of ongoing stress, often independent from volume resuscitation status.[77]

Current guidelines in septic shock call for early source control, appropriate antibiotics, and norepinephrine as the first-line vasopressor, vasopressin as a second-line agent, and stress dose steroids considered in cases of refractory shock.[71] Older age by itself is not a contraindication to surgical intervention; however, if the patient's comorbidities and acute illness make them a poor surgical candidate, a frank discussion with the patient and family should be had regarding alternative options such as potential interventional radiology involvement.

MANAGEMENT OF RESPIRATORY FAILURE IN THE OLDER ADULT

Standard management of respiratory failure should be pursued in older patients with escalation from supplemental oxygen to high-flow nasal cannula to noninvasive ventilation, and finally to invasive mechanical ventilation as appropriate, depending on the level of oxygenation and ventilatory support needed and the patient's advance

Table 2
Difficulties associated with intubation in the older patient

Physiology	Significance	Mitigation Strategy
Increased incidence of poor dentition, edentulousness[78]	Increased risk of dental injury/ aspiration Poor seal with bag-valve-mask	Consider leaving dentures in during bagging (with care to avoid aspiration and removal before laryngoscopy)
Decreased muscle mass[78]	Poor seal with bag-valve-mask	
Decreased hypoepiglottic ligament integrity[79]	Floppier epiglottis, more difficult to "lift" during DL	Consider using Miller blade for DL or hyperangulated blade with VL
Cervical spine arthritis and/or prior fusion[78]	Limited atlantooccipital joint extension for vocal cord visualization	Use VL or FB as primary method[78]
Decreased:[14] • Baseline oxygen tension • Chemoreceptor sensitivity • Functional reserve • Chest wall compliance	More effort to preoxygenate Faster desaturation when apneic	Use apneic oxygenation[80] • Stable saturations: maintain level of respiratory support (NIV, HFNC)[81] until RSI • Refractory hypoxia: escalate to NIV[a] for preoxygenation[81] until RSI or place SGD[82]
Higher Mallampati scores Decreased thyromental distance	Difficult vocal cord visualization	Have backup airway adjuncts (eg, bougie, VL) ready[78]

Abbreviations: DL, direct laryngoscopy; FB, fiberoptic bronchoscopy; HFNC, high-flow nasal cannula; NIV, noninvasive ventilation; RSI, rapid sequence induction; SGD, supraglottic device; VL, video laryngoscopy.
[a] If not contraindicated.

directives. Should intubation be necessary, the emergency physician should be aware of inherent difficulties and have a plan for their management (**Table 2**).

Rapid sequence induction (RSI) is generally safe in older patients[83,84] as long as hemodynamics are stabilized before induction. Etomidate, a commonly used medication touted for its hemodynamically stable profile, can still cause or exacerbate hypotension in under-resuscitated patients,[85] and using half the standard dose (0.15 mg/kg rather than 0.3 mg/kg) should be considered. A similar dose adjustment is recommended with propofol, which is known to have hypotensive and negative inotropic effects. Ketamine has been demonstrated to be as safe as or safer than etomidate in critically ill patients requiring intubation,[86,87] owing to its positive effects on blood pressure via sympathomimetic effect. This sympathetic activity also includes, however, secondary tachycardia, which can worsen arrhythmias or cause increased myocardial demand and potential ischemia in the elderly heart. It should be noted that in patients with refractory shock and catecholamine-depleted states, the administration of ketamine can lead to cardiovascular collapse.[88,89]

After intubation, ventilator settings should be adjusted to lower the fraction of inspired oxygen (Fio_2) to less than 60% as soon as possible to avoid oxygen toxicity. An initial positive end-expiratory pressure (PEEP) setting of 5 to 8 cmH_2O is reasonable, with a higher range (8–12 cmH2O, for example) for obese patients. Higher PEEP strategies targeting lower driving pressures are recommended as the starting point for patients with moderate to severe ARDS, but these recommendations are conditional on maintaining plateau pressures less than 30 cmH_2O.[90,91] In general, lung protective ventilation strategies per the ARDSNet trial are also recommended[92] although the more recent PReVENT trial supports the safety of intermediate tidal volumes in patients without ARDS,[93] which would be preferable to inducing heavy sedation for the sole purpose of ventilator synchrony.

ADVANCE DIRECTIVES AND GOALS OF CARE

Older patients may request limits on invasive life-prolonging treatments. In one study of octogenarians living independently, more than a quarter refused noninvasive positive pressure ventilation, nearly half declined invasive mechanical ventilation, and 63% declined renal replacement therapy after intubation.[94] Early identification of advance directives in the critically ill older patient is crucial for physicians to determine appropriate management strategies going forward.

If predefined advance directives do not exist, it is important to learn what level of personal function and capability would be in line with their priorities should they survive. Focusing on the patient's wishes unburdens family members and directs the conversation toward concrete goals rather than vague possibilities. An informed determination by the medical team as to whether reaching the desired goal is likely and whether it will involve immediate or future invasive interventions, possible ventilator dependence, or prolonged institutionalization can inform patient and family decision making. If the prognosis is not apparent, it remains imperative that the discussion is at least initiated to ensure that care going forward continues to center on the patient's ultimate happiness and personal goals of care.

When discussing treatment plans, it is important that they are not characterized as "doing everything" versus providing less care, but rather that the team's maximum effort will be made to achieve the patient's personal goals, whether the goal is to live as long as possible or to die with comfort prioritized. There should be no judgment of which goals of care are appropriate, but it is the physician's responsibility to communicate which goals are unattainable.

SUMMARY

Older patients make up an increasing portion of the population and have both a physiologic predisposition to illness and comorbidities that increase the odds of critical illness and death. The presentation of acute severe illness may be subtle and special attention must be paid to changes in mental status, the shock index, capillary refill time, and tachypnea to detect critical illness and intervene early. Resuscitation should be guided by frequent physical reassessment augmented by ultrasound and an understanding of aging physiology. Patients' advanced directives and personal goals of care should be sought early, with guidance offered to patients and their families regarding the risks and long-term effects of intensive care.

CLINICS CARE POINTS

- Advance directives and goals of care should be discussed early, basing the focus of care on the patient's wishes for themselves.
- The lack of fever, tachycardia, hypotension, or severe pain is unhelpful to rule out acute severe illness. Assessment of mental status, the shock index, and capillary refill time are better indicators of perfusion status and potential shock state.
- Management of the various shock states is *generally* the same; geriatric patients are at higher risk for pulmonary edema and arrhythmias in response to fluid resuscitation and intravenous catecholamines, and may require less aggressive options if they are too sick for otherwise-recommended surgical intervention.
- Aggressive fluid resuscitation for shock should be neither proscriptive nor solely based on lactate clearance. Use additional markers of perfusion and POCUS to determine need for additional IV fluids versus peripheral vasopressor or inotrope administration.
- Older patients have a decreased functional reserve and can rapidly decompensate to respiratory failure, with inherent roadblocks to successful intubation. Anticipation of these roadblocks with ready mitigation strategies is key.
- The standard medications for RSI are generally safe in older patients, but decreased dosing of sedative agents is recommended and patients should be hemodynamically stabilized as much as possible before RSI is initiated.

DISCLOSURE

The authors have nothing to disclose.

REFERENCES

1. Ortman JM, Velkoff VA, Hogan H. An aging nation: the older population in the United States. Current Population Reports. US Department of Commerce, Economics and Statistics Administration. US Census Bureau; May 2014. Report P25–1140. Available at: https://www.census.gov/library/publications/2014/demo/p25-1140.html.
2. Laporte L, Hermetet C, Jouan Y, et al. Ten-year trends in intensive care admissions for respiratory infections in the elderly. Ann Intensive Care 2018;8(1):84.
3. Sjoding M, Prescott H, Wunsch H, et al. Longitudinal changes in ICU admissions among elderly patients in the United States. Crit Care Med 2016;44(7):1353–60.
4. Flaatten H, de Lange D, Artigas A, et al. The status of intensive care medicine research and a future agenda for very old patients in the ICU. Intensive Care Med 2017;43(9):1319–28.

5. Pearse R, Harrison D, James P, et al. Identification and characterisation of the high-risk surgical population in the United Kingdom. Crit Care 2006;10(3):R81.
6. Barnett K, Mercer S, Norbury M, et al. Epidemiology of multimorbidity and implications health care, research, and medical education: a cross sectional study. Lancet 2012;380(9836):37–43.
7. Stavem K, Hoel H, Skjaker S, et al. Charlson comorbidity index derived from chart review or administrative data: agreement and prediction of mortality in intensive care patients. Clin Epidemiol 2017;9:311–20.
8. Peigne V, Somme D, Guérot E, et al. Treatment intensity, age and outcome in medical ICU patients: results of a French administrative database. Ann Intensive Care 2016;6(1):7.
9. da Costa J, Vitorino R, Silva G, et al. A synopsis on aging—theories, mechanisms and future prospects. Ageing Res Rev 2016;29:90–112.
10. Cheitlin MD. Cardiovascular physiology-changes with aging. Am J Geriatr Cardiol 2003;12(1):9–13.
11. Oxenham H, Sharpe N. Cardiovascular aging and heart failure. Eur J Heart Fail 2003;5:427–34.
12. Mirza M, Strunets A, Shen WK, et al. Mechanisms of arrhythmias and conduction disorders in older adults. Clin Geriatr Med 2012;28(4):555–73.
13. Zoni-Berisso M, Lercari F, Carazza T, et al. Epidemiology of atrial fibrillation: European perspective. Clin Epidemiol 2014;6:213–20.
14. Janssens JP, Pache JC, Nicod LP. Physiological changes in respiratory function associated with ageing. Eur Respir J 1999;13(1):197–205.
15. Marik P. Aspiration pneumonitis and pneumonia: a clinical review. N Engl J Med 2001;344:665–72.
16. Gekle M. Kidney and aging – a narrative review. Exp Gerontol 2017;87(Pt B): 153–5.
17. McLean AJ, Le Couteur DG. Aging biology and geriatric clinical pharmacology. Pharmacol Rev 2004;56(2):163.
18. Sotaniemi EA, Arranto AJ, Pelkonen O, et al. Age and cytochrome P450-linked drug metabolism in humans: an analysis of 226 subjects with equal histopathologic conditions. Clin Pharmacol Ther 1997;61(3):331.
19. van den Beld AW, Kaufman JM, Zillikens MC, et al. The physiology of endocrine systems with ageing. Lancet Diabetes Endocrinol 2018;6(8):647–58.
20. Wagner M, Jurcoane A, Volz S, et al. Age-related changes of cerebral autoregulation: new insights with quantitative T2'-mapping and pulsed arterial spin-labeling MR imaging. AJNR Am J Neuroradiol 2012;33(11):2081–7.
21. Tam HM, Lam CL, Huang H, et al. Age-related difference in relationships between cognitive processing speed and general cognitive status. Appl Neuropsychol Adult 2015;22(2):94–9.
22. Eeles E, Hubbard R, White S, et al. Hospital use, institutionalisation, and mortality associated with delirium. Age Ageing 2010;39(4):470–5.
23. Tripathy S, Mishra JC, Dash SC. Critically ill elderly patients in a developing world - Mortality and functional outcome at 1 year: a prospective single-center study. J Crit Care 2014;29:474.e7-13.
24. Master A, Lasser R. The relationship of pulse pressure and diastolic pressure to systolic pressure in healthy subjects, 20-94 years of age. Am Heart J 1965;70(2): 163–71.
25. Berger T, Green J, Horeczko T, et al. Shock index and early recognition of sepsis in the emergency department: pilot study. West J Emerg Med 2013;14(2):168–74.

26. Chung JY, Hsu CC, Chen JH, et al. Shock index predicted mortality in geriatric patients with influenza in the emergency department. Am J Emerg Med 2019; 37(3):391–4.
27. Kim S, Hong K, Shin S, et al. Validation of the shock index, modified shock index, and age shock index for predicting mortality of geriatric trauma patients in emergency departments. J Korean Med Sci 2016;31(12):2026–32.
28. McFadden J, Price R, Eastwood H, et al. Raised respiratory rate in elderly patients: a valuable physical sign. Br Med J 1982;284(6316):626–7.
29. Roghmann MC, Warner J, Mackowiak PA. The relationship between age and fever magnitude. Am J Med Sci 2001;322(2):68–70.
30. Norman D. Fever in the elderly. Clin Infect Dis 2000;31(1):148–51.
31. Ely E, Siegel M, Inouye S. Delirium in the intensive care unit: an under-recognized syndrome of organ dysfunction. Semin Respir Crit Care Med 2001;22(2):115–26.
32. Van de Meeberg E, Festen S, Kwant M, et al. Improved detection of delirium, implementation and validation of the CAM-ICU in elderly emergency department patients. Eur J Emerg Med 2017;24(6):411–6.
33. Ait-Oufella H, Bige N, Boelle P, et al. Capillary refill time exploration during septic shock. Intensive Care Med 2014;40:958–64.
34. Hernández G, Ospina-Tascon G, Petri L, et al. Effect of a resuscitation strategy targeting peripheral perfusion status vs serum lactate levels on 28-day mortality among patients with septic shock. The ANDROMEDA-SHOCK randomized clinical trial. JAMA 2019;321(7):654–64.
35. Ait-Oufella H, Lemoinne S, Boelle P, et al. Mottling score predicts survival in septic shock. Intensive Care Med 2011;37(5):801–7.
36. Dumas G, Lavillegrand JR, Joffre J, et al. Mottling score is a strong predictor of 14-day mortality in septic patients whatever vasopressor doses and other tissue perfusion parameters. Crit Care 2019;23(1):211.
37. Jin K, Murugan R, Sileanu FE, et al. Intensive monitoring of urine output is associated with increased detection of acute kidney injury and improved outcomes. Chest 2017;152(5):972–9.
38. Ghane MR, Gharib M, Ebrahimi A, et al. Accuracy of early rapid ultrasound in shock (RUSH) examination performed by emergency physician for diagnosis of shock etiology in critically ill patients. J Emerg Trauma Shock 2015;8(1):5–10.
39. Cecconi M, De Backer D, Antonelli M, et al. Consensus on circulatory shock and hemodynamic monitoring. Task force of the European Society of Intensive Care Medicine. Intensive Care Med 2014;40(12):1795–815.
40. Mercado P, Maizel J, Beyls C, et al. Transthoracic echocardiography: an accurate and precise method for estimating cardiac output in the critically ill patient. Crit Care 2017;21:136.
41. Cherpanath T, Hirsch A, Geerts B, et al. Predicting fluid responsiveness by passive leg raising: a systematic review and meta-analysis of 23 clinical trials. Crit Care Med 2016;44(5):981–91.
42. Ma IWY, Caplin JD, Azad A, et al. Correlation of carotid blood flow and corrected carotid flow time with invasive cardiac output measurements. Crit Ultrasound J 2017;9(1):10.
43. Scheinfeld M, Bilali A, Koenigsberg M. Understanding the spectral Doppler waveform of the hepatic veins in health and disease. Radiographics 2009; 29(7):2081–98.
44. Denault A, Beaubien-Souligny W, Elmi-Sarabi M, et al. Clinical significance of portal hypertension diagnosed with bedside ultrasound after cardiac surgery. Anesth Analg 2017;124(4):1109–15.

45. Marr K, Jakimovski D, Mancini M, et al. Jugular venous flow quantification using doppler sonography. Ultrasound Med Biol 2018;44(8):1762–9.
46. Self W, Semler M, Wanderer JP, et al. Balanced crystalloids versus saline in non-critically ill adults. N Engl J Med 2018;378(9):819–28.
47. Holcomb JB, Tilley BC, Baraniuk S, et al. Transfusion of plasma, platelets, and red blood cells in a 1:1:1 vs a 1:1:2 ratio and mortality in patients with severe trauma: the PROPPR randomized clinical trial. JAMA 2015;313(5):471–82.
48. Lim G, Harper-Kirksey K, Parekh R, et al. Efficacy of a massive transfusion protocol for hemorrhagic trauma resuscitation. Am J Emerg Med 2018;36(7):1178–81.
49. Murry JS, Zaw AA, Hoang DM, et al. Activation of massive transfusion for elderly trauma patients. Am Surg 2015;81(10):945–9.
50. Beekley AC. Damage control resuscitation: a sensible approach to the exsanguinating surgical patient. Crit Care Med 2008;36(7 Suppl):S267–74.
51. Owattanapanich N, Chittawatanarat K, Benyakorn T, et al. Risks and benefits of hypotensive resuscitation in patients with traumatic hemorrhagic shock: a meta-analysis. Scand J Trauma Resusc Emerg Med 2018;26(1):107.
52. Chaikof EL, Dalman RL, Eskandari MK, et al. The Society for Vascular Surgery practice guidelines on the care of patients with an abdominal aortic aneurysm. J Vasc Surg 2018;67(1):2–77.e2.
53. Hranjec T, Sawyer RG, Young JS, et al. Mortality factors in geriatric blunt trauma patients: creation of a highly predictive statistical model for mortality using 50,765 consecutive elderly trauma admissions from the National Sample Project. Am Surg 2012;78(12):1369–75.
54. Bridges LC, Waibel BH, Newell MA. Permissive hypotension: potentially harmful in the elderly? a national trauma data bank analysis. Am Surg 2015;81(8):770–7.
55. Hébert P, Wells G, Blajchman M, et al. A multicenter, randomized, controlled clinical trial of transfusion requirements in critical care. N Engl J Med 1999;340:409–17.
56. Holst LB, Haase N, Wetterslev J, et al. Lower versus higher hemoglobin threshold for transfusion in septic shock. N Engl J Med 2014;371(5):1381–91.
57. Simon G, Craswell A, Thom O, et al. Outcomes of restrictive versus liberal transfusion strategies in older adults from nine randomized controlled trials: a systematic review and meta analysis. Lancet 2017;4(10):e465–74.
58. Benjamin E, Muntner P, Alonso A, et al. Heart disease and stroke statistics—2019 update: a report from the American Heart Association. Circulation 2019;139(10):e56–528.
59. Vasan R, Xanthakis V, Lyass A, et al. Epidemiology of left ventricular systolic dysfunction and heart failure in the Framingham Study: an echocardiographic study over 3 decades. JACC Cardiovasc Imaging 2018;11(1):1–11.
60. Muir A, Kirby B, King A, et al. Mixed venous oxygen saturation in relation to cardiac output in myocardial infarction. Br Med J 1970;4(5730):276–8.
61. Marik P, Kaufman D. The effects of neuromuscular paralysis on systemic and splanchnic oxygen utilization in mechanically ventilated patients. Chest 1996;109:1038–42.
62. Krafft P, Steltzer H, Hiesmayr M, et al. Mixed venous oxygen saturation in critically ill septic shock patients. The role of defined events. Chest 1993;103(3):900–6.
63. Hartog C, Bloos F. Venous oxygen saturation. Best Pract Res Clin Anaesthesiol 2014;28(4):419–28.
64. Levy B, Clere-Jehl R, Legras A, et al. Epinephrine versus norepinephrine for cardiogenic shock after acute myocardial infarction. J Am Coll Cardiol 2018;72:173–82.

65. Tisdale JE, Patel RV, Webb CR, et al. Proarrhythmic effects of intravenous vasopressors. Ann Pharmacother 1995;29(3):269–81.

66. Bosch NA, Cimini J, Walkey AJ. Atrial fibrillation in the ICU. Chest 2018;154(6): 1424–34.

67. Boriani G, Fauchier L, Aguinaga L, et al. European Heart Rhythm Association (EHRA) consensus document on management of arrhythmias and cardiac electronic devices in the critically ill and post-surgery patient, endorsed by Heart Rhythm Society (HRS), Asia Pacific Heart Rhythm Society (APHRS), Cardiac Arrhythmia Society of Southern Africa (CASSA), and Latin American Heart Rhythm Society (LAHRS). Europace 2019;21(1):7–8.

68. Hamzaoui O, Georger JF, Monnet X, et al. Early administration of norepinephrine increases cardiac preload and cardiac output in septic patients with life-threatening hypotension. Crit Care 2010;14(4):R142.

69. Marik P. Iatrogenic salt water drowning and the hazards of a high central venous pressure. Ann Intensive Care 2014;4:21.

70. Permpikul C, Tongyoo S, Viarasilpa T, et al. Early use of norepinephrine in septic shock resuscitation (CENSER). A randomized trial. Am J Respir Crit Care Med 2019;199(9):1097–105.

71. Levy MM, Evans LE, Rhodes A. The surviving sepsis campaign bundle: 2018 update. Crit Care Med 2018;46(6):997–1000.

72. Lamontagne F, Richards-Belle A, Thomas K, et al. Effect of reduced exposure to vasopressors on 90-day mortality in older critically ill patients with vasodilatory hypotension. JAMA 2020;323(10):938–49.

73. Teboul J, Monnet X, Chemla D, et al. Arterial pulse pressure variation with mechanical ventilation. Am J Respir Crit Care Med 2018;199(1):22–31.

74. Hjortrup P, Haase N, Bundgaard H, et al. Restricting volumes of resuscitation fluid in adults with septic shock after initial management: the CLASSIC randomised, parallel-group, multicentre feasibility trial. Intensive Care Med 2016;42(11): 1695–705.

75. Andrews B, Semler M, Muchemwa L, et al. Effect of an early resuscitation protocol on in-hospital mortality among adults with sepsis and hypotension: a randomized clinical trial. JAMA 2017;318(13):1233–40.

76. Levy B, Desebbe O, Montemont C, et al. Increased aerobic glycolysis through beta2 stimulation is a common mechanism involved in lactate formation during shock states. Shock 2008;30(4):417–21.

77. Spiegel R, Gordon D, Marik P. The origins of the lacto-bolo reflex: the mythology of lactate in sepsis. J Thorac Dis 2020;12(Suppl 1):S48–53.

78. Johnson KN, Botros DB, Groban L, et al. Anatomic and physiopathologic changes affecting the airway of the elderly patient: implications for geriatric-focused airway management. Clin Interv Aging 2015;10:1925–34.

79. Sawatsubashi M, Umezaki T, Kusano K, et al. Age-related changes in the hyoepiglottic ligament: functional implications based on histopathologic study. Am J Otolaryngol 2010;31(6):448–52.

80. Binks MJ, Holyoak RS, Melhuish TM, et al. Apneic oxygenation during intubation in the emergency department and during retrieval: a systematic review and meta-analysis. Am J Emerg Med 2017;35(10):1542–6.

81. Fong KM, Au SY, Ng GWY. Preoxygenation before intubation in adult patients with acute hypoxemic respiratory failure: a network meta-analysis of randomized trials. Crit Care 2019;23(1):319.

82. Wu C, Wei J, Cen Q, et al. Supraglottic jet oxygenation and ventilation-assisted fibre-optic bronchoscope intubation in patients with difficult airways. Intern Emerg Med 2017;12(5):667–73.

83. Theodosiou CA, Loeffler RE, Oglesby AJ, et al. Rapid sequence induction of anesthesia in elderly patients in the emergency department. Resuscitation 2011;82(7):881–5.

84. Imamura T, Brown CA III, Ofuchi H, et al. Emergency airway management in geriatric and younger patients: analysis of a multicenter prospective observational study. Am J Emerg Med 2013;31:190–6.

85. Benson M, Junger A, Fuchs C, et al. Use of an anesthesia information management system (AIMS) to evaluate the physiologic effects of hypnotic agents used to induce anesthesia. J Clin Monit Comput 2000;16(3):183–90.

86. Jabre P, Combes X, Lapostolle F, et al. Etomidate versus ketamine for rapid sequence intubation in acutely ill patients: a multicenter randomised controlled trial. Lancet 2009;374(9686):293–300.

87. Van Berkel MA, Exline MC, Cape KM, et al. Increased incidence of clinical hypotension with etomidate compared to ketamine for intubation in septic patients: A propensity matched analysis. J Crit Care 2017;38:209–14.

88. Waxman K, Shoemaker WC, Lippmann M. Cardiovascular effects of anesthetic induction with ketamine. Anesth Analg 1980;59(5):355–8.

89. Dewhirst E, Frazier W, Leder M, et al. Cardiac arrest following ketamine administration for rapid sequence intubation. J Intensive Care Med 2013;28(6):375–9.

90. Amato MB, Meade MO, Slutsky AS, et al. Driving pressure and survival in the acute respiratory distress syndrome. N Engl J Med 2015;372(8):747–55.

91. Fan E, Del Sorbo L, Goligher E, et al. An Official American Thoracic Society/European Society of Intensive Care Medicine/Society of Critical Care Medicine Clinical practice guideline: mechanical ventilation in adult patients with acute respiratory distress syndrome. Am J Respir Crit Care Med 2017;195(9):1253–63.

92. Acute Respiratory Distress Syndrome Network, Brower RG, Matthay MA, et al. Ventilation with lower tidal volumes as compared with traditional tidal volumes for acute lung injury and the acute respiratory distress syndrome. N Engl J Med 2000;342(18):1301–8.

93. Writing Group for the PReVENT Investigators, Simonis FD, Serpa Neto A, et al. Effect of a low vs intermediate tidal volume strategy on ventilator-free days in intensive care unit patients without ARDS: a randomized clinical trial. JAMA 2018;320(18):1872–80.

94. Philippart F, Vesin A, Bruel C, et al. The ETHICA study (Part 1): elderly's thoughts about intensive care unit admission for life-sustaining treatments. Intensive Care Med 2013;39(9):1565–73.

Rapid Fire

Acute Brain Failure in Older Emergency Department Patients

Debra Eagles, MD, MSc[a,b,c],*, Danya Khoujah, MBBS, MEHP[d,e,1]

KEYWORDS

- Emergency department • Delirium • Mental status • Screening • Infection
- Polypharmacy

KEY POINTS

- Delirium is common and associated with significant morbidity and mortality.
- Evaluate mental status in all older patients presenting to the emergency department; do not rely on gestalt—use a validated tool to assess for delirium.
- Obtain a thorough medication list (including over-the-counter medications), paying special attention to medications with anticholinergic properties.
- Utilize nonpharmacologic measures, such as reorientation and decreasing unfamiliar stimuli, for high-risk individuals to prevent and treat delirium.
- Consider using low-dose antipsychotics in agitated delirious patients who are at imminent risk of harm.

CASE

Mrs Penelope Jones, an 86-year-old woman, presents to the emergency department (ED) after falling. She is brought in by ambulance after being found on the floor in her apartment. Her past medical history includes hypertension, hypothyroidism, and remote stroke. Her medications include hydrochlorothiazide, levothyroxine, and clopidogrel.

On assessment, Mrs Jones is asleep in the bed. She rouses to voice and states she tripped on the carpet. She denies hitting her head. Her only complaint is right wrist

[a] Department of Emergency Medicine, University of Ottawa, Ottawa, Ontario, Canada; [b] School of Epidemiology and Public Health, University of Ottawa, Ottawa, Ontario, Canada; [c] Ottawa Hospital Research Institute, Ottawa, Ontario, Canada; [d] Emergency Medicine, MedStar Franklin Square Medical Center, 9000 Franklin Square Dr, Baltimore, MD 21237, USA; [e] Department of Emergency Medicine, University of Maryland School of Medicine, Baltimore, MD, USA
[1] Present address: 110 S Paca St, 6th Floor, Suite 200, Baltimore, MD 21201, USA
* Corresponding author. Epidemiology Program, The Ottawa Hospital, Civic Campus, F658a, 1053 Carling Avenue, Ottawa, Ontario K1Y 4E9, Canada.
E-mail address: deagles@toh.ca
Twitter: @DanyaKhoujah (D.K.)

Emerg Med Clin N Am 39 (2021) 287–305
https://doi.org/10.1016/j.emc.2020.12.002
0733-8627/21/© 2020 Elsevier Inc. All rights reserved.

pain. Further review of systems is unremarkable. Throughout the interview, she is noted to lose focus on the conversation, occasionally closing her eyes and requiring prompting to answer questions. Her physical examination is unremarkable aside from an obviously deformed right wrist. A radiograph is ordered and some collateral history gathered from Mrs Jones' daughter.

LEARNING POINTS
Definition of Delirium

The American Psychiatric Association *Diagnostic and Statistical Manual of Mental Disorders* (Fifth Edition) classifies delirium as a minor neurocognitive disorder.[1] To be diagnosed with delirium, a patient must meet the 5 criteria outlined in **Table 1**.

Delirium has been described using various phenotypes, including the psychomotor impact, arousal state, and severity. Psychomotor subtypes include hyperactive, hypoactive, or mixed.[1] Hypoactive is the most common, least likely to be identified,[2] and associated with worse outcomes in hospitalized patients.[3] Patients with delirium may exhibit increased, decreased, or normal level of arousal. Delirious older ED patients with normal levels of arousal have an increased risk of six-month mortality.[4] The measurement of delirium severity may be useful to monitor clinical course and treatment response.[5–7] Increased delirium severity is associated with increased mortality and subsequent cognitive impairment.[3,8,9]

Delirium Prevalence in the Emergency Department

Delirium is common in older patients presenting to the ED. Prevalence may be as high as 17%.[10–12] Literature consistently has shown that health care providers are poor at recognizing delirium in older ED patients despite the development of multiple validated tools to identify delirium over the past two decades.[11,13,14] A recent study showed that delirium was missed in 84.6% of older ED patients.[15] Up to 28% of patients with undiagnosed delirium are discharged home from the ED,[16–18] and, for those who are admitted, it remains unrecognized in the majority.[2]

Table 1 Diagnostic criteria for delirium	
Criteria A	A disturbance in attention (ie, reduced ability to direct, focus, sustain, and shift attention) and awareness (reduced orientation to the environment)
Criteria B	The disturbance develops over a short period of time (usually hours to a few days), represents a change from baseline attention and awareness, and tends to fluctuate in severity during the course of a day.
Criteria C	An additional disturbance in cognition (eg, memory deficit, disorientation, language, visuospatial ability, or perception)
Criteria D	The disturbances in criteria A and C are not better explained by another preexisting, established, or evolving neurocognitive disorder and do not occur in the context of a severely reduced level of arousal, such as coma
Criteria E	There is evidence from the history, physical examination, or laboratory findings that the disturbance is a direct physiologic consequence of another medical condition, substance intoxication or withdrawal (ie, due to a drug of abuse or to a medication), or exposure to a toxin, or is due to multiple etiologies.

Sequelae of Delirium

Delirium is an acute medical emergency. It has a devasting impact on patients, their families, and the health care system. Delirium in older ED patients is associated with an increase in hospital admission,[19] intensive care unit admission,[20] hospital length of stay,[18,20] likelihood of discharge to a higher level of care,[19–21] and death.[4,12,17,20,22] Delirium has been shown to cause significant psychological distress to patients and their families.[23,24] Additionally, the economic impact of delirium is huge; in 2011 it was estimated to be greater than $164 billion per year in the United States.[10,25]

Delirium results from acute brain failure; however, its sequelae may have more prolonged consequences than originally thought. There is mounting evidence that it results in adverse long-term outcomes. Delirium has been shown to persist up to twelve months[26] in up to 50% of patients and furthermore is known to be a risk factor for subsequent cognitive[8,21,27–29] and functional decline.[29–31]

Physiology/Pathophysiology of Delirium

Multiple hypotheses have been proposed regarding the pathophysiology of delirium, including neuronal aging; oxidative stress; neuroinflammatory, neuroendocrine, and neurotransmitter dysfunction; and circadian rhythm dysregulation.[6,32–34] The investigation of neurotransmitters and biomarkers that can validate the underlying basis of these theoretic models is an area of rapidly expanding research.[35–37] Advanced neuroimaging also may have a role to play in identifying structural abnormalities of the brain in patients suffering from delirium.[38,39]

Given the multiple proposed hypotheses, it is likely that delirium is the end result of multiple abnormalities that are unique to that individual, based on predisposing factors and precipitating insults.[32,40] The expression of delirium is as unique and variable as the pathophysiologic basis from which it arose in that specific individual.

PREDISPOSING FACTORS AND PRECIPITATING INSULTS FOR DELIRIUM

Predisposing Factors

Delirium occurs in vulnerable patients who possess underlying predisposing factors and subsequently are exposed to a precipitating insult. There are many underlying risk factors predisposing older patients to delirium development (**Table 2**). The most common predisposing factor is dementia, which is present in at least half of the patients presenting with delirium.[2]

Precipitating Insults

Precipitating insults are summarized in **Table 2**. The resultant delirium may be delayed by 24 hours or more and often is multifactorial.[10,41–43] The most common precipitating insult is infection, accounting for approximately 50% of presentations.[2,10] An underlying infection may be missed in older adults because they often present atypically and may lack a fever, leukocytosis, or localizing symptoms.[44–46]

Medications, whether prescribed or over the counter, are implicated in up to 30% of patients presenting with delirium.[41,47] Medications with anticholinergic properties are particularly deliriogenic.[42,48] Older adults are more susceptible to adverse drug events due to altered pharmacokinetics and pharmacodynamics; this is compounded by the presence of polypharmacy.[49] Commonly implicated medications are listed in **Table 3**. Alcohol use and illicit drug use are relatively common in older adults,[50] and intoxication and withdrawal syndromes should be considered as causes of delirium.

Table 2
Predisposing factors and precipitating insults in delirium[2,10,41,47,48,52]

Predisposing Factors	Precipitating Insults
Dementia	Infections, for example, UTI and pneumonia
Age	
Premorbid functional impairment	Medications and toxins
Visual or hearing impairment	Intracranial diseases, for example, stroke, meningitis/encephalitis, seizures, neoplasm, and hypertensive encephalopathy
Preexisting psychiatric illness (bipolar disorder, schizophrenia	
Underlying stroke or seizure disorder	
Chronic use of medications, for example, narcotics and benzodiazepines	Cardiovascular disease, for example, ACS and CHF
Alcohol or drug use disorder	Metabolic disorders, for example, electrolyte abnormalities, hepatic and uremic encephalopathy, and thiamine deficiency
	Endocrine disorders, for example, thyroid disorders and adrenal disorders
	Dehydration and malnutrition
	Iatrogenic, for example, prolonged ED stay, restraints, pain

Abbreviations: ACS, acute coronary syndrome; CHF, congestive heart failure; UTI, urinary tract infection.
Data from: Cheung ENM, Benjamin S, Heckman G, et al. Clinical characteristics associated with the onset of delirium among long-term nursing home residents. *BMC Geriatr.* 2018;18(1):39; and Canto JG, Rogers WJ, Goldberg RJ, et al. Association of age and sex with myocardial infarction symptom presentation and in-hospital mortality. *JAMA.* 2012;307(8):813-822.

Iatrogenic causes that precipitate delirium, in addition to medications, include prolonged ED length of stay (>10 hours),[51] use of physical restraints,[41] sleep deprivation, undergoing a procedure,[41] and under-treatment of pain.[52] Pain, which may result from an acute medical condition or injury, urinary retention, constipation, or hunger,[52] frequently is undertreated in the geriatric population.[53] Furthermore, eliciting the presence of pain may be challenging in patients with cognitive impairment, necessitating the utilization of a standardized scale, such as the Pain Assessment in Advanced Dementia.[54]

Clinician recognize that Mrs. Jones is vulnerable to delirium given her age and history of stroke. Clinician suspect that the pain from the fracture and the long wait in the ED may increase her risk. Clinician wonder what other elements of the history and physical examination are relevant and whether clinician should order any additional tests.

Table 3
Medication classes frequently implicated in delirium[47,48]

Antihistamines[a]	Muscle relaxants
Antiemetics	Opioids[a]
Dihydropyridines[a]	Sedative-hypnotics[a]
Diuretics	

[a] Highest risk.
Data from: Clegg A, Young JB. Which medications to avoid in people at risk of delirium: a systematic review. *Age Ageing.* 2011;40(1):23-29.

HISTORY

The clinician should use the interview as an opportunity to observe the patient's mental status. Many patients with altered mental status may deny the existence of a problem, whether due to lack of insight, stoicism, or fear of losing independence. Obtaining collateral history provides the clinician with a better understanding of a patient's baseline mental status, an appreciation for the time course and progression of the current illness, and clues to the precipitating insult(s). Obtaining an accurate medication list (including over-the-counter medications), in addition to recent changes or the possibility of an overdose, is essential.

PHYSICAL EXAMINATION
General Examination

Apparently normal vital signs should not falsely reassure the emergency practitioner, because fever, tachycardia, and hypotension may be attenuated in older adults despite being critically ill.[55] An accurate respiratory rate should be obtained, because tachypnea is the most sensitive vital sign for infection.[44]

Fully undressing patients is necessary to perform a thorough examination. Subtle signs of trauma should be sought out because history of injury may not be apparent, due to stoicism or elder abuse. A skin examination looking for signs of infection, medication patches, or indwelling catheters is prudent. Localizing signs of infection, such as abdominal tenderness[56] or neck stiffness,[57] may be absent and should not deter the astute emergency physician from pursuing the appropriate diagnosis.

Mental Status Evaluation

Multiple guidelines advocate for the evaluation of mental status in all older patients presenting to the ED to assess for the presence of delirium.[58–61] A complete mental status evaluation includes assessment of consciousness, perception (such as hallucinations and delusions), and cognition (orientation, attention, memory, executive function, language, and visuospatial ability).

MAKING THE DIAGNOSIS

More than twenty delirium screening tools have been developed; however, not all are suitable for the ED.[62] Several tools have been validated in the ED and are summarized in **Table 4**.[63,64] The Geriatric Emergency Department Guidelines, a research-based and consensus-based best practices report, advocates the use of the Delirium Triage Screen (DTS) and Brief Confusion Assessment Method (bCAM) for mental status evaluation.[58] Flowsheets, training manual, and videos can be accessed at http://eddelirium. org/delirium-assessment/dts/ and http://eddelirium.org/delirium-assessment/bcam/

Table 4	
Delirium screening tools validated in the emergency department[66]	
4AT	Modified CAM for the ED
Brief CAM	Month of the year backward test
CAM for the intensive care unit	Ottawa 3DY
Four-item Abbreviated Mental Test	RASS

Abbreviation: CAM, confusion assessment method.
Data from Refs.[96–102]

for the DTS and bCAM, respectively. Their diagnostic characteristics are presented in **Table 5**.

The DTS (**Fig. 1**) is highly sensitive (98%),[65] takes less than twenty seconds to administer, and does not require the use of additional instruments, making it ideal as a screening test to rule out delirium. It is composed of two parts: the Richmond Agitation-Sedation Scale (RASS) and spelling "lunch" backwards. The RASS (**Table 6**) is a ten-point scale that measures patient arousal.[66] The score is determined by observing a patient's response to verbal or physical stimulation. If a patient scores anything other than zero, then the patient screens positive for delirium. If the patient is alert and calm (RASS = 0), then the patient is asked to spell the word "lunch" backwards. If the patient is able to do so with only one error or less, then delirium has been ruled out and no further testing is required. If the screen is positive, the diagnosis of delirium should be confirmed with a highly specific formal test for delirium, such as the bCAM.

The bCAM (**Fig. 2**) was adapted from the confusion assessment method for the intensive care unit and contains the four cardinal features of delirium.[67] Its algorithmic approach, with objective questions to test inattention and disorganized thinking, makes it simple to perform in less than two minutes. Tips on scoring are summarized in **Table 7**.

Clinician gather collateral history from Mrs Jones' daughter, who tells clinician that her mother, whom she last spoke with two days ago, is normally "sharp as a tack." Evaluating her now, clinician find her confused to place, unable to correctly name the months of the year backwards, and drowsy. Mrs. Jones scores positive on the bCAM. Clinician think she has delirium but clinician are not sure why.

WORK-UP

Once delirium has been identified, a comprehensive evaluation to determine the underlying etiology must be undertaken. At a minimum, a complete blood cell count, basic metabolic panel to assess electrolytes, renal function, blood glucose, and an electrocardiogram (ECG) should be obtained.[43,68,69] A urine analysis and a chest radiograph usually are done as well.[69] This initial work-up may uncover a common precipitant of delirium, such as infection or electrolyte abnormality, or an emergent precipitant, such as myocardial ischemia. Atypical presentations in older adults and the propensity of adverse drug events necessitate a relatively liberal initial work-up. Care must be taken to not misinterpret asymptomatic bacteriuria or pyuria as a urinary tract infection, leading to unnecessary treatment or, even worse, premature diagnostic closure about the precipitating insult of the delirious episode.[44,69,70] Further work-up, such as liver function tests, ammonia levels, cardiac biomarkers, thyroid-stimulating hormone, head computed tomography (CT), arterial blood gas for hypercarbia,

Table 5 Diagnostic characteristics of the Delirium Triage Screen and Brief Confusion Assessment Method[66]				
Test	Sensitivity (95% CI)	Specificity (95% CI)	Negative Likelihood Ratio (95% CI)	Positive Likelihood Ratio (95% CI)
DTS	98.0% (89.5–99.5)	54.8% (49.6–59.9)	0.04 (0.01–0.25)	2.17 (1.92–2.45)
bCAM	84.0% (71.5–91.7)	95.8% (93.2–97.4)	0.17 (0.09–0.32)	19.94 (11.97–33.19)

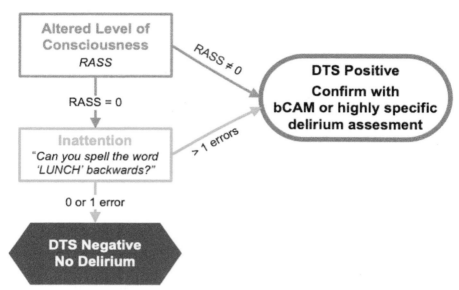

Fig. 1. DTS. (Available at http://eddelirium.org/wp-content/uploads/2015/07/DTS-Flowsheet-07-09-2015-Revision-RASS-CORRECTED.pdf. Accessed May 1, 2020; with permission.)

electroencephalogram, or a lumbar puncture (LP), should be tailored for each patient according to the clinical situation. Indiscriminate test ordering can be harmful because it may trigger a clinical cascade of further testing and unnecessary procedures or admission. A head CT should be performed only in a patient presenting with a decreased level of consciousness, focal neurologic deficit, or history of trauma on anticoagulants.[71–73] Its yield in the undifferentiated delirious patient is low; hence, it should not be performed indiscriminately.[69] The decision to obtain an LP in altered older adults is a difficult one, because telltale signs of meningitis/encephalitis, such as fever[46] and neck stiffness,[57] frequently are absent. Therefore, an LP should be considered when no other cause of altered mental status can be found.

While awaiting her laboratory tests and radiograph results, Mrs Jones pulls out her intravenous line and becomes agitated. She gets out of her bed and starts pacing down the hallway. Clinician are worried about her falling and would rather she stay in her room. What are possible treatment options for her hyperactive delirium?

PREVENTION AND MANAGEMENT
Treatment of the Inciting Cause

The management of delirium lays in the treatment of the inciting cause; this may include administering fluids, treating pain and infection, or discontinuing offending agents.[43,68,74–76] When a delirious patient becomes agitated, however, a more immediate intervention may be necessary to facilitate care and ensure the safety of the patient and staff.

Nonpharmacologic Management

Management of delirium should start with nonpharmacologic measures (**Table 8**) that aim at decreasing unfamiliar stimuli and improving orientation.[43,76–79] Verbal de-

Score	Term	Description
Table 6 **Richmond agitation-sedation scale**		
+4	Combative	Overtly combative or violent; immediate danger to staff
+3	Very agitated	Pulls on or removes tube(s) or catheters) or has aggressive behavior toward staff
+2	Agitated	Frequent nonpurposeful movement or patient-ventilator dyssynchrony
+ 1	Restless	Anxious or apprehensive but movements not aggressive or vigorous
0	Alert and calm	
−1	Drowsy	Not fully alert, but has sustained (more than 10 s) awakening, with eye contact, to voice
−2	Light sedation	Briefly (<10 s) awakens with eye contact to voice
−3	Moderate sedation	Any movement (but no eye contact) to voice
−4	Deep sedation	No response to voice, but any movement to physical stimulation
−5	Unarousable	No response to voice or physical stimulation

Procedure
1. Observe patient. Is patient alert and calm (score 0)?
    Does patient have behavior that is, consistent with restlessness or agitation (score +1 to +4 using the criteria listed under DESCRIPTION)?
2. If patient is not alert, in a loud speaking voice state patient's name and direct patient to open eyes and look at speaker. Repeat once if necessary. Can prompt patient to continue looking at speaker.
    Patient has eye opening and eye contact, which is sustained for more than 10 s (score −1).
    Patient has eye opening and eye contact, but this is not sustained for 10 s (score −2).
    Patient has any movement in response to voice, excluding eye contact (score −3).
3. If patient does not respond to voice, physically stimulate patient by shaking shoulder and then rubbing sternum if there is no response to shaking shoulder.
    Patient has any movement to physical stimulation (score −4).
    Patient has no response to voice or physical stimulation (score −5).

From Sessler CN, Gosnell MS, Grap MJ, et al. The Richmond Agitation-Sedation Scale: validity and reliability in adult intensive care unit patients. American journal of respiratory and critical medicine. 2002;166(10):1338-1344; Permission granted for reproduction from CN Sessler.

escalation is a valuable tool that can be used to identify wants and feelings, set clear limits, and offer choices and optimism.[80] Nonpharmacologic interventions are effective at preventing delirium in high-risk individuals[43,68,81] and should be implemented when caring for older adults in the ED.[58]

Another model of care for the older patient is T-A-DA: tolerate, anticipate, and don't agitate. The key concepts are summarized in **Table 9**.[78] Implementing T-A-DA appears to be associated with decreases in delirium, functional decline, and hospital length of stay without an increase in falls.[78]

Pharmacologic Treatment

The use of medications to prevent delirium is not recommended.[82] If nonpharmacologic interventions have been ineffective in preventing the escalation of a delirious patient's behavior, however, putting themselves or others at risk of harm, pharmacologic agents may be necessary.[43,58,83] Patients on chronic antipsychotics or benzodiazepines should have their home medications continued so as not to precipitate

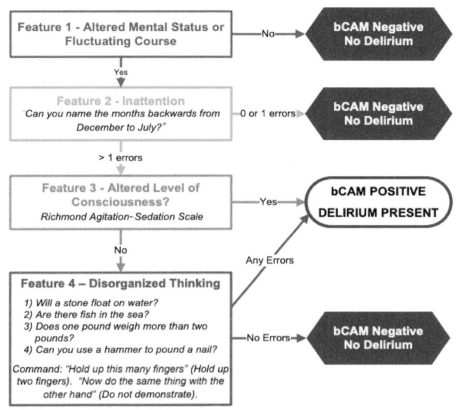

Fig. 2. bCAM. (Available at http://eddelirium.org/wp-content/uploads/2015/06/bCAM-FLOWSHEET-Color.pdf. Accessed May 1, 2020; with permission. Permission granted by Dr. Jin Han and the American Geriatric Society, 2020.)

withdrawal unless it is thought that their presentation is secondary to these medicines.[69] Antipsychotics appear superior to benzodiazepines.[58,68,69,81,84] Medications and recommendations regarding their use are summarized in **Table 10**.

For most delirious patients, the goal is to achieve calmness, with true sedation reserved for the most violent and physically destructive individuals. Most experts recommend starting at the lower end of dosing spectrum, often using half the usual dose and slowly increasing, to minimize side effects, including oversedation.[69,81] Oral administration is preferred because it preserves a patient's autonomy and has fewer side effects while retaining effectiveness.[83,85] Intramuscular (IM) routes of administration generally have fewer side effects than intravenous and, therefore, are preferred if oral is not a viable option.[69,84–86]

Antipsychotics
There is no evidence that the use of antipsychotics decreases hospital length of stay or the duration of the delirium itself.[87] All antipsychotics have a black-box warning by the Food and Drug Administration about increased mortality in older patients with dementia-related psychosis,[69] a concern echoed by the Beers Criteria list.[48] Another significant effect is dose-related short-lived QTc prolongation and possible resulting

Table 7
Scoring tips for the Brief Confusion Assessment Method

Feature	Scoring Tips
Altered mental status of fluctuating course	Altered mental status from baseline is determined by collateral history. If altered and unable to get collateral history, assume this feature is positive.
Inattention	If patient perseverates on a month or takes longer than 15 s to respond, this is considered an error. If the patient refuses to answer, this is considered positive for inattention.
Altered level of consciousness	If the patient is not alert and calm (RASS = 0), then this feature is positive. If the patient is RASS −4 or −5, the patient is considered stuporous or comatose and delirium cannot be determined.
Disorganized thinking	Any incorrect answer or refusal to answer is considered positive.

Data From: Han JH. Brief Confusion Assessment Method, Instruction Manual V1. October 15, 2015, Vanderbilt University.

torsades de pointes. Some experts recommend obtaining an ECG prior to antipsychotic administration.[48,81]

A few studies compared typical and atypical antipsychotics for delirium in head-to-head studies with unclear superiority.[87] Expert consensus, however, recommends atypical antipsychotics,[84] such as low-dose olanzapine or risperidone, over typical

Table 8
Nonpharmacologic management for the prevention and treatment of delirium[41,62,70,77–79]

Things to Do	Things to Avoid
Ensure patients have their glasses and hearing aids	Unnecessary tethering (Foley catheters, telemetry monitors, and oxygen and pulse oximetry tubing)
Disimpact ear wax (if applicable)	Bright artificial light at night
Reduce ambient noise	Dehydration
Allow people who are familiar to the patient to be at the bedside (eg, caregivers)	Prolonged ED length of stay
Use easily visible clocks and calendars	Unnecessary physical restraints
Ambulate frequently with supervision	
Cover saline lock with gauze wrap or a cast sleeve	
Administer home medications on schedule (unless contraindicated)	
Normalize daily function by providing food and hydration	
Play a video-recorded message of family members greeting the patient	

Data from Refs.[103–105]

Table 9
Tolerate, anticipate, and don't agitate: T-A-DA concept[79]

Element	Explanation	Example
Tolerate	Tolerating some of the behaviors of delirium and allowing patients to respond to their environment while monitoring them closely to prevent harm	Allow patient to get out of the bed independently under close supervision; consider what this behavior may mean (eg, request for toileting).
Anticipate	Anticipating which actions will worsen delirium and consider alternatives	Anticipate that Foley catheter placement may worsen delirium and obtain a urine sample, placing a straight catheter and then discontinuing it immediately.
Don't Agitate	Avoiding agitating the patient which often is unintentional	Have all members of the care team see the patient at once to decrease the number of unfamiliar interactions and physical examinations.

ones.[69] Physicians preferentially may start with a medication the patient has been pre-scribed in the past. A summary of antipsychotics and their recommended doses is depicted in **Table 11**, as based on expert consensus given the lack of high-quality studies in this population.

Typical (first-generation) antipsychotics

Haloperidol is the most commonly used and studied of all antipsychotics. Start with a low dose (0.5–2 mg) to minimize risk of QTc prolongation and extrapyramidal

Table 10
Pharmacologic management of delirium[48,84]

Medication Class	Relevant Mechanism of Action	Recommendation
Antipsychotics	Dopamine receptor antagonists	May be used with caution if necessary, for safety[a]
Benzodiazepines	γ-Aminobutyric acid agonists	First choice if withdrawal from alcohol/benzodiazepines or with seizures Avoid in other agitated older adults
Diphenhydramine	Antihistamine	Avoid due to strong anticholinergic properties
Ketamine	N-methyl-D-aspartate antagonist	Scarce data in older adults May be most useful in patients who are agitated secondary to pain Avoid if underlying schizophrenia
Cholinesterase inhibitors	Cholinesterase inhibitors	Not recommended outside of experimental studies

[a] Based on consensus and low-quality data

Data from: Yu A, Wu S, Zhang Z, et al. Cholinesterase inhibitors for the treatment of delirium in non-ICU settings. *Cochrane Db Syst Rev.* 2018;6(6):Cd012494; Erstad BL, Patanwala AE. Ketamine for analgosedation in critically ill patients. *J Crit Care.* 2016;35:145-149.

Table 11
Antipsychotics for treatment of delirium[70,90–92]

Type	Medication	Dose Oral	Dose Intramuscular	Dosing Frequency (as Needed)	Common Side Effect(s)
Typical	Haloperidol	0.5–2 mg	0.5–1 mg	q1h PRN; maximum of 3–5 mg in 24 h	Extrapyramidal symptoms
	Droperidol	N/A	5 mg	May repeat once	QT prolongation
Atypical	Risperidone	0.5–1 mg	N/A	BID PRN	Orthostatic
	Olanzapine	2.5–5 mg	2.5–5 mg	BID PRN	hypotension
	Ziprasidone	N/A	10 mg	q2h PRN; maximum of 40 mg in 24 h	Worsening heart disease or heart
	Quetiapine	12.5–25 mg	N/A	BID PRN or QHS PRN	failure[a]

Abbreviations: BID, twice daily; IM, intramuscular; PRN, as needed; QHS, at bedtime.
[a] Unique to Ziprasidone.
Data from: Harrigan EP, Miceli JJ, Anziano R, et al. A randomized evaluation of the effects of six antipsychotic agents on QTc, in the absence and presence of metabolic inhibition. J Clin Psychopharmacol. 2004;24(1):62-69; and Berkowitz AL. Ziprasidone therapy in elderly patients with psychotic mood disorders and Parkinson's disease. Psychiatry. 2006;3(11):59-63.

effects.[69,81] Doses greater than or equal to 5 mg IM, which typically are used in younger individuals, should be avoided.[69]

Droperidol, another potent typical antipsychotic, fell out of favor earlier this century, due to presumed side effects, yet appears safe to use.[81,88,89] Although QT prolongation may occur in doses greater than or equal to 2.5 mg in a dose-related fashion, torsades de pointes does not appear to develop in patients receiving less than or equal to 10 mg IM, if at all.[88–91]

Given their propensity for extrapyramidal symptoms, typical antipsychotics are best avoided in patients with Parkinson disease and dementia with Lewy bodies (DLB).

Atypical (second-generation) antipsychotics
Atypical antipsychotics, such as risperidone, ziprasidone, olanzapine, and quetiapine, differ from typical antipsychotics in their effect on norepinephrine and serotonin receptors, leading to lower rates of extrapyramidal side effects. They should be used preferentially in patients with Parkinson disease and DLB.[48,68]

Benzodiazepines
Benzodiazepines are the mainstay of treatment of most younger agitated patients[84] but should not be the first drug of choice in agitated older adults.[68,81,84] There are no adequate studies that demonstrate their efficacy or safety in this patient population,[92] and they may worsen and prolong the delirium[48] or even cause a paradoxic effect.[69] If used, start with a smaller dose (eg, lorazepam, 0.5 mg) and increase as needed.[69]

Physical restraints
Physical restraints are the last resort in managing an agitated delirious older adult who is at imminent risk of severe injury to self or others. They may be necessary only while waiting for chemical sedation to take effect.[58]

Mrs Jones is calmer after employing nonpharmacologic methods and treating her pain. She does not require any psychotropic or hypnotic medications. Her radiograph reveals a Colles fracture. Her ED work-up is otherwise negative. She is able to ambulate steadily with her cane. Can clinician discharge Mrs. Jones home, or should clinician admit her to the hospital?

DISPOSITION: DOES EVERYBODY NEED TO BE ADMITTED?

Most delirious patients benefit from admission to the hospital for further work-up and management of the precipitating insult. Admission also ensures their safety because they may be unable to care for themselves while altered. The decision to admit is complicated by the factor that admission itself can precipitate or worsen delirium.[69]

Discharge may be considered if (1) there is a reliable caregiver who can monitor the patient closely; (2) the cause of the patient's delirium was identified and treated; and (3) the patient's symptoms are improving.[69] Other alternatives to admission include home health care and hospital-at-home models.[93,94] It is prudent to remember that a delay in disposition worsens delirium.[51] Should a patient request to be discharged independently or leave against medical advice, their decision-making capacity should be assessed and documented thoroughly, because lack of capacity frequently is missed.[95] Capacity is not permanent and can be affected temporarily by delirium.

CASE CONCLUSION

Mrs Jones wishes to be discharged home. She is discharged in the care of her daughter, who has agreed to stay with her for several days to ensure that she is safe and does not become confused again. She has been provided with a prescription for analgesia and a bowel regimen, follow-up with the orthopedic surgeon, and a referral for cognitive evaluation as an outpatient.

SUMMARY: IMPLEMENTING CHANGE

The key to improving the detection and management of delirium in older ED patients is to adopt a systematic approach at both the individual and hospital levels. There are several available resources, including the Geriatric Emergency Department Guidelines and the ADEPT tool, which provides an evidence-based framework to assess, diagnose, evaluate, prevent, and treat delirium in geriatric patients.[58,69]

CLINICS PEARLS

- Delirium is common and associated with significant morbidity and mortality.
- Evaluate mental status in all older patients presenting to the ED; do not rely on gestalt—use a validated tool to assess for delirium.
- Obtain a through medication list (including over-the-counter medications), paying special attention to medications with anticholinergic properties.
- Utilize nonpharmacologic measures, such as reorientation and decreasing unfamiliar stimuli, for high-risk individuals to prevent and treat delirium.
- Consider using low-dose atypical antipsychotics in agitated delirious patients who are at imminent risk of harm.

DISCLOSURE

The authors have nothing to disclose.

REFERENCES

1. American Psychiatric Association. In: Diagnostic and statistical manual of mental disorders. Fifth Edition. Arlington (VA): American Psychiatric Association; 2013. Accessed June 1, 2013.

2. Han JH, Zimmerman EE, Cutler N, et al. Delirium in older emergency department patients: recognition, risk factors, and psychomotor subtypes. Acad Emerg Med 2009;16(3):193–200.

3. Jackson TA, Wilson D, Richardson S, et al. Predicting outcome in older hospital patients with delirium: a systematic literature review. Int J Geriatr Psychiatry 2016;31(4):392–9.

4. Han JH, Brummel NE, Chandrasekhar R, et al. Exploring delirium's heterogeneity: association between arousal subtypes at initial presentation and 6-month mortality in older emergency department patients. Am J Geriatr Psychiatry 2017;25(3):233–42.

5. Oh ES, Fong TG, Hshieh TT, et al. Delirium in older persons: Advances in diagnosis and treatment. JAMA 2017;318(12):1161–74.

6. Hshieh TT, Inouye SK, Oh ES. Delirium in the elderly. Clin Geriatr Med 2020; 36(2):183–99.

7. Jones RN, Cizginer S, Pavlech L, et al. Assessment of instruments for measurement of delirium severity: a systematic review. JAMA Intern Med 2019;179(2): 231–9.

8. Vasunilashorn SM, Fong TG, Albuquerque A, et al. Delirium severity postsurgery and its relationship with long-term cognitive decline in a cohort of patients without dementia. J Atten Disord 2018;61(1):347–58.

9. Vasunilashorn SM, Marcantonio ER, Gou Y, et al. Quantifying the severity of a delirium episode throughout hospitalization: the combined importance of intensity and duration. J Gen Intern Med 2016;31(10):1164–71.

10. Inouye SK, Westendorp RG, Saczynski JS. Delirium in elderly people. Lancet 2014;383(9920):911–22.

11. Elie M, Rousseau F, Cole M, et al. Prevalence and detection of delirium in elderly emergency department patients. CMAJ 2000;163(8):977–81.

12. Han JH, Shintani A, Eden S, et al. Delirium in the emergency department: an independent predictor of death within 6 months. Ann Emerg Med 2010;56(3): 244–52.e1.

13. Lewis LM, Miller DK, Morley JE, et al. Unrecognized delirium in ED geriatric patients. Am J Emerg Med 1995;13(2):142–5.

14. Hustey FM, Meldon S, Palmer R. Prevalence and documentation of impaired mental status in elderly emergency department patients. Acad Emerg Med 2000;7(10):1166.

15. Boucher V, Lamontagne ME, Nadeau A, et al. Unrecognized Incident Delirium in Older Emergency Department Patients. J Emerg Med 2019;57(4):535–42.

16. Hustey FM, Meldon SW, Smith MD, et al. The effect of mental status screening on the care of elderly emergency department patients. Ann Emerg Med 2003; 41(5):678–84.

17. Kakuma R, du Fort GG, Arsenault L, et al. Delirium in older emergency department patients discharged home: effect on survival. J Am Geriatr Soc 2003;51(4): 443–50.

18. Han JH, Eden S, Shintani A, et al. Delirium in older emergency department patients is an independent predictor of hospital length of stay. Acad Emerg Med 2011;18(5):451–7.

19. Naughton BJ, Moran MB, Kadah H, et al. Delirium and other cognitive impairment in older adults in an emergency department. Ann Emerg Med 1995; 25(6):751–5.

20. Kennedy M, Enander RA, Tadiri SP, et al. Delirium risk prediction, healthcare use and mortality of elderly adults in the emergency department. J Am Geriatr Soc 2014;62(3):462–9.

21. Witlox J, Eurelings LS, de Jonghe JF, et al. Delirium in elderly patients and the risk of postdischarge mortality, institutionalization, and dementia: a meta-analysis. JAMA 2010;304(4):443–51.

22. Sri-on J, Tirrell GP, Vanichkulbodee A, et al. The prevalence, risk factors and short-term outcomes of delirium in Thai elderly emergency department patients. Emerg Med J 2016;33(1):17–22.

23. Schmitt EM, Gallagher J, Albuquerque A, et al. Perspectives on the delirium experience and its burden: common themes among older patients, their family caregivers, and nurses. Gerontologist 2019;59(2):327–37.

24. Bohart S, Merete Møller A, Forsyth Herling S. Do health care professionals worry about delirium? Relatives' experience of delirium in the intensive care unit: A qualitative interview study. Intensive Crit Care Nurs 2019;53:84–91.

25. Leslie DL, Inouye SK. The importance of delirium: economic and societal costs. J Am Geriatr Soc 2011;59(Suppl 2):S241–3.

26. McCusker J, Cole M, Dendukuri N, et al. The course of delirium in older medical inpatients: a prospective study. J Gen Intern Med 2003;18(9):696–704.

27. Girard TD, Jackson JC, Pandharipande PP, et al. Delirium as a predictor of long-term cognitive impairment in survivors of critical illness. Crit Care Med 2010; 38(7):1513–20.

28. Pandharipande PP, Girard TD, Ely EW. Long-term cognitive impairment after critical illness. N Engl J Med 2014;370(2):185–6.

29. Han JH, Vasilevskis EE, Chandrasekhar R, et al. Delirium in the Emergency Department and Its Extension into Hospitalization (DELINEATE) Study: Effect on 6-month Function and Cognition. J Am Geriatr Soc 2017;65(6):1333–8.

30. Hshieh TT, Saczynski J, Gou RY, et al. Trajectory of functional recovery after postoperative delirium in elective surgery. Ann Surg 2017;265(4):647–53.

31. Shi Z, Mei X, Li C, et al. Postoperative delirium is associated with long-term decline in activities of daily living. Anesthesiology 2019;131(3):492–500.

32. Hughes CG, Patel MB, Pandharipande PP. Pathophysiology of acute brain dysfunction: what's the cause of all this confusion? Curr Opin Crit Care 2012; 18(5):518–26.

33. Maldonado JR. Delirium pathophysiology: An updated hypothesis of the etiology of acute brain failure. Int J Geriatr Psychiatry 2018;33(11):1428–57.

34. Shafi MM, Santarnecchi E, Fong TG, et al. Advancing the Neurophysiological Understanding of Delirium. J Am Geriatr Soc 2017;65(6):1114–8.

35. Hall RJ, Watne LO, Cunningham E, et al. CSF biomarkers in delirium: a systematic review. Int J Geriatr Pyschiatry 2018;33(11):1479–500.

36. Amgarth-Duff I, Hosie A, Caplan G, et al. Toward best practice methods for delirium biomarker studies: An international modified Delphi study. Int J Geriatr Pyschiatry 2020;35(7):737–48.

37. Michels M, Michelon C, Damásio D, et al. Biomarker predictors of delirium in acutely ill patients: a systematic review. J Geriatr Psychiatry Neurol 2019; 32(3):119–36.

38. Fong TG, Bogardus ST Jr, Daftary A, et al. Cerebral perfusion changes in older delirious patients using 99mTc HMPAO SPECT. J Gerontol A Biol Sci Med Sci 2006;61(12):1294–9.

39. Cavallari M, Dai W, Guttmann CRG, et al. Neural substrates of vulnerability to postsurgical delirium as revealed by presurgical diffusion MRI. Brain 2016; 139(4):1282–94.

40. Han JH, Wilber ST. Altered mental status in older patients in the emergency department. Clin Geriatr Med 2013;29(1):101–36.

41. Inouye SK, Charpentier PA. Precipitating factors for delirium in hospitalized elderly persons. Predictive model and interrelationship with baseline vulnerability. JAMA 1996;275(11):852–7.

42. Han L, McCusker J, Cole M, et al. Use of medications with anticholinergic effect predicts clinical severity of delirium symptoms in older medical inpatients. Arch Intern Med 2001;161(8):1099–105.

43. Davis D, Searle SD, Tsui A. The Scottish Intercollegiate Guidelines Network: risk reduction and management of delirium. Age Ageing 2019;48(4):485–8.

44. Caterino JM. Evaluation and management of geriatric infections in the emergency department. Emerg Med Clin North Am 2008;26(2):319–43, viii.

45. Fontanarosa PB, Kaeberlein FJ, Gerson LW, et al. Difficulty in predicting bacteremia in elderly emergency patients. Ann Emerg Med 1992;21(7):842–8.

46. Shah K, Richard K, Edlow JA. Utility of lumbar puncture in the afebrile vs. febrile elderly patient with altered mental status: a pilot study. J Emerg Med 2007; 32(1):15–8.

47. Alagiakrishnan K, Wiens CA. An approach to drug induced delirium in the elderly. Postgrad Med J 2004;80(945):388–93.

48. American Geriatrics Society 2019 Updated AGS Beers Criteria® for potentially inappropriate medication use in older adults. J Am Geriatr Soc 2019;67(4): 674–94.

49. Davies EA, O'Mahony MS. Adverse drug reactions in special populations - the elderly. Br J Clin Pharmacol 2015;80(4):796–807.

50. CBHSQ. 2015 National survey on drug use and health: detailed tables. Rockville (MD): Substance Abuse and Mental Health Services Administration; 2016.

51. Bo M, Bonetto M, Bottignole G, et al. Length of stay in the emergency department and occurrence of delirium in older medical patients. J Am Geriatr Soc 2016;64(5):1114–9.

52. Feast AR, White N, Lord K, et al. Pain and delirium in people with dementia in the acute general hospital setting. Age Ageing 2018;47(6):841–6.

53. Platts-Mills TF, Esserman DA, Brown DL, et al. Older US emergency department patients are less likely to receive pain medication than younger patients: results from a national survey. Ann Emerg Med 2012;60(2):199–206.

54. Warden V, Hurley AC, Volicer L. Development and psychometric evaluation of the Pain Assessment in Advanced Dementia (PAINAD) scale. J Am Med Dir Assoc 2003;4(1):9–15.

55. Khoujah D, Martinelli AN, Winters ME. Resuscitating the critically ill geriatric emergency department patient. Emerg Med Clin North Am 2019;37(3):569–81.

56. Spangler R, Van Pham T, Khoujah D, et al. Abdominal emergencies in the geriatric patient. Int J Emerg Med 2014;7:43.

57. Choi C. Bacterial meningitis in aging adults. Clin Infect Dis 2001;33(8):1380–5.

58. National Institute of Neurological D. Stroke. NIH stroke scale. Bethesda (MD): National Institute of Neurological Disorders and Stroke, Dept. of Health and Human Services; 2011.

59. The Geriatrics Emergency Department Guidelines. Ann Emerg Med 2014; 63(5):e5.

60. NICE Guidelines on Delirium: Diagnosis, Prevention and Managment. In. United Kingdom: National Institute for Health and Care Excellence Clinical Guidelines; 2010. Available at: https://www.nice.org.uk/guidance/cg103.

61. Cooke M, Burns A, Oliver D. The Silver Book: Quality Care for Older People with Urgent and Emergency Care Needs. United Kingdom: 2012. Available at: https://www.bgs.org.uk/sites/default/files/content/attachment/2018-05-01/Silver %20Book%202012%20Complete.pdf.

62. Kilshaw L. Australian, New Zealand Society for Geriatric M. Australian and New Zealand Society for Geriatric Medicine position statement no. 14 guidelines for the management of older persons presenting to emergency departments 2008. Australas J Ageing 2009;28(3):153–7.

63. De J, Wand AP. Delirium screening: a systematic review of delirium screening tools in hospitalized patients. Gerontologist 2015;55(6):1079–99.

64. LaMantia MA, Messina FC, Hobgood CD, et al. Screening for delirium in the emergency department: a systematic review. Ann Emerg Med 2014;63(5): 551–60.e2.

65. Mariz J, Costa Castanho T, Teixeira J, et al. Delirium diagnostic and screening instruments in the emergency department: an up-to-date systematic review. Geriatrics (Basel) 2016;1(3):22.

66. Han JH, Wilson A, Vasilevskis EE, et al. Diagnosing delirium in older emergency department patients: validity and reliability of the delirium triage screen and the brief confusion assessment method. Ann Emerg Med 2013;62(5):457–65.

67. Sessler CN, Gosnell MS, Grap MJ, et al. The Richmond Agitation-Sedation Scale: validity and reliability in adult intensive care unit patients. Am J Respir Crit Care Med 2002;166(10):1338–44.

68. Ely EW, Inouye SK, Bernard GR, et al. Delirium in mechanically ventilated patients: validity and reliability of the confusion assessment method for the intensive care unit (CAM-ICU). JAMA 2001;286(21):2703–10.

69. Australian and New Zealand Society for Geriatric Medicine Position Statement Abstract: Delirium in older people. Australas J Ageing 2016;35(4):292.

70. Shenvi C, Kennedy M, Austin CA, et al. Managing delirium and agitation in the older emergency department patient: the ADEPT tool. Ann Emerg Med 2020; 75(2):136–45.

71. Shimoni Z, Cohen R, Froom P. Prevalence, impact, and management strategies for asymptomatic bacteriuria in the acute care elderly patient: a review of the current literature. Expert Rev Anti Infect Ther 2020;18(5):453–60.

72. Hardy JE, Brennan N. Computerized tomography of the brain for elderly patients presenting to the emergency department with acute confusion. Emerg Med Australas 2008;20(5):420–4.

73. Naughton BJ, Moran M, Ghaly Y, et al. Computed tomography scanning and delirium in elder patients. Acad Emerg Med 1997;4(12):1107–10.

74. Lai MM, Wong Tin Niam DM. Intracranial cause of delirium: computed tomography yield and predictive factors. Intern Med J 2012;42(4):422–7.

75. Husebo BS, Ballard C, Sandvik R, et al. Efficacy of treating pain to reduce behavioural disturbances in residents of nursing homes with dementia: cluster randomised clinical trial. BMJ 2011;343:d4065.

76. Björkelund KB, Hommel A, Thorngren KG, et al. Reducing delirium in elderly patients with hip fracture: a multi-factorial intervention study. Acta Anaesthesiol Scand 2010;54(6):678–88.

77. Yue J, Tabloski P, Dowal SL, et al. NICE to HELP: operationalizing National Institute for Health and Clinical Excellence guidelines to improve clinical practice. J Am Geriatr Soc 2014;62(4):754–61.

78. Rivosecchi RM, Smithburger PL, Svec S, et al. Nonpharmacological interventions to prevent delirium: an evidence-based systematic review. Crit Care Nurse 2015;35(1):39–50.

79. Flaherty JH, Little MO. Matching the environment to patients with delirium: lessons learned from the delirium room, a restraint-free environment for older hospitalized adults with delirium. J Am Geriatr Soc 2011;59(Suppl 2):S295–300.

80. Johnson K, Curry V, Steubing A, et al. A non-pharmacologic approach to decrease restraint use. Intensive Crit Care Nurs 2016;34:12–9.

81. Richmond JS, Berlin JS, Fishkind AB, et al. Verbal De-escalation of the Agitated Patient: Consensus Statement of the American Association for Emergency Psychiatry Project BETA De-escalation Workgroup. West J Emerg Med 2012;13(1): 17–25.

82. Trzepacz P, Breitbart W, Franklin J, et al. Practice guideline for the treatment of patients with delirium. 2010.

83. Siddiqi N, Harrison JK, Clegg A, et al. Interventions for preventing delirium in hospitalised non-ICU patients. Cochrane Database Syst Rev 2016;(3):CD005563.

84. Gottlieb M, Long B, Koyfman A. Approach to the agitated emergency department patient. J Emerg Med 2018;54(4):447–57.

85. Wilson MP, Pepper D, Currier GW, et al. The psychopharmacology of agitation: consensus statement of the american association for emergency psychiatry project Beta psychopharmacology workgroup. West J Emerg Med 2012;13(1): 26–34.

86. New A, Tucci VT, Rios J. A modern-day fight club? the stabilization and management of acutely agitated patients in the Emergency Department. Psychiatr Clin North Am 2017;40(3):397–410.

87. Kalish VB, Gillham JE, Unwin BK. Delirium in older persons: evaluation and management. Am Fam Physician 2014;90(3):150–8.

88. Burry L, Mehta S, Perreault MM, et al. Antipsychotics for treatment of delirium in hospitalised non-ICU patients. Cochrane Database Syst Rev 2018;6(6): Cd005594.

89. Khokhar MA, Rathbone J. Droperidol for psychosis-induced aggression or agitation. Cochrane Database Syst Rev 2016;12(12):Cd002830.

90. Perkins J, Ho JD, Vilke GM, et al. American Academy of Emergency Medicine Position Statement: Safety of Droperidol Use in the Emergency Department. J Emerg Med 2015;49(1):91–7.

91. Page CB, Parker LE, Rashford SJ, et al. Prospective study of the safety and effectiveness of droperidol in elderly patients for pre-hospital acute behavioural disturbance. Emerg Med Australas 2020;32(5):731–6.

92. Calver L, Isbister GK. Parenteral sedation of elderly patients with acute behavioral disturbance in the ED. Am J Emerg Med 2013;31(6):970–3.

93. Li Y, Ma J, Jin Y, et al. Benzodiazepines for treatment of patients with delirium excluding those who are cared for in an intensive care unit. Cochrane Database Syst Rev 2020;2(2):Cd012670.

94. Leff B, Burton L, Mader SL, et al. Hospital at home: feasibility and outcomes of a program to provide hospital-level care at home for acutely ill older patients. Ann Intern Med 2005;143(11):798–808.

95. Sessums LL, Zembrzuska H, Jackson JL. Does this patient have medical decision-making capacity? JAMA 2011;306(4):420–7.
96. O'Sullivan D, Brady N, Manning E, et al. Validation of the 6-item cognitive impairment test and the 4AT test for combined delirium and dementia screening in older Emergency Department attendees. Age Ageing 2018;47(1):61–8.
97. Grossmann FF, Hasemann W, Graber A, et al. Screening, detection and management of delirium in the emergency department - a pilot study on the feasibility of a new algorithm for use in older emergency department patients: the modified Confusion Assessment Method for the Emergency Department (mCAM-ED). Scand J Trauma Resusc Emerg Med 2014;22(1):19.
98. Hasemann W, Grossmann FF, Bingisser R, et al. Optimizing the month of the year backwards test for delirium screening of older patients in the emergency department. Am J Emerg Med 2019;37(9):1754–7.
99. Han JH, Wilson A, Graves AJ, et al. Validation of the Confusion Assessment Method for the Intensive Care Unit in older emergency department patients. Acad Emerg Med 2014;21(2):180–7.
100. Yadav K, Boucher V, Carmichael PH, et al. Serial Ottawa 3DY assessments to detect delirium in older emergency department community dwellers. Age Ageing 2019;49(1):130–4.
101. Dyer AH, Briggs R, Nabeel S, et al. The abbreviated mental test 4 for cognitive screening of older adults presenting to the emergency department. Eur J Emerg Med 2017;24(6):417–22.
102. Han JH, Vasilevskis EE, Schnelle JF, et al. The diagnostic performance of the richmond agitation sedation scale for detecting delirium in older emergency department patients. Acad Emerg Med 2015;22(7):878–82.
103. Cohen-Mansfield J, Werner P. Management of verbally disruptive behaviors in nursing home residents. J Gerontolog 1997;52(6):M369–77.
104. Fong TG, Tulebaev SR, Inouye SK. Delirium in elderly adults: diagnosis, prevention and treatment. Nat Rev Neurol 2009;5(4):210–20.
105. Waszynski CM, Milner KA, Staff I, et al. Using simulated family presence to decrease agitation in older hospitalized delirious patients: a randomized controlled trial. Int J Nurs Stud 2018;77:154–61.

Chronic Brain Failure

James P. Wolak, MD[a,b]

KEYWORDS

• Dementia • Neurocognitive • Neuropsychiatric • Emergency • Agitation

KEY POINTS

- Chronic brain failure is also known as dementia or major neurocognitive disorder. Like other organ failure syndromes, its impact on quality of life can be mitigated with proper management.
- In addition to cognitive symptoms such as memory loss, chronic brain failure involves neuropsychiatric symptoms such as psychosis, mood lability, and agitation.
- The symptoms of chronic brain failure can mimic those of acute brain failure (delirium), but there are major distinctions to help guide diagnostic thinking.
- Neuropsychiatric symptoms are best managed nonpharmacologically. Medications to treat agitation should be used only as a last resort.
- The use of logic and reason are rarely successful when attempting to redirect someone with advanced dementia. Interactions that offer a sense of choice are more likely to succeed.

CASE

Pertinent history: A 78-year-old man with a history of Alzheimer's disease (AD) was sent to the emergency department (ED) after becoming aggressive toward staff at his assisted living facility (ALF). Over the prior week, he had been leaving the facility repeatedly, accusing staff of stealing his belongings and poisoning his food. On the day of presentation, he struck a staff member while she was attempting to redirect him. He has had no recent medical illness.

Past medical history: Hypertension, osteoarthritis, and benign prostatic hyperplasia. AD diagnosed by his primary care provider approximately 5 years ago. Currently, he receives his primary care through the ALF's nurse practitioner.

Surgical history: Left total hip arthroplasty 6 months prior

Medications: Hydrochlorothiazide 25 mg twice daily, tamsulosin 0.4 mg daily, trazodone 25 mg nightly, quetiapine 100 mg nightly (started 1 week prior), lorazepam topical gel 2 mg twice daily as needed for anxiety/agitation (started 2 days prior)

Family history: Mother died of AD at age 80, father died of myocardial infarction at age 54

[a] Department of Psychiatry, Maine Medical Center, 22 Bramhall Street, Portland, ME 04102, USA; [b] Tufts University School of Medicine, Boston, MA, USA
E-mail address: wolakj@mmc.org

Emerg Med Clin N Am 39 (2021) 307–322
https://doi.org/10.1016/j.emc.2021.01.008
0733-8627/21/© 2021 Elsevier Inc. All rights reserved.

Social history: 10th grade education, retired assembly-line worker, divorced, one daughter who lives out of state and is designated as his power of attorney; 30 pack-year history of smoking

Pertinent physical examination: Temperature: 37.2C; blood pressure: 141/93; heart rate: 110; respiratory rate: 20; oxygen saturation by pulse oximetry: 99% on room air

General: Alert, thin, disheveled, smelling of urine. Oriented to self only. Minimally cooperative, attempting to leave ED, states that there is nothing wrong with him.

Skin: No rashes or petechiae

HEENT: Pupils equal, round, reactive to light, mucous membranes dry, conjunctivae pale

Neck: Full range of movement (ROM), neck veins flat

Cardiovascular: Regular rhythm, tachycardic, no murmurs/rubs/gallops, distal pulses equal bilaterally

Pulmonary: Rate increased, lungs clear with no wheezes, rales, or rhonchi

Abdominal: Soft, nontender, nondistended, normal bowel sounds

Musculoskeletal: Normal pulses throughout, full ROM of all extremities, no peripheral edema

Neurologic: 5/5 strength and normal sensation throughout, gait slightly unsteady

Psychiatric: Dysphoric mood, irritable affect, paranoid delusions, no hallucinations

Montreal Cognitive Assessment (MoCA) = 11/30

Diagnostic testing: A delirium workup was initiated.

WBC	6.6 k/μL
Hgb	13.2 g/dL
Hct	39.5%
Plt	190 k/μL
Na	128 mmol/L
Potassium	4.2 mmol/L
Cl	97 mmol/L
CO_2	19 mmol/L
Glucose	139 mg/dL
BUN	20 mg/dL
Creatinine	1.51 mg/dL

Abbreviations: BUN, blood urea nitrogen; Cl, chloride; CO_2, carbon dioxide; Hct, hematocrit; Hgb, hemoglobin; Na, sodium; Plt, platelet; WBC, white blood cell.

Electrocardiogram: Sinus tachycardia, normal axis and intervals, no ST elevation or depression, T waves normal

Chest radiograph: Normal

Head CT: There is global parenchymal volume loss. The ventricles are enlarged commensurate with parenchymal loss. No acute intracranial process is identified.

Clinical course: The patient was thought to be at high risk for falls given his agitation and minimal cooperation with staff. He was also physically threatening. He repeatedly asked for his wife and was told that she was "out of town." After several failed attempts to administer oral medication for acute agitation, the patient received olanzapine 5 mg intramuscularly. He remained agitated after 15 minutes so was assigned a one-to-one staff companion for constant monitoring. After approximately 40 minutes, he was awake and alert, remaining seated in a recliner.

The patient was a poor historian, so collateral history was obtained from a nurse at the ALF. She reported that she had known the patient since he moved there 2 years ago. He had some moderate memory loss that worsened precipitously 6 months ago following an extended hospitalization for a hip replacement with postoperative delirium. He was ordinarily quiet and "a loner," but over the past few months he had become more anxious and irritable. He was frequently restless, especially late in the day, and began accusing staff of stealing clothing and personal items from his room. He had difficulty falling asleep, and awoke several times throughout the night, usually to urinate. Within the past few weeks, he was sleeping very little overall. He normally had a good appetite but was eating and drinking less over the past few weeks, accusing staff of poisoning his food. The ALF medical provider had prescribed quetiapine and lorazepam gel without any benefit. The patient had wandered away from the ALF several times recently, but always returned willingly. On the day of presentation, however, he struck a staff member who attempted to direct him back inside the building.

The nurse reported that she had consulted with the ALF Director; they felt that the patient required a "higher level of care" and thus would be discharged from their facility.

Several attempts to contact the patient's daughter were unsuccessful.

INTRODUCTION AND BACKGROUND

- Chronic brain failure is a complex, acquired syndrome characterized by progressive and usually irreversible decline in multiple areas of higher mental function, resulting in a gradual loss of independent daily living activities. This loss of independent function has a wide-ranging impact on individuals, families, and health care systems.[1]
- Chronic brain failure is an umbrella term, used to describe a class of disorders more commonly known as dementias and major neurocognitive disorders (these terms are used interchangeably in this article, reflecting their use in the literature). These terms emphasize consequences rather than causes; the syndrome can result from a number of different disease processes.
- Chronic brain failure is predominantly, although not exclusively, a disorder of later life, typically affecting persons older than 65 years.
- Older adults with dementia are frequent ED visitors who have greater comorbidity, incur higher costs, are admitted to hospitals at higher rates, return to EDs at higher rates, and have higher mortality after an ED visit than patients without dementia.[2] They are also associated with higher rates of delirium, falls, behavioral problems, and physical decline.[3]
- Patients with dementia are viewed as particularly challenging to ED clinicians.[4] Although most patients do not present with a chief complaint of dementia, their dementia and related symptoms often overshadow the primary reason for the ED visit.
- Chronic brain failure is distinct from acute brain failure (ie, delirium); the initial diagnosis cannot be made if delirium is present. Nevertheless, dementia and delirium are frequently encountered in tandem. As illustrated by the preceding case example, dementia is a risk factor for delirium, and delirium can accelerate the progression of dementia.

- Diagnosis and management of major neurocognitive disorder spans multiple medical specialties, including neurology, psychiatry, geriatrics, and general internal medicine, yet no one specialty clearly "owns" the diagnostic class. This can complicate treatment and disposition planning.
- The nature of their symptoms makes people with dementia more dependent and vulnerable, both socially and in terms of physical and mental health.

Prevalence/Incidence

- Within the United States, approximately 5.7 million people are living with dementia.[5]
- As the population worldwide continues to age, the number of individuals at risk will also increase, particularly among the very old.
  - The prevalence doubles every 5 years after the age of 65, with more than 20% of 80-year-olds having moderate-to-severe dementia.[6]
- AD is the most prevalent subtype of dementia, accounting for 60% to 80% of cases.[5]
- ED-based studies of cognitive impairment report that up to 70% of older adults seen with cognitive impairment have undiagnosed dementia.[7]

Physiology/Pathophysiology

The clinical syndrome of major neurocognitive disorder can be caused by several different pathophysiological processes that alter or damage nerve cells and synapses in the brain. The diagnostic category is broken down into corresponding subtypes based on clinical, genetic, and neuropathological features. The most common of these is AD, followed by vascular dementia, dementia with Lewy bodies, and frontotemporal dementia (**Table 1**). Less common causes include Huntington disease, normal pressure hydrocephalus, Parkinson disease, traumatic brain injury, substance/medication use, human immunodeficiency infection, and prion disease.[8]

The clinical symptoms and pathophysiological processes of these diseases overlap significantly. For example, research indicates that at least one-third of AD cases are complicated by some degree of vascular pathology.[9] Determining what specific subtype of major neurocognitive disorder a patient has can be important for prognosis and long-term treatment planning. For the emergency physician evaluating a patient with cognitive impairment in the ED, however, it is more important to differentiate between acute/potentially reversible causes and chronic/irreversible ones.

Clinical Characteristics

Dementia subtypes can be difficult to diagnose clinically because of their multifactorial causes, overlapping symptoms, and inconsistent clinical presentations. Within the category, the most commonly used diagnosis code is Dementia Not Otherwise Specified,[10] which likely reflects these diagnostic challenges.

Fortunately, patients usually present to the ED with an existing diagnosis of dementia; the initial diagnosis is not commonly made by emergency physicians. Nevertheless, an understanding of the clinical characteristics of dementia can aid the emergency physician in managing the patient with chronic brain failure.

Although the hallmark of dementia is memory loss, symptoms typically involve multiple domains of brain function:

1. Complex attention
   - Experiences difficulty processing multiple stimuli (television, radio, conversation)
   - Gets easily distracted by competing events in the environment

Table 1
The most common causes of major neurocognitive disorder

Disease	Pathology	Time Course	Clinical Features
Alzheimer's disease	Characterized by plaques, tangles, and neuronal loss.	Insidious onset. Slow progressive cognitive and functional decline.	Almost always includes neuropsychiatric symptoms in later stages.
Vascular dementia	Results from cerebrovascular disease.	Stepwise progression with variable rates of decline.	Often associated with focal neurologic signs such as spasticity, hemiparesis, and extrapyramidal signs. Apathy and depression are common.
Dementia with Lewy bodies	α-Synuclein aggregates in neurons.	Progressive cognitive decline.	Includes fluctuating cognition, visual hallucinations, parkinsonism, rapid-eye movement sleep disorder, and hypersensitivity to antipsychotics.
Frontotemporal dementia (includes Pick disease)	Focal degeneration of frontal and temporal lobes. Involves hyperphosphorylated tau protein inclusion bodies. Knife-edge atrophy on MRI.	Typically a more rapid rate of decline than with Alzheimer's disease.	Progressive change in personality, behavior, and language. Motor impairment syndromes co-occur.

- Is unable to perform mental calculations
2. Executive functioning
   - Abandons complex projects
   - Needs to focus on one task at a time
   - Needs assistance with activities of daily living and making basic decisions
3. Learning and memory
   - Repeats self in conversation, often within the same conversation
   - Cannot keep track of short lists of items such as shopping lists or plans for the day
   - Requires frequent reminders to orient to task at hand
4. Language
   - Experiences significant difficulties with expressive and/or receptive language
   - Often uses vague, general phrases such as "that thing" and "you know what I mean"
   - Prefers general pronouns rather than names
   - With severe impairment, may not recall names of friends and family, and may lose fluent language
5. Perceptual-motor

- Struggles with previously familiar activities (using tools, driving a car)
- Gets lost in familiar environments
- Often gets more confused at dusk, when shadows and lowering levels of light change perceptions

6. Social cognition
    - Exhibits behavior clearly out of acceptable social range
    - Demonstrates lack of sensitivity to social standards of modesty in dress and restraint in political, religious, or sexual topics of conversation

In addition to impairments in the preceding cognitive domains, dementia can involve noncognitive neuropsychiatric symptoms, which include the following:

1. Mood disturbance (depression, irritability)
2. Psychosis (hallucinations, delusions)
3. Agitation
4. Aggression
5. Apathy
6. Sleep disturbance
7. Disinhibition

Despite being almost universally present in chronic brain failure, noncognitive neuropsychiatric symptoms have not been included in the diagnostic criteria for dementia in the current classification system (**Box 1**).

Box 1
Major neurocognitive disorder, DSM-5 diagnostic criteria[8]

A. Evidence of significant cognitive decline from a previous level of performance in one or more cognitive domains (complex attention, executive function, learning and memory, language, perceptual-motor, or social cognition) based on
   1. Concern of the individual, a knowledgeable informant, or the clinician that there has been a significant decline in cognitive function; and
   2. A substantial impairment in cognitive performance, preferably documented by standardized neuropsychological testing or, in its absence, another quantified clinical assessment.

B. The cognitive deficits interfere with independence in everyday activities (ie, at a minimum, requiring assistance with complex instrumental activities of daily living such as paying bills or managing medications).

C. The cognitive deficits do not occur exclusively in the context of a delirium.

D. The cognitive deficits are not better explained by another mental disorder (eg, major depressive disorder, schizophrenia).

ASSESSING PATIENTS
Rule Out Delirium

Delirium can be life-threatening, and patients with dementia are at increased risk for delirium.[12] The acute symptoms of delirium may be similar to the chronic symptoms of dementia. Therefore, the emergency physician must rule out delirium, starting by determining whether a patient's cognitive impairment is acute or chronic.

- Delirium is a syndrome characterized by the following:
    - Disorientation (confusion, inability to name time or place)

- Impaired attention (easily distracted, unable to complete simple tasks)
- A fluctuating state of consciousness (periods of alertness alternating with somnolence)
- Delirium usually results from *acute* conditions, such as the following:
  - Medication adverse effects
  - Acute medical disorders, such as infections or metabolic abnormalities
  - Substance intoxication or withdrawal
- Delirium can include neurocognitive symptoms, such as the following:
  - Depressed mood and affect
    - Slowed movement and appearance
    - Limited range of emotional expression
  - Psychosis
    - Delusions (firmly held false beliefs, such as paranoia)
    - Hallucinations (the perception of an external stimulus, such as a sound or a vision, without an actual external stimulus)
  - Agitation
    - Excited behavioral activity, usually accompanied by fear, anger, or extreme anxiety

Distinguishing between acute and chronic etiologies of neurocognitive impairment can be challenging.[13] The major clinical distinctions between delirium and dementia are summarized in **Table 2**.

It is rare for geriatric patients to present with a new-onset primary psychotic disorder, such as schizophrenia. In an older patient with no prior history of neuropsychiatric symptoms, a medical cause should be assumed until proven otherwise.[14]

Assess for Pain

The inability to successfully communicate pain in severe dementia is a major barrier to effective treatment.[15] The behavioral indicators of pain have long been recognized, and many clinical tools have been developed to assess pain in older patients, including those with dementia. Behaviors including agitation and aggression can be considered as signs of pain.[16] However, in patients with major neurocognitive disorder, these signs may be interpreted as neuropsychiatric symptoms of dementia rather

Table 2
Major distinctions between delirium and dementia

Characteristic	Delirium	Dementia
Symptom onset	Rapid, over hours or days	Gradual, over months or years
Disease course	Transient, usually limited	Chronic, persistent
Attention	Impaired, distracted	Usually intact, but may be impaired in advanced disease
Consciousness, sensorium	Altered, fluctuating	Usually alert and stable
Hallucinations	Often present, typically visual	Usually absent, but can be present in advanced disease
Prognosis	Usually reversible	Progressively deteriorating, no known cure

Adapted from The Geriatric Emergency Department Guidelines, 2013.

than of pain.[17] In order to avoid missing this diagnosis, pain should always be considered as a potential precipitant in any patient with dementia who presents with neuropsychiatric symptoms.

Consider other Diagnoses

After the patient has been assessed for delirium and pain, other reversible causes of dementia should be considered. Dementia of relatively recent onset has a higher likelihood of a potentially reversible etiology, underscoring the importance of obtaining a careful history. Some of these conditions include the following:

1. Medications that may affect mentation (sedatives, some anticholinergics, and hormone replacement)
2. Major depressive disorder (the term "pseudodementia" refers to neurocognitive impairment that results from major depression)
3. Normal pressure hydrocephalus
4. Vitamin B12 and folate deficiency
5. Thyroid disease
6. Benign tumors
7. Subdural hematoma
8. Infectious diseases (eg, syphilis)

It should be noted that the concept of "reversible dementia" is controversial in the literature. Some clinicians consider these conditions to be a form of delirium. One study estimated that only 1.5% of all dementias are reversible,[18] and routine screening for uncommon reversible causes of dementia is considered by some to be low yield.[19]

Clinical Tools and Scales

Despite its prevalence in the ED, neurocognitive impairment frequently goes unrecognized.[20] This has led some investigators to call for greater use of cognitive assessment tools in the ED, including the use of dementia screens after delirium has been ruled out.[21]

The Mini Mental State Examination (MMSE) and the MoCA are the most widely used brief screening tools for cognitive impairment, but because they require approximately 15 minutes to administer, they are impractical for routine use in the ED.

The Abbreviated Mental Test 4 (AMT-4), Short Blessed Test, Brief Alzheimer's Screen (BAS), the Six Item Screener, and Ottowa 3DY (O3DY) are some of the ultrabrief screening instruments developed to identify geriatric patients with cognitive dysfunction in the ED.[22] The AMT-4 has been shown to be the most accurate ED screening instrument to rule in the diagnosis of dementia, whereas the BAS is the most accurate screener to rule it out.[23]

The ADEPT tool was developed as an easy-to-use, point-of-care tool to assist emergency physicians in the care of older patients with confusion and agitation.[11] It is an open-access, Web-based tool available on the American College of Emergency Physicians emPOC mobile device app. It was designed to be used by clinicians on shift. To help ensure thorough consideration of the multiple etiologies of neurocognitive symptoms in older patients, it highlights 5 core concepts: assess, diagnose, evaluate, prevent, and treat (**Box 2**). However, none of the preceding tools can be used to definitively diagnose dementia, and none of them differentiate the severity of cognitive impairment. Many require special training to administer, involve complex calculations in the scoring process, assume a cooperative patient, or have other barriers to their widespread use in the ED setting. In addition, some cognitive assessment instruments may not be valid across lower socioeconomic and limited health literacy populations.[24] Further refinement of clinical instruments and the application of technology to the assessment process may accelerate the use of standardized tools to reduce the rate of unrecognized neurocognitive impairment in the ED.

Box 2
Principles of the ADEPT tool

ASSESS
- Perform a thorough evaluation to determine the underlying cause.
- The history, medication review, and collateral information are crucial.
- Perform a thorough physical examination.

DIAGNOSE
- Screen for delirium in any agitated or confused older patient.
- Screen for underlying major neurocognitive disorder (dementia).

EVALUATE
- Perform a thorough, focused medical workup for agitation or confusion.
- General tests for most patients
- Specific, targeted testing and evaluation

PREVENT
- Individual patient measures to prevent or manage delirium
- Hospital and systems-based measures to prevent or manage delirium

TREAT
- Take a multimodal approach to treatment.
- Use verbal de-escalation principles.
- If needed, start with oral medications.
- Carefully consider the use of intramuscular or intravenous medications.
- Avoid benzodiazepines if possible unless in withdrawal.
- Be cautious to prevent harm and minimize side effects.

From Shenvi C, Kennedy M, Austin CA, Wilson MP, Gerardi M, Schneider S. Managing Delirium and Agitation in the Older Emergency Department Patient: The ADEPT Tool. Ann Emerg Med. 2020;75(2):136-145.

TREATING PATIENTS

Emergency physicians frequently struggle with management of the acutely agitated patient with dementia. Because of the increased risks associated with use of medications in older patients, clinicians should consider using nonpharmacological interventions as first-line therapy.

The best initial approach is to prevent agitation before it starts. This begins with identification of any potentially modifiable precipitants to agitation.[25] These include the following:

- Delirium
- Medication side effects
- Pain
- Physical needs (hunger, need for toileting)
- Emotional needs (separation from family, need for support)
- Environmental factors (noise, overcrowding, understimulation)
- Caregivers (including family) who are inflexible in their approach to the patient

Preventive measures include the following:

- Gentle verbal redirection, tailored to the patient's personality and emotional state

- Frequent reorientation to their surroundings
- Staff members reintroducing themselves at each encounter
- Well-lit rooms to minimize misperceptions
- One-to-one bedside companions
- Manual activities (coloring, folding, jigsaw puzzle)

TREATMENT OF ACUTE AGITATION

No drug is approved by the Food and Drug Administration (FDA) to treat agitation associated with dementia, and medications should be used only as a last resort. Antipsychotics are the most frequently prescribed medications for this purpose,[26] despite an FDA black-box warning of increased mortality when used in older adults with dementia (odds ratio 1.7).[27] Other serious side effects include the following: extrapyramidal symptoms (EPS), sedation, tardive dyskinesia (TD), gait disturbances, falls, anticholinergic side effects, and cerebrovascular events.

Antipsychotics

Despite the FDA warning, most clinicians recognize that antipsychotics are effective psychotropic agents for controlling severe agitation, aggressive behavior, and psychosis. Second-generation antipsychotics (SGA) have the best evidence to support their use in the treatment of agitation associated with dementia. Evidence suggests that risperidone and olanzapine are useful in reducing aggression, and that risperidone reduces psychosis.[28] Haloperidol, a first-generation antipsychotic, has been shown to be useful in reducing aggression,[29] but is more likely to cause EPS and TD than the SGAs. Despite their modest efficacy, none of these drugs should be used routinely to treat patients with dementia with aggression or psychosis unless there is severe distress or risk of physical harm, and only after case-by-case consideration of benefits versus risks.

Special care should be taken when using antipsychotics in patients with Lewy body dementia or Parkinson dementia. These diseases both involve dopamine dysfunction. Because all antipsychotics have some degree of dopamine blockade, their use could worsen or precipitate extrapyramidal symptoms.[30] Antipsychotics with the least amount of dopamine blockade, such as quetiapine, may be better tolerated by these patients. A newer antipsychotic, pimavanserin, may reduce psychosis symptoms without worsening motor function and is FDA approved for use in Parkinson disease.[31]

Benzodiazepines

Care must be taken when prescribing benzodiazepines to older persons. The half-life of benzodiazepines may be increased dramatically in late life, with diazepam having a half-life nearing 4 days in persons in their 80s.[32] Older persons are also more susceptible to the potential side effects of benzodiazepines, such as memory impairment, fatigue, drowsiness, motor dysfunction, and falls. Some investigators argue that short-acting benzodiazepines may be used temporarily for acute agitation or agitation associated with anxiety.[26] In general, however, they are best avoided.[33]

TREATMENT OF CHRONIC SYMPTOMS

The following medications are not typically used on an as needed basis for control of acute neuropsychiatric symptoms, but they are frequently prescribed to help manage chronic symptoms.

Cholinesterase Inhibitors

Donepezil, galantamine, and rivastigmine are cholinesterase inhibitors (ChEI) that are FDA approved for use in mild to moderate AD but are commonly used in nearly all dementia subtypes. When taken daily, they can enhance cognition, reduce behavioral changes, and delay functional decline in persons with major neurocognitive impairment; however, they do not affect the progression of disease. Common side effects include nausea, vomiting, and diarrhea.

Memantine

Memantine is an N-methyl-D-aspartate (NMDA) receptor antagonist that can also have beneficial effects on cognition, behavior, and function in dementia. It is frequently prescribed in combination with a ChEI. It generally has few adverse effects.

Antidepressants

Depression is a common neuropsychiatric symptom of dementia, and use of antidepressants among patients with major neurocognitive disorder is widespread. Despite limited evidence for the efficacy of these medications in treatment of depression in patients with dementia, some investigators and clinical organizations recommend their use.[34] Selective serotonin reuptake inhibitors, such as sertraline and citalopram, are most commonly used because of their favorable side-effect profile. Trazodone, an antidepressant with mixed serotonin, histamine, and α-adrenergic activity, is sometimes used to treat agitation in chronic brain failure, despite little supporting evidence.[35] Trazodone and mirtazapine are often prescribed for sleep.

DECISION-MAKING CAPACITY

The cognitive deficits of chronic brain failure often impair a patient's decision-making capacity and ability to provide informed consent. Before administering any medication or treatment, an effort to obtain informed consent should be made to the extent possible. Many patients have a designated decision-maker, such as a guardian or power of attorney; however, all patients with dementia cannot be assumed to have impaired capacity. To demonstrate decision-making capacity, the patient must (1) communicate a consistent choice, (2) understand the relevant information, (3) appreciate the current situation and its consequences, and (4) manipulate information rationally.[36] Decision-making capacity is situation-specific, and some patients who carry a diagnosis of major neurocognitive disorder may still be able to meet those 4 criteria in a given situation.

Treatment decisions and disposition planning for patients with advanced dementia should take into consideration the severity of their neurocognitive impairment and ideally should be guided by the goals of care for that individual. Unfortunately, the goals of care are often unclear when making disposition plans; 56% to 99% of older adults do not have advance directives available at ED presentation.[37]

DISPOSITION

Despite the potential to optimize a patient's quality of life during the disease course, dementia remains a progressively debilitating disorder that ultimately results in death. Of persons in the United States who die with dementia, approximately 16% die in hospitals.[38] In one study, 19% of nursing home patients who died with advanced dementia had a burdensome transition near the end of life (hospitalization in the last 3 days of life, multiple hospitalizations in the last 90 days of life, or care in multiple nursing homes after hospitalization in the last 90 days of life).[39]

Patients with dementia are at increased risk of hospitalization, despite no true medical indication. This may be due to a decrease in community supports and resources to safely care for persons with major neurocognitive impairments.[40] It has also been associated with "caregiver burnout," which occurs when someone caring for a patient with dementia is overwhelmed by the agitation, psychosis, and other neuropsychiatric symptoms of the disease.[41] As seen in the preceding case example, an entire residential care facility also can be overwhelmed by the severity of a patient's symptoms to the point where they no longer feel capable of safely caring for that patient. Without any clear discharge options, many patients with dementia are admitted to inpatient medical services despite lacking medical necessity.[42]

Effective treatment of neuropsychiatric symptoms can help facilitate the patient's return to their home or care facility. This may include appropriate pain management. Surveys have indicated that the goal of care for most patients is comfort.[43] If available and appropriate, a palliative care consultation or hospice referral can be considered. Patients with advanced dementia who are enrolled in hospice have been shown to have a lower risk of dying in the hospital[44] and of being hospitalized in the last 30 days of life.[45] In addition, their families have greater satisfaction with care.[46]

DISCUSSION

The term *chronic brain failure* has been used here in an attempt to better represent the condition to which it refers. The term emerged in the 1970s as an alternative to *dementia*, which was thought to be imprecise and, when used as a lay term, stigmatizing and potentially pejorative.[47] More recently, the term *neurocognitive disorders* has been officially adopted,[8] but it excludes the emotional, behavioral, and other noncognitive aspects of brain function that can be part of the syndrome. Like chronic heart and kidney failure, chronic brain failure describes a progressive loss of organ function that is typically irreversible but whose symptoms can be mitigated with proper management.

Unlike with other organ failure syndromes, however, little progress has been made to advance our understanding of dementia, despite tremendous research efforts. No new AD therapies have won federal approval since 2003, and AD clinical trials have had a 99% failure rate. Since the introduction of tacrine in 1993, only 5 drugs have been approved by the FDA to treat AD, and those merely alleviate symptoms, such as memory loss and confusion; they do not prevent, slow, or reverse the disease.[48]

Some promising developments have been made in nonpharmacologic approaches to chronic brain failure. Some of the most significant of these have been in the area of prevention: for example, linking aerobic exercise to lower rates of AD.[49] Others involve conceptualizing dementia as a spectrum syndrome, with interventions tailored to the degree of impairment, and to the personality and preferences of each individual patient. Interactions that give a patient a sense of choice and independence are more likely to be successful.[50] The diagnosis of dementia does not imply specific functional impairments, and many individuals with chronic brain failure live rich, active lives. Treatment goals should be focused on helping patients cope with the negative aspects of their illness so that they can live the best life that they can.

Chronic brain failure involves physical changes in the brain that can degrade a person's ability to modulate the behavioral expression of emotion. For example, a person with dementia who is receiving personal hygiene care might feel embarrassed or threatened and react aggressively. Fear, anxiety, and insecurity in someone with severe neurocognitive impairment are often expressed as paranoia and/or aggression.

Effective communication, therefore, requires an understanding of the patient's underlying emotional state and an adaptation to their internal experience of reality.

Use of logic and reason is rarely successful when attempting to redirect a patient with severe neurocognitive impairment. Efforts to alter their reality can create frustration and confusion and lead to unsafe behaviors. Should a patient become agitated, the clinician should identify what the patient sees as their own needs in the moment and adapt their approach to the underlying emotion. Distraction or redirection of the patient's thoughts can also be effective; for example, gently changing the subject or asking about something or someone from their past.

The use of deceit in dementia care, also known as "therapeutic lying," is widespread but controversial. One survey of nursing home staff showed that 96% of respondents (n = 112) across disciplines lied to cognitively impaired residents.[51] Despite this widespread practice, many caregivers feel uncomfortable or guilty about deceiving patients, even if it is perceived to be in their best interests.[52] It can be viewed as demeaning and disrespectful to the patient, and inconsistent with the principle of patient autonomy. In the preceding case example, the patient asked for his wife and was told that she was out of town; however, if he was told that she was dead each time he asked for her, he might experience recurrent grief. Thus, deception can be used to the patient's benefit. In the absence of clear ethical guidelines, the provider is left to use his or her clinical judgment in deciding whether to use deception as part of the management approach. When making that decision, consideration should be given to the patient's degree of memory impairment, and the deception should occur only respectfully and in the best interest of the patient.

The stress of caring for patients with chronic brain failure is well documented.[53] The neuropsychiatric symptoms of severe dementia have a profound physical and psychological impact on both professional and informal caregivers. Psychological distress and burnout are common.[54] This in turn can have negative effects on the caregiver's relationship with the patient and is the primary driver of long-term placement.[55] Emergency physicians can play a role in identifying caregiver burnout, encouraging healthy stress-release practices among caregivers, and directing them to appropriate resources, such as those offered by the Alzheimer's Association (www.alz.org) and the Family Caregiver Alliance (www.caregiver.org).

DISCLOSURE

The author has nothing to disclose.

REFERENCES

1. Plassman BL, Langa KM, Fisher GG, et al. Prevalence of dementia in the United States: the aging, demographics, and memory study. Neuroepidemiology 2007; 29(1–2):125–32.
2. LaMantia MA, Stump TE, Messina FC, et al. Emergency department use among older adults with dementia. Alzheimer Dis Assoc Disord 2016;30(1):35–40.
3. Fernando E, Fraser M, Hendriksen J, et al. Risk factors associated with falls in older adults with dementia: a systematic review. Physiother Can 2017;69(2): 161–70.
4. Jacobsohn GC, Hollander M, Beck AP, et al. Factors influencing emergency care by persons with dementia: stakeholder perceptions and unmet needs. J Am Geriatr Soc 2019;67(4):711–8.
5. Alzheimer's Association. 2018 Alzheimer's disease facts and figures. Alzheimer's Dement 2018;14(3):367–429.

6. Qiu C, Kivipelto M, von Strauss E. Epidemiology of Alzheimer's disease: occurrence, determinants, and strategies toward intervention. Dialogues Clin Neurosci 2009;11(2):111–28.

7. Abraham G, Zun L. *Delirium and dementia* in Rosen's emergency medicine: concepts and clinical practice. 8th edition. Philadelphia: Elsevier/Saunders; 2014.

8. American Psychiatric Association. In: Diagnostic and statistical manual of mental disorders, 5th ed (DSM-5). Arlington (VA): American Psychiatric Publishing; 2013.

9. Sadowski M, Pankiewicz J, Scholtzova H, et al. Links between the pathology of Alzheimer's disease and vascular dementia. Neurochem Res 2004;29(6):1257–66.

10. Goodman RA, Lochner KA, Thambisetty M, et al. Prevalence of dementia subtypes in United States Medicare fee-for-service beneficiaries, 2011-2013. Alzheimers Dement 2017;13(1):28–37.

11. Shenvi C, Kennedy M, Austin CA, et al. Managing delirium and agitation in the older emergency department patient: The ADEPT Tool. Ann Emerg Med 2020;75(2):136–45.

12. Morandi A, Davis D, Bellelli G, et al. The diagnosis of delirium superimposed on dementia: an emerging challenge. J Am Med Dir Assoc 2017;18(1):12–8.

13. Siafarikas N, Selbaek G, Fladby T, et al. Frequency and subgroups of neuropsychiatric symptoms in mild cognitive impairment and different stages of dementia in Alzheimer's disease. Int Psychogeriatr 2018;30:103–13.

14. Targum SD, Abbott JL. Psychoses in the elderly: a spectrum of disorders. J Clin Psychiatry 1999;60:4–10.

15. Hadjistavropoulos T, Herr K, Prkachin KM, et al. Pain assessment in elderly adults with dementia. Lancet Neurol 2014;13(12):1216–27.

16. Burfield AH, Wan TT, Sole ML, et al. Behavioral cues to expand a pain model of the cognitively impaired elderly in long-term care. Clin Interv Aging 2012;7:207–23.

17. Horgas AL. Assessing pain in persons with dementia. Medsurg Nurs 2008;16:207–8.

18. Michel JM, Sellal F. Les démences « curables » en 2011 ["Reversible" dementia in 2011]. Geriatr Psychol Neuropsychiatr Vieil 2011;9(2):211–25.

19. Boustani M, Peterson B, Harris R, et al. Screening for dementia. Rockville (MD): Agency for Healthcare Research and Quality (US); 2003.

20. Boucher V, Lamontagne ME, Nadeau A, et al. Unrecognized incident delirium in older emergency department patients. J Emerg Med 2019;57(4):535–42.

21. Han JH, Suyama J. Delirium and dementia. Clin Geriatr Med 2018;34(3):327–54.

22. Carpenter CR, Bassett ER, Fischer GM, et al. Four sensitive screening tools to detect cognitive dysfunction in geriatric emergency department patients: brief Alzheimer's Screen, Short Blessed Test, Ottawa 3DY, and the caregiver-completed AD8. Acad Emerg Med 2011;18(4):374–84.

23. Carpenter CR, Banerjee J, Keyes D, et al. Accuracy of dementia screening instruments in emergency medicine: a diagnostic meta-analysis. Acad Emerg Med 2019;26(2):226–45.

24. Scazufca M, Almeida OP, Vallada HP, et al. Limitations of the Mini-Mental State Examination for screening dementia in a community with low socioeconomic status: results from the Sao Paulo Ageing & Health Study. Eur Arch Psychiatry Clin Neurosci 2009;259:8–15.

25. Piechniczek-Buczek J. Psychiatric emergencies in the elderly population. Emerg Med Clin North Am 2006;24(2):467–viii.

26. Azermai M. Dealing with behavioral and psychological symptoms of dementia: a general overview. Psychol Res Behav Manag 2015;8:181–5.
27. U.S. Food and Drug Administration. Available at: https://www.fda.gov/drugs/drug-safety-and-availability/. Accessed May 14, 2020.
28. Ballard CG, Waite J, Birks J. Atypical antipsychotics for aggression and psychosis in Alzheimer's disease. Cochrane Database Syst Rev 2006;(1):CD003476.
29. Lonergan E, Luxenberg J, Colford JM, et al. Haloperidol for agitation in dementia. Cochrane Database Syst Rev 2002;(2):CD002852.
30. McKeith I, Fairbairn A, Perry R, et al. Neuroleptic sensitivity in patients with senile dementia of Lewy body type. BMJ 1992;305(6855):673–8.
31. Cummings J, Isaacson S, Mills R, et al. Pimavanserin for patients with Parkinson's disease psychosis: a randomised, placebo-controlled phase 3 trial. Lancet 2014; 383(9916):8–14.
32. Blazer DG, Steffens DC. Older adults. In: Roberts LW, Yudofsky SC, Hales RE, editors. The American Psychiatric Association Publishing Textbook of Psychiatry. 7th edition. Washington, DC: American Psychiatric Publishing; 2019.
33. Geriatric emergency department guidelines. American College of Emergency Physicians; American Geriatrics Society; Emergency Nurses Association; Society for Academic Emergency Medicine; Geriatric Emergency Department Guidelines Task Force. Ann Emerg Med. 2014 May;63(5):e7-25. doi: 10.1016/j. annemergmed.2014.02.008.
34. Kimchi EZ, Lyketsos CG. Dementia and mild neurocognitive disorders. In: Steffens DC, Blazer DG, Thakur ME, editors. The American psychiatric publishing textbook of geriatric psychiatry. 5th edition. Washington, DC: American Psychiatric Publishing; 2016. p. 177–242.
35. Martinon-Torres G, Fioravanti M, Grimley EJ. Trazodone for agitation in dementia. Cochrane Database Syst Rev 2004;(4):CD004990.
36. Appelbaum PS, Grisso T. Assessing patients' capacities to consent to treatment [published correction appears in N Engl J Med 1989 Mar 16;320(11):748]. N Engl J Med 1988;319(25):1635–8.
37. Wissow LS, Belote A, Kramer W, et al. Promoting advance directives among elderly primary care patients. J Gen Intern Med 2004;19(9):944–51.
38. Mitchell SL, Teno JM, Miller SC, et al. A national study of the location of death for older persons with dementia. J Am Geriatr Soc 2005;53:299–305.
39. Gozalo P, Teno JM, Mitchell SL, et al. End-of-life transitions among nursing home residents with cognitive issues. N Engl J Med 2011;365:1212–21.
40. Torjesen I. Figures show big increase in emergency admissions for dementia patients. BMJ 2020;368:m249.
41. Phelan EA, Borson S, Grothaus L, et al. Association of incident dementia with hospitalizations. JAMA 2012;307:165–72.
42. Givens JL, Selby K, Goldfeld KS, et al. Hospital transfers of nursing home residents with advanced dementia. J Am Geriatr Soc 2012;60:905–9.
43. Mitchell SL, Teno JM, Kiely DK, et al. The clinical course of advanced dementia. N Engl J Med 2009;361:1529–38.
44. Miller SC, Lima JC, Looze J, et al. Dying in U.S. nursing homes with advanced dementia: how does health care use differ for residents with, versus without, end-of-life Medicare skilled nursing facility care? J Palliat Med 2012;15:43–50.
45. Miller SC, Gozalo P, Mor V. Hospice enrollment and hospitalization of dying nursing home patients. Am J Med 2001;111:38–44.
46. Kiely DK, Givens JL, Shaffer ML, et al. Hospice use and outcomes in nursing home residents with advanced dementia. J Am Geriatr Soc 2010;58:2284–91.

47. Isaacs B, Caird FI. Brain failure": a contribution to the terminology of mental ab-normality in old age. Age Ageing 1976;5(4):241–4.
48. Baily M. After many disappointments, the search for Alzheimer's drugs is more urgent than ever. The Washington Post 2017. Health & Science.
49. Valenzuela PL, Castillo-García A, Morales JS, et al. Exercise benefits on Alz-heimer's disease: State-of-the-science [published online ahead of print, 2020 Jun 17]. Ageing Res Rev 2020;62:101108.
50. Lanctôt KL, Amatniek J, Ancoli-Israel S, et al. Neuropsychiatric signs and symp-toms of Alzheimer's disease: new treatment paradigms. Alzheimers Dement (N Y) 2017;3(3):440–9.
51. James IA, Wood-Mitchell AJ, Waterworth AM, et al. Lying to people with demen-tia: developing ethical guidelines for care settings. Int J Geriatr Psychiatry 2006; 21(8):800–1.
52. Mental Health Foundation. Dementia – what is truth?. 2014. Available at: https://www.mentalhealth.org.uk/projects/dementia-and-truth-telling. Accessed May 21, 2020.
53. Brodaty H, Draper B, Low LF. Nursing home staff attitudes towards residents with dementia: strain and satisfaction with work. J Adv Nurs 2003;44(6):583–90.
54. Schulz R, Martire LM. Family caregiving of persons with dementia: prevalence, health effects, and support strategies. Am J Geriatr Psychiatry 2004;12(3):240–9.
55. Wuest J, Ericson PK, Stern PN. Becoming strangers: the changing family care-giving relationship in Alzheimer's disease. J Adv Nurs 1994;20(3):437–43.

Cardiopulmonary Emergencies in Older Adults

Rebecca Theophanous, MD[a], Wennie Huang, PharmD, BCPS[a],
Luna Ragsdale, MD, MPH[a,b],*

KEYWORDS

- Atrial fibrillation • Congestive heart failure • Pneumonia • Pulmonary embolism
- COVID-19 • Older adults

KEY POINTS

- Older adults have age-related changes that make them more susceptible to cardiopulmonary disease.
- Older adults have higher morbidity and mortality.
- Older adults can present with atypical symptoms.
- Treatment should be decided through shared decision making with patients and their families.

INTRODUCTION

The number of Americans aged 65 years and older will nearly double to 95 million over the next 40 years.[1] As patients age, they undergo physiologic changes that make them more susceptible to certain diseases. This article discusses 4 common cardiopulmonary emergency department (ED) presentations with a focus on the unique considerations of older adult patients, namely atrial fibrillation (AF), congestive heart failure (HF), pulmonary embolism (PE), and pneumonia.

ATRIAL FIBRILLATION
Epidemiology and Pathophysiology

AF is the most common cardiac arrhythmia, affecting nearly 2.5 million people in the United States. Older adults are disproportionately affected by this condition, and 70% of all patients who have AF are between the ages of 65 and 85 years.[2]

With aging, the heart undergoes structural remodeling as well as changes in neural regulation. Enlargement of the left atrium, autonomic neural dysregulation, ion channel

[a] Department of Surgery, Division of Emergency Medicine, Duke University Hospital, 2301 Erwin Road, Durham, NC 27710, USA; [b] Emergency Department, Durham VA Health Care System, Durham, NC 27710, USA
* Corresponding author. Durham VA Health Care System, 508 Fulton Street, Durham, NC 27705.
E-mail address: luna.ragsdale@va.gov
Twitter: @rbectheo (R.T.); @pharmd_aware (W.H.); @lunaragsdale (L.R.)

Emerg Med Clin N Am 39 (2021) 323–338
https://doi.org/10.1016/j.emc.2021.01.010
0733-8627/21/Published by Elsevier Inc.

emed.theclinics.com

dysfunction, and reduced left ventricular diastolic filling from hypertrophy can all increase an older adult's risk of developing AF.[3]

Patients with AF are at high risk for stroke, with a significantly increased risk in older adults (up to 23.5% in patients aged 80–90 years).[4] Furthermore, older adults are more likely to have severe functional deficits from a stroke affecting their daily living and placing them at higher risk for falls.

Anticoagulation therapy is the main preventive method for thromboembolic stroke; however, increased bleeding risk, frequent falls, and medication interactions are major considerations in older patients.[5]

Management

In the ED, treatment of AF in older patients with a rapid ventricular rate is similar to other patients. If the patient is unstable (has hypotension, altered mental status, active chest pain, shortness of breath, or signs of acute congestive HF), treatment should be targeted toward stabilizing the patient with synchronized electrical cardioversion. If the patient is clinically stable, practitioners can choose to treat AF with rate control (β-blocker or calcium channel blocker) or rhythm control (ie, chemical or electrical cardioversion) therapy, with studies showing an overall similar success rate but a decreased ED length of stay in those patients who are cardioverted.[6,7]

Another consideration in ED patients who are presenting with AF is the duration of symptoms. In the past, studies have suggested that patients in rapid AF for less than 48 hours have a much lower risk for venous thromboembolic events (VTEs) within 30 days after electrical cardioversion (1.1%).[8] However, more recent studies have recommended an even shorter electrical cardioversion window of less than 12 hours, with a risk for VTE of only 0.3%.[8] In addition, the calculation of a CHA2DS2-Vasc (congestive HF; hypertension; age $\geq$75 years; diabetes mellitus; prior stroke, TIA, or thromboembolism; vascular disease; age 65–74 years; sex category) score is useful in determining risk of VTEs after cardioversion and in deciding on anticoagulation in patients with AF. Lip and colleagues[9] showed zero thromboembolic events in patients with a CHA_2DS_2-VASc score of 0, less than 1% with a score of 1, and a rate of 1.9% to 3.9% events in patients with a score of 2 to 5.

Considerations for anticoagulation in older patients

Anticoagulation for prevention of VTEs in patients with AF has been a controversial topic, especially in older patients who have an increased risk of falls and bleeding. The 2 mainstays of anticoagulation therapy are vitamin K antagonists (VKAs; eg, warfarin), which require frequent International Normalized Ratio (INR) checks, and direct oral anticoagulants (DOACs; eg, rivaroxaban, apixaban, dabigatran). An important age-related change is impairment in renal function, which leads to decreased elimination of VKA and DOACs and thus an increased bleeding risk, as reflected in bleeding prediction scores such as HAS-BLED (hypertension, abnormal renal/liver function, stroke, bleeding history or predisposition, labile INR, elderly, drugs/alcohol concomitantly) or HEMORR$_2$HAGES (hepatic or renal disease, ethanol abuse, malignancy history, older [age>75 y], reduced platelet count or function, rebleeding risk, hypertension [uncontrolled], anemia, genetic factors, excessive fall risk, stroke history, maximum score)[10,11] (**Tables 1** and **2**).

Cost of therapy is an important consideration when choosing a therapy because the DOACs are significantly more expensive than warfarin. However, transportation to laboratory draws must also be considered. In low-risk patients with a CHA_2DS_2-VASc score of 0 to 1, 81 mg of aspirin is an option.

Multiple clinical trials and meta-analyses have shown a relative risk reduction for aspirin versus placebo of 21%, with an even larger risk reduction of 62% seen for

Table 1
HAS-BLED[9]

Risk Factor	Score
Hypertension Uncontrolled, >160 mm Hg systolic	1
Renal disease Dialysis, Cr>2.26 mg/dL or >200 μmol/L	1
Liver disease Cirrhosis or bilirubin >2× normal or with ALT/AST/AP>3× normal	1
Stroke history	1
Prior major bleeding	1
Labile INR Unstable/high INR; time in therapeutic range <60%	1
Age>65 y	1
Medication predisposing to bleeding Aspirin, clopidogrel, NSAIDs	1
Alcohol use ≥8 drinks/wk	1
Maximum score	9

A score of 0 to 2 indicates low risk of bleeding; a score of ≥3 indicates high risk of bleeding.
  Abbreviations: ALT, alanine aminotransferase; AP, alkaline phosphatase; AST, aspartate transaminase; Cr, creatinine; NSAIDs, nonsteroidal antiinflammatory drugs.

warfarin versus placebo.[12,13] However, older patients also have a higher risk for life-threatening or fatal bleeding, with an anticoagulation-intensity adjusted relative risk of 4.6 in patients older than 80 years.[14]

Clinicians should use caution in prescribing anticoagulation therapy in patients who are at high risk for falls and should have a risk-versus-benefit discussion with all patients. Recent studies on fall-related hemorrhage events in patients on VKA are mixed, with some studies showing no difference in rates of acute intracranial hemorrhage, whereas others do show increased rates of bleeding. Patients with a higher

Table 2
HEMORR₂HAGES[11]

Clinical Characteristic	Score
Hepatic or renal disease	1
Ethanol abuse	1
Malignancy history	1
Older (age >75 y)	1
Reduced platelet count or function	1
Rebleeding risk	2
Hypertension (uncontrolled)	1
Anemia	1
Genetic factors	1
Excessive fall risk	1
Stroke history	1
Maximum score	12

A score of 0 to 1 indicates low risk of bleeding; a score of 2 to 3 indicates intermediate risk; a score ≥4 indicates high risk of bleeding.

CHA_2DS_2-VASc score of 2 or greater, indicating an increased risk for stroke and myocardial infarction (MI), seem to benefit overall from anticoagulation, even in the setting of an increased risk of hemorrhage.[15]

A meta-analysis by Deng and colleagues[16] included 5 phase III randomized control trials to evaluate the efficacy and safety of VKA versus DOACs in the prophylaxis of stroke or systemic embolism in older patients (>75 years old). They found that DOACs resulted in a lower incidence of stroke/systemic embolism and major bleeding compared with warfarin (hazard ratio, 0.71; 95% confidence interval, 0.33–1.50), with apixaban ranking the best (rank probabilities, 71.4%).[16]

Summary

AF is a common condition in older patients and treatment varies depending on the duration of symptoms and clinical presentation. Acute treatment options include electrical cardioversion or medical treatment with rate versus rhythm control. An important factor to consider in patients newly diagnosed in the ED is anticoagulation for prevention of VTEs and stroke. Because older adults are often at high risk for falls or severe bleeding events, physicians should have a risk-versus-benefit discussion with their patients and should use clinical tools to assist in their decisions. Treatment options include VKAs (warfarin) or DOACs. DOACs may have a safer bleeding risk profile. Overall, treatment should be tailored to each patient using shared decision making.

CONGESTIVE HEART FAILURE
Pathophysiology and Clinical Presentation

Congestive HF is the most common cause of hospital admissions and readmissions in older adults. With increasing survival rates from MI and a growing geriatric population, acute HF is prevalent and requires prompt recognition and treatment. Survival rates for decompensated HF have not improved in recent decades despite advances in diagnosis and treatment.[17]

Aging causes decreased elasticity of blood vessels, leading to increased afterload, left ventricular hypertrophy (LVH), and increased coronary oxygen consumption. Ischemia and fibrosis can occur when oxygen requirements are not met, causing systolic and diastolic HF. Concurrently, decreased cardiac output leads to decreased renal perfusion, which in turn activates the renin-angiotensin pathway. This increase in circulating catecholamine levels causes potent vasoconstriction and increased renal absorption that can exacerbate HF.

HF can be broadly categorized into 2 types: (1) diastolic HF, also known as HF with preserved ejection fraction; and (2) systolic HF, also known as HF with reduced ejection fraction. HFpEF accounts for approximately 50% of all patients with HF and is the most common type of HF in older adults.[18]

The classic symptoms of HF are shortness of breath, abdominal distension, leg swelling, orthopnea, and dyspnea on exertion. Older patients often present with atypical symptoms, such as decreased appetite, confusion, and fatigue. Infection is the most common instigating cause of decompensated HF, along with medication and dietary noncompliance, cardiac arrhythmias, and anemia.

Aortic stenosis is another important consideration in older adults, with a prevalence of 2% to 7% in patients aged 65 years and older having severe aortic stenosis.[19] In this age group, it is typically caused by diffuse atherosclerotic disease and the presentation is late because symptoms such as dyspnea, angina, and syncope can be attributed to other comorbidities.[19] Care should be taken with vasodilators and with aggressive fluid resuscitation in those patients with a systolic murmur because this may be the only indicator. Definitive treatment in severely symptomatic patients include open surgical versus transcatheter aortic valve replacement.[20]

Diagnosis

Acute HF is primarily a clinical diagnosis based on the patient's history and physical examination. The patient may appear volume overloaded with abdominal distension and leg edema, or may simply have tachypnea with shortness of breath, bibasilar rales, wheezing, reduced breath sounds, and jugular venous distension.

Point-of-care ultrasonography (POCUS) is useful in evaluating for a reduced ejection fraction, a dilated and minimally collapsible inferior vena cava (>2.5 cm, <50% change in diameter), pericardial effusion, or LVH. Bedside thoracic ultrasonography can help distinguish between a volume-overloaded state and a primary pulmonary process such as obstructive lung disease. Diffuse pulmonary B lines indicate an acute interstitial process, such as pulmonary edema in the case of HF (**Fig. 1**). Pleural effusions at the lung bases are detected with a higher sensitivity than with chest radiographs.[21] A study by Zanobetti and colleagues[22,23] showed excellent concordance between POCUS and ED diagnosis in patients with acute HF, with a kappa of 0.81.

Laboratory values

Age-adjusted pro–brain natriuretic protein (pro-BNP) for patients more than 85 years old includes a higher gray zone of 250 to 590 pg/mL and should be compared with the patient's baseline for the most useful interpretation. High-sensitivity troponin level may be increased secondary to underlying myocardial ischemia caused by the HF state rather than acute coronary syndrome. These patients often have acute renal failure

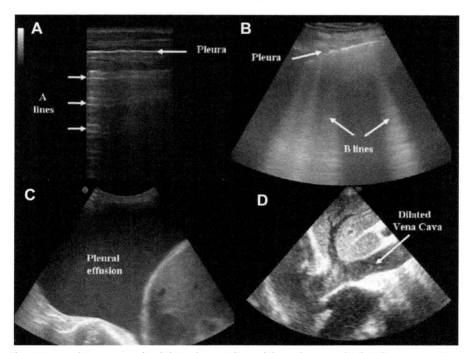

Fig. 1. Lung ultrasonography. (A) Dry lung, A lines; (B) wet lung, multiple B lines in a patient with decompensated HF (appearance of comet tails with ≥3 in each lung field); (C) large pleural effusion; (D) a dilated inferior vena cava.[22]

and transaminitis, which is caused by cardiorenal and cardiohepatic syndromes, respectively, from cardiac congestion and decreased blood flow to end organs.[20]

Management

In the acute setting, rapid diagnosis and treatment are paramount to improving mortality and morbidity in older patients. Each episode of decompensation substantially worsens the long-term course of these patients.[24] Patients should be positioned upright to improve their respiration. Oxygen therapy should only be used in patients who are hypoxic (oxygen saturation <90%). If the patient is in acute respiratory distress with pulmonary edema, noninvasive positive pressure ventilation (NIPPV) should be initiated if possible. NIPPV consistently decreases intubation rates and improves early outcomes of patients with acute cardiogenic pulmonary edema.[25]

Initiation of a vasodilator such as nitroglycerin is first-line treatment of decompensated HF and should be titrated aggressively to reduce afterload. Options include sublingual tablets or spray, or intravenous (IV) infusion. Patients who are taking a phosphodiesterase inhibitor such as sildenafil, have severe aortic stenosis, or have an acute inferior MI should not receive vasodilators.

Angiotensin-converting enzyme inhibitors reduce preload and afterload and are useful in patients with chronic HF. Their role in acute decompensation is controversial. Inotropes should not be used unless the patient is in cardiogenic shock, because they cause increased mortality.[26] Morphine is also associated with increased mortality.[27] Diuresis with IV loop diuretics (eg, furosemide) should be initiated in patients with fluid overload. The Diuretic Optimization Strategies Evaluation trial showed no significant difference in patient symptoms with bolus versus continuous-infusion dosing or low-dose versus high-dose diuretics. The high-dose strategy was associated with greater relief of dyspnea, fluid loss, weight loss, and fewer serious adverse events.[28]

Palliative care in patients with advanced HF focuses on management of symptoms rather than improving survival; oxygen is used in relieving dyspnea if the patient is hypoxic and small-dose opioids assist with air hunger and breathlessness.[29,30]

Summary

Acute HF is the leading cause of hospital admissions and readmissions in the older population. Symptoms in the older population are often atypical. Treatments include rapid reduction of blood pressure with nitroglycerin, diuresis, and supplemental oxygen if hypoxic. Patients in severe respiratory distress benefit greatly from NIPPV.

Palliative care should be considered in frail older patients presenting with multiple readmissions for HF.

PULMONARY EMBOLISM
Pathophysiology

VTE is caused by a triad of venous stasis, activation of the blood coagulation cascade, and endothelial vein damage. Older patients are at increased risk of VTE likely secondary to enhancement of coagulation activation, increased incidence of comorbid conditions, and immobilization.[31]

Clinical Presentation

The presentation of PE can be atypical in older patients.[32] Syncope is a common presentation, whereas pleuritic chest pain and shortness of breath are less common. Some patients may be completely asymptomatic, leading to a delayed diagnosis.[33]

Fewer older adults present with tachycardia and tachypnea. Furthermore, leg pain and swelling are less common.[34] Other clinical findings, such as hypoxia, right heart strain on electrocardiogram, and chest radiograph findings, are neither sensitive nor specific for the diagnosis of PE.

Diagnostic Testing

The Wells score for VTE is valid in older patients and stratifies clinical probability for thrombus as low, intermediate, or high. The use of D-dimer testing is highly sensitive for clot rule out in patients with a low pretest probability. In the past, a 500-mg/L cutoff was used for patients at low risk for clot. More recent studies have shown that an age-adjusted D-dimer with a higher cutoff for patients as they age (age × 10 μg/L in patients >50 years old) has higher specificity in all age categories, with the most pronounced difference in patients more than 80 years old (specificity 35.2%), without adversely affecting sensitivity.[34]

The diagnostic gold standard for PE is a chest computed tomography (CT) angiogram. Clinicians must consider renal impairment in older patients because a normal creatinine level does not always signify normal creatinine clearance. The utility of ventilation and perfusion scan is limited because it requires normal underlying lung tissue, which may not be present in older patients.[35]

Ultrasonography Findings

POCUS is a useful diagnostic tool in patients who are critically ill. A meta-analysis shows that transthoracic echocardiogram has a high specificity (83%) and low sensitivity (53%) in the diagnosis of PE.[36] A summary of ultrasonography findings in PE is given in **Box 1**.

Management

Patients who have a low PESI (Pulmonary Embolism Severity Index) score (<85 points) are at low risk for severe morbidity and thus may be safe to discharge home with anticoagulation. Because every year of age adds 10 points to the score, older patients are not usually in this low-risk category.

Anticoagulation is the primary treatment modality for patients with VTE/PE. Outpatient treatment options include low-molecular-weight heparin (LMWH) in patients without chronic renal failure, LMWH bridge to VKA (requires frequent INR checks), and DOACs. Unstable patients are typically started on IV heparin for more rapid clot breakdown, with consideration for potential intracatheter thrombolysis or clot retrieval.[37]

Although older patients may have increased bleeding risk given comorbidities and risk of falls, the benefit of anticoagulation still outweighs the risks associated with PE (2.2% risk of fatal bleeding vs 5.9% risk of fatal PE).[38] Creatinine clearance should be calculated before initiation of treatment, because many older patients have renal insufficiency, which affects clearance of LMWH, VKA, and DOACs.[39,40]

For patients in whom anticoagulation is contraindicated (eg, intracranial hemorrhage; large acute stroke; severe bleeding, such as gastrointestinal bleeding), an inferior vena cava filter can be placed to prevent extension or migration of clots from the pelvis and lower extremities to the heart and lungs.[41]

Summary

Older patients are at increased risk of VTE and often present with insidious symptoms such as fatigue but can also be asymptomatic. Age-adjusted D-dimers may be used to rule out VTE in patients who are at low risk for clots. POCUS is useful in evaluating for signs of right heart strain at the bedside and the diagnosis is confirmed with a CT angiogram. The benefits of treating PE in older patients usually outweigh the risks. Treatment options include anticoagulation with LMWH in patients with normal renal

> **Box 1**
> **Signs of right heart strain on ultrasonography**
>
> Dilated RV (1:1 ratio RV to LV) on AP4 or PSAX views
>
> Septal wall flattening or D sign on PSAX views
>
> McConnell sign (RV wall hypokinesis with apical sparing) on AP4 view
>
> Other findings:
> - Abnormal septal motion
> - Tricuspid regurgitation
> - 60/60 sign
> - Right heart thrombus
> - RV hypokinesis
> - Pulmonary hypertension
> - RV end-diastolic diameter
> - Tricuspid annular plane systolic excursion
> - RV systolic pressure
>
> *Abbreviations:* AP4, apical 4-chamber view; LV, left ventricle; PSAX, parasternal short axis; RV, right ventricle.
>
> *Data from* Fields JM, Davis J, Girson L, et al. Transthoracic Echocardiography for Diagnosing Pulmonary Embolism: A Systematic Review and Meta-Analysis. *J Am Soc Echocardiogr* 2017;30:714-23.

function, LMWH bridge to warfarin, or DOACs for outpatient management. Intracatheter thrombolysis or clot retrieval is used in patients in extremis.

PNEUMONIA
Epidemiology

More than 100 years ago, Sir William Osler called pneumonia a "friend of the aged" because there was little that could be done for treatment and it was viewed as a fast, painless death. Despite advances in vaccines and antimicrobial therapies, community-acquired pneumonia (CAP) is the fourth most common cause of death in older adults.

The incidence of pneumonia is 4 times greater in older adults than in younger, with 1 in 20 adults aged 85 years and older diagnosed with CAP annually.[42] Furthermore, older adults are 5 times more likely to be hospitalized with CAP than their younger counterparts.[43,44] The disproportionate risks of CAP in the geriatric population are multifactorial and secondary to the physiology of aging as well as underlying comorbidities.

Pathophysiology

Age-related decrease in chest wall compliance and a weakened diaphragm diminish respiratory reserve. Changes to the lung parenchyma and lung function lead to so-called senile emphysema.[45] Because of these changes, older adults are more susceptible to respiratory failure when acutely ill. Preceding viral infection, particularly influenza A, is a risk factor for bacterial pneumonia. Comorbidities such as cardiovascular disease, lung disease, malignancy, and diabetes increase the risk of pneumonia in older adults.[46] Neurologic conditions such as Parkinson disease, stroke, or dementia may cause a reduced ability to cough and can contribute to silent aspiration.

Polypharmacy is common in older adults and is another contributing factor.[47] Certain medications, such as antipsychotics, anticholinergics, and inhaled corticosteroids, have been associated with a higher risk of pneumonia.[48,49]

Clinical Presentation

Fever, chills, and shortness of breath are common presentations but are not always present. Symptom onset can be insidious or abrupt. Older patients may have atypical symptoms such as fatigue, vomiting, diarrhea, or delirium and may be hypothermic rather than febrile.[50,51] Patients may or may not have a cough.

Diagnostic Testing

Patients should have a chest radiograph to look for focal opacities. However, in some patients, opacities may be subtle because of poor imaging technique, difficulty in positioning, or underlying lung disease or chest wall abnormalities. In a study by Haga and colleagues,[52] CT scans detected up to 47% of pneumonia not seen on chest radiographs. Another study reported that up to one-third of patients admitted with clinical signs of pneumonia did not have evidence of pneumonia on chest radiograph.[53] Although CT is more sensitive, costs and incidental findings may limit its use in the diagnosis of CAP. In addition, severely ill patients who are hypoxic may not be able to lie flat.

Lung Ultrasonography Findings

Lung ultrasonography findings in pneumonia include more focal B lines, and are usually defined as a lung consolidation plus air bronchograms (scattered dotlike and branching hyperechoic dots) that are dynamic (centrifugal movements caused by breathing).[52] Other findings can also be seen, such as the shred sign (or fractal sign), which is an irregular pattern seen in nontranslobar or small consolidations (**Fig. 2**).[55]

POCUS has a sensitivity and specificity of 94% and 96%, respectively, for pneumonia when performed by an experienced user, compared with chest radiograph or CT chest.[56]

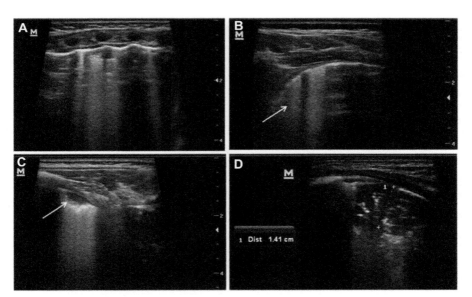

Fig. 2. Lung ultrasonography images in a patient with bronchiolitis complicated by pneumonia. (A) Multiple B lines, consistent with bronchiolitis. (B) Irregular pleural surface and confluent B lines (arrow). (C) Small subpleural consolidation without sonographic air bronchograms (arrow) plus focally confluent B lines arising from the margin of the consolidation (left posterior lung). (D) Consolidation with hyperechoic air bronchograms suggestive of pneumonia (right posterior lung).[54]

Prognosis

Not all older adults with pneumonia require admission. Severity prediction scales can help identify low-risk patients who can be discharged from the ED, such as the Pneumonia Severity Index score.[57] The score is heavily weighted toward age and comorbidities, and should be used, along with clinical judgment, to determine need for hospital admission.[57] Patients who are not able to maintain oral intake or who have severe comorbid illnesses, impaired functional status, or psychosocial or cognitive barriers to follow-up may require admission regardless of their scores on these tools.[58]

Management

The most common pathogens causing CAP in older patients are *Streptococcus pneumoniae* and *Haemophilus influenzae*. Additional therapies can be added based on the patient's risk for methicillin-resistant *Staphylococcus aureus* (MRSA) or *Pseudomonas*. Patients should receive antibiotics in a timely fashion.[59] Supportive treatment may include antipyretics, IV fluids, and pressors for septic shock.[60] Steroids are not recommended.[58] Antibiotic therapy for pneumonia is summarized in **Table 3**.

Summary

Pneumonia is common in older adults and can present with atypical symptoms. A chest radiograph is the initial imaging modality to evaluate for focal opacities, and some patients may require additional imaging with a CT scan. Bedside lung ultrasonography is useful to evaluate for lung abnormalities. Treatment should be tailored to the patient's comorbidities and risk factors for multidrug-resistant organisms.

CORONAVIRUS INFECTIOUS DISEASE 2019 CONSIDERATIONS

Coronavirus infectious disease 2019 (COVID-19) is an active pandemic that has been rapidly evolving within the past year. This disease has especially affected the older population, who have the highest mortality.[60] The incidence among those aged 85 years or older was 1138 per 100,000, compared with 403 per 100,000 in the general population.[61] Patients at high risk for severe illness are those with diabetes, hypertension, cardiovascular disease, and cerebrovascular disease.[62] A study of 1099 patients with COVID-19 pneumonia found that 27% of those who are severely ill are aged 60 years and older.[63] The mortality of patients more than 60 years of age is significantly higher than that of younger patients, 5.3% versus 1.4%, with increased rates of hospitalization and intensive care unit admission.[64] In patients with COVID-19, the most common symptoms are fever, followed by cough and increased sputum production.

Many long-term care facilities (LTCFs) have experienced COVID-19 outbreaks, which have been difficult to manage because older patients often have impaired immune responses and comorbidities. Older adults may not have typical symptoms as with influenza, thus delaying diagnosis and contributing to transmission.[65] Furthermore, more than 50% who test positive may be asymptomatic, making it difficult to separate symptomatic from asymptomatic patients.[65] As a result, many LTCFs have taken precautions to restrict nonessential visitors and adopt universal masking.

Table 3
Treatment of pneumonia in older adults

Outpatient Antibiotic Therapies	
Patients with no comorbidities and no risk factors for MRSA or *Pseudomonas*	Amoxicillin or doxycycline or azithromycin
Patients with comorbidities (COPD, structural lung disease, immunosuppression, recent influenzalike illness) or risk factors for MRSA or *Pseudomonas*, such as patients from LTCFs	• Amoxicillin/clavulanate or cephalosporin (cefpodoxime or cefuroxime) plus doxycycline or a macrolide • Or monotherapy with a respiratory fluoroquinolone (levofloxacin or moxifloxacin)
Inpatient Antibiotic Therapies	
Patients who are to be admitted and who do not have risk factors for MRSA or *Pseudomonas aeruginosa*	• Monotherapy with a respiratory fluoroquinolone (levofloxacin or moxifloxacin) • Or combination therapy with a β-lactam (ampicillin + sulbactam, cefotaxime, ceftriaxone, or ceftaroline) and a macrolide (azithromycin or clarithromycin). Or a β-lactam with doxycycline (patients with contraindications to fluoroquinolones or macrolides)
Patients with risk factors for multidrug-resistant organisms[a]	Vancomycin (for MRSA) and piperacillin-tazobactam, a fourth-generation cephalosporin, aztreonam, meropenem, or imipenem (for *P aeruginosa*)

Abbreviations: COPD, chronic obstructive pulmonary disease; LTCF, long-term care facility.
[a] Anaerobic coverage is only indicated for suspected or confirmed lung abscess or empyema.
Data from Metlay JP, Waterer GW, Long AC, et al. Diagnosis and Treatment of Adults with Community-acquired Pneumonia. An Official Clinical Practice Guideline of the American Thoracic Society and Infectious Diseases Society of America. *Am J Respir Crit Care Med.* 2019;200(7):e45-e67.

There are many ramifications of this highly infectious disease in older patients. Patients with cognitive impairment are at even higher risk for delirium because of isolation from family members, universal masking requirements, and contact restrictions.

As the COVID-19 pandemic continues to evolve, many hospitals have incorporated palliative care early in affected patients. More studies will need to be conducted to help guide clinical practice.

SUMMARY

The percentage of older adults is increasing worldwide. Older adults are susceptible to serious illness, including AF, congestive HF, PE, and pneumonia. AF is the most common arrhythmia in this group and can cause complications such as stroke. Clinical tools including the CHA_2DS_2-VASc score, along with patient-centered shared decision making, should guide decisions on anticoagulation in the prevention of VTE. Congestive HF is the most common cause of hospital admission and readmission in the older adult population. Rapid diagnosis and treatment decreases morbidity and increases survival. Palliative care should be incorporated early into discussions with patients who have end-stage disease.

Older adults are also at high risk for PE because of age-related changes and comorbidities. The use of age-adjusted D-dimer can help stratify low-risk patients. Anticoagulation is standard treatment and is recommended despite increased falls and bleeding risk in older adults.

Pneumonia is also prevalent and is one of the leading causes of death. Early antibiotic administration and supportive care are critical. Patients are at risk for viral coinfections such as influenza and the current pandemic of COVID-19.

In conclusion, older adults require special consideration in terms of diagnosis and treatment. Informed discussions with patients and families regarding goals of care should be included in any treatment plan.

CLINICS CARE POINTS

- Older adults can present with atypical symptoms.
- In AF, use clinical tools such as the CHA2D2S-Vasc score and HAS-BLED scores, along with patient-centered shared decision making to guide decisions on anticoagulation in the prevention of VTE.
- Congestive HF requires rapid diagnosis and treatment to decrease morbidity and mortality. Palliative care discussions should begin in the ED for those who have recurrent exacerbations and with end-stage disease.
- As with the other cardiopulmonary emergencies, PE is more prevalent in the older adult population. The use of age-adjusted D-dimer can be helpful for low-risk patients. The benefits of anticoagulation outweigh the risks of bleeding.
- Ultrasonography can be a helpful diagnostic tool for pneumonia, especially in critically ill patients. Antibiotics for pneumonia should be tailored to patients' risk factors. Early administration of antibiotics and supportive care decreases mortality from infection.
- COVID-19 is a geriatric emergency. Patients can be asymptomatic or can present with atypical symptoms. Early discussions on goals of care with the patient and patient's family should be started in the ED.

DISCLOSURE STATEMENT

The authors have nothing to disclose.

REFERENCES

1. 2017 National Population Projections Tables: Main Series. Available at: https://www.census.gov/data/tables/2017/demo/popproj/2017-summary-tables.html. Accessed May 29, 2020.
2. Feinberg WM, Blackshear JL, Laupacis A, et al. Prevalence, age distribution, and gender of patients with atrial fibrillation. Analysis and implications. Arch Intern Med 1995;155:469–73.
3. Andrade J, Khairy P, Dobrev D, et al. The clinical profile and pathophysiology of atrial fibrillation: relationships among clinical features, epidemiology, and mechanisms. Circ Res 2014;114(9):1453–68.
4. Garwood CL, Corbett TL. Use of anticoagulation in older patients with atrial fibrillation who are at risk for falls. Ann Pharmacother 2008;42:523–32.
5. Dharmarajan TS, Varma S, Akkaladevi S, et al. To anticoagulate or not to anticoagulate? A common dilemma for the provider: physicians' opinion poll based on a case study of an older long-term care facility resident with dementia and atrial fibrillation. J Am Med Dir Assoc 2006;7:23–8.

6. Kelly P, Devore A, Wu J, et al. Rhythm control versus rate control in patients with atrial fibrillation and heart failure with preserved ejection fraction: insights from get with the guidelines-heart failure. J Am Heart Assoc 2019;8(24):e011560.

7. Jacoby J, Cesta M, Heller M, et al. Synchronized emergency department cardioversion of atrial dysrhythmias saves time, money and resources. J Emerg Med 2005;28(1):27–30.

8. Nuotio I, Hartikainen J, Gronberg T, et al. Time to cardioversion for acute atrial fibrillation and thromboembolic complications. JAMA 2014;312(6):647–9.

9. Lip GY, Nieuwlaat R, Pisters R, et al. Refining clinical risk stratification for predicting stroke and thromboembolism in atrial fibrillation using a novel risk factor-based approach: the euro heart survey on atrial fibrillation. Chest 2010;137(2): 263–72.

10. Camm AJ, Kirchhof P, Lip GY, et al. European Heart Rhythm Association; European Association for Cardio-Thoracic Surgery. Guidelines for the management of atrial fibrillation: the Task Force for the Management of Atrial Fibrillation of the European Society of Cardiology (ESC). Eur Heart J 2010;31(19):2369–429.

11. Gage BF, Yan Y, Milligan PE, et al. Clinical classification schemes for predicting hemorrhage: results from the National Registry of Atrial Fibrillation (NRAF). Am Heart J 2006;151(03):713–9.

12. The efficacy of aspirin in patients with atrial fibrillation. Analysis of pooled data from 3 randomized trials. The Atrial Fibrillation Investigators. Arch Intern Med 1997;157:1237–40.

13. Hart RG, Benavente O, McBride R, et al. Antithrombotic therapy to prevent stroke in patients with atrial fibrillation: a meta-analysis. Ann Intern Med 1999;131: 492–501.

14. Fihn SD, Callahan CM, Martin DC, et al. The risk for and severity of bleeding complications in older patients treated with warfarin. The National Consortium of Anticoagulation Clinics. Ann Intern Med 1996;124:970–9.

15. Gage BF, Birman-Deych E, Kerzner R, et al. Incidence of intracranial hemorrhage in patients with atrial fibrillation who are prone to fall. Am J Med 2005;118:612–7.

16. Deng K, Cheng J, Rao S, et al. Efficacy and safety of direct oral anticoagulants in older patients with atrial fibrillation: a network meta-analysis. Front Med 2020; 7:107.

17. Abdelhafiz AH. Heart failure in older people: causes, diagnosis and treatment. Age Ageing 2002;31:29–36.

18. Butrous H, Hummel SL. Heart failure in older adults. Can J Cardiol 2016;32(9): 1140–7.

19. Chrysohoou C, Tsiachris D, Stefanadis C. Aortic stenosis in the elderly: challenges in diagnosis and therapy. Maturitas 2011;70(4):349–53.

20. Richard G, Jose J. My approach to management of aortic stenosis in the elderly. Trends Cardiovasc Med 2016;26(5):479–80.

21. Melgarejo S, Schaub A, and Noble V. Point of care ultrasound: an overview. American College of Cardiology, October 31, 2017.

22. Zanobetti M, Scorpiniti M, Gigli C, et al. Point-of-care ultrasonography for evaluation of acute dyspnea in the ED. Chest 2017;151(6):1295–301.

23. Zanatta M, Benato P, Cianci V. Pre-hospital ultrasound: current indications and future perspectives. Int J Crit Care Emerg Med 2016;2:019.

24. Gheorghiade M, De Luca L, Fonarow GC, et al. Pathophysiologic targets in the early phase of acute heart failure syndromes. Am J Cardiol 2005;96(6A):11G–7G.

25. Masip J, Roque M, Sanchez B, et al. Noninvasive ventilation in acute cardiogenic pulmonary edema: systematic review and meta-analysis. JAMA 2005;294: 3124–30.

26. McMurray JJ, Adamopoulos S, Anker SD, et al. ESC guidelines for the diagnosis and treatment of acute and chronic heart failure 2012: The Task Force for the Diagnosis and Treatment of Acute and Chronic Heart Failure 2012 of the European Society of Cardiology. Developed in collaboration with the Heart Failure Association (HFA) of the ESC. Eur J Heart Fail 2012;14:803–69.

27. Peacock WF, Hollander JE, Diercks DB, et al. Morphine and outcomes in acute decompensated heart failure: an ADHERE analysis. Emerg Med J 2008;25: 205–9.

28. Felker GM, Lee KL, Bull DA, et al. Diuretic strategies in patients with acute decompensated heart failure. N Engl J Med 2011;364:797–805.

29. Kelley AS, Morrison RS. Palliative care for the seriously ill. N Engl J Med 2015; 373:747–55.

30. Booth S, Wade R, Johnson M, et al. The use of oxygen in the palliation of breathlessness. A report of the expert working group of the Scientific Committee of the Association of Palliative Medicine. Respir Med 2004;98:66–77.

31. Nurmohamed MT, Büller HR, ten Cate JW. Physiological changes due to age. Implications for the prevention and treatment of thrombosis in older patients. Drugs Aging 1994;5(1):20–33.

32. Zwierzina D, Limacher A, Mean M, et al. Prospective comparison of clinical prognostic scores in older patients with pulmonary embolism. J Thromb Haemost 2012;10:2270–6.

33. Stein PD, Beemath A, Matta F, et al. Clinical characteristics of patients with acute pulmonary embolism: data from PIOPED II. Am J Med 2007;120:871–9.

34. Righini M, Es JV, Exter PD, et al. Age-adjusted D-dimer cutoff levels to rule out pulmonary embolism the ADJUST-PE study. JAMA 2014;311:1117–24.

35. Perrier A, Desmarais S, Miron MJ, et al. Non-invasive diagnosis of venous thromboembolism in outpatients. Lancet 1999;353:190–5.

36. Fields JM, Davis J, Girson L, et al. Transthoracic echocardiography for diagnosing pulmonary embolism: a systematic review and meta-analysis. J Am Soc Echocardiogr 2017;30:714–23.

37. Kearon C, Akl EA, Comerota AJ, et al. Antithrombotic therapy for VTE disease: antithrombotic therapy and prevention of thrombosis, 9th ed: American College of Chest Physicians Evidence-Based Clinical Practice Guidelines. Chest 2012; 141:e419S–96S.

38. Monreal M, Lopez-Jimenez L. Pulmonary embolism in patients over 90 years of age. Curr Opin Pulm Med 2010;16:432–6.

39. Schwartz JB. The current state of knowledge on age, sex, and their interactions on clinical pharmacology. Clin Pharmacol Ther 2007;82:87–96.

40. Cockcroft DW, Gault MH. Prediction of creatinine clearance from serum creatinine. Nephron 1976;16:31–41.

41. Falatko JM, Dalal B, Qu L. Impact of anticoagulation in older patients with pulmonary embolism that undergo IVC filter placement: a retrospective cohort study. Heart Lung Circ 2017;26:1317–22.

42. Janssens JP, Krause KH. Pneumonia in the very old. Lancet Infect Dis 2004;4(2): 112–24.

43. Kaplan V, Clermont G, Griffin MF, et al. Pneumonia: still the old man's friend? Arch Intern Med 2003;163(3):317–23.

44. Kaplan V, Angus DC, Griffin MF, et al. Hospitalized community-acquired pneumonia in the older: age- and sex-related patterns of care and outcome in the United States. Am J Respir Crit Care Med 2002;165(6):766–72.

45. Sharma G, Goodwin J. Effect of aging on respiratory system physiology and immunology. Clin Interv Aging 2006;1(3):253–60.

46. Henig O, Kaye KS. Bacterial pneumonia in older adults. Infect Dis Clin North Am 2017;31(4):689–713.

47. Charlesworth CJ, Smit E, Lee DS, et al. Polypharmacy among adults aged 65 years and older in the United States: 1988-2010. J Gerontol A Biol Sci Med Sci 2015;70(8):989–95.

48. Eurich DT, Lee C, Marrie TJ, et al. Inhaled corticosteroids and risk of recurrent pneumonia: a population based, nested case-control study. Clin Infect Dis 2013;57:1138–44.

49. Paul KJ, Walker RL, Dublin S. Anticholinergic medications and risk of community-acquired pneumonia in older adults: a population based case-control study. J Am Geriatr Soc 2015;63:476–85.

50. Marrie TJ, File TM Jr. Bacterial pneumonia in older adults. Clin Geriatr Med 2016; 32(3):459–77.

51. El-Solh AA, Niederman MS, Drinka P. Nursing home acquired pneumonia: a review of risk factors and therapeutic approaches. Curr Med Res Opin 2010;26: 2707–14.

52. Haga T, Fukuoka M, Morita M. Computed tomography for the diagnosis and evaluation of the severity of community-acquired pneumonia in the older. Intern Med 2016;55(5):437–41.

53. Basi SK, Marrie TJ, Huang JQ, et al. Patients admitted to hospital with suspected pneumonia and normal chest radiographs: epidemiology, microbiology, and outcomes. Am J Med 2004;117(5):305–11.

54. Biagi C, Pierantoni L, Baldazzi M, et al. Lung ultrasound for the diagnosis of pneumonia in children with acute bronchiolitis. BMC Pulm Med 2018;18:191.

55. Lichtenstein D. Novel approaches to ultrasonography of the lung and pleural space: where are we now? Breathe (Sheff) 2017;13(2):100–11.

56. Chavez MA, Shams N, Ellington L, et al. Lung ultrasound for the diagnosis of pneumonia in adults: a systematic review and meta-analysis. Respir Res 2014; 15(1):50.

57. Fine MJ, Auble TE, Yealy DM, et al. A prediction rule to identify low-risk patients with community-acquired pneumonia. N Engl J Med 1997;336(4):243–50.

58. Metlay JP, Waterer GW, Long AC, et al. Diagnosis and treatment of adults with community-acquired pneumonia. An official clinical practice guideline of the American Thoracic Society and Infectious Diseases Society of America. Am J Respir Crit Care Med 2019;200(7):e45–67.

59. Kumar A, Roberts D, Wood KE, et al. Duration of hypotension before initiation of effective antimicrobial therapy is the critical determinant of survival in human septic shock. Crit Care Med 2006;34(6):1589–96.

60. Li J-Y, You Z, Wang Q, et al. The epidemic of 2019-novel-coronavirus (2019-nCoV) pneumonia and insights for emerging infectious diseases in the future. Microbes Infect 2020;22(2):80–5.

61. Stokes EK, Zambrano LD, Anderson KN, et al. Coronavirus disease 2019 case surveillance — United States, January 22–May 30, 2020. MMWR Morb Mortal Wkly Rep 2020;69:759–65.

62. Guan WJ, Ni ZY, Hu Y, et al. China Medical Treatment Expert Group for Covid-19. Clinical Characteristics of Coronavirus Disease 2019 in China. N Engl J Med 2020;382(18):1708–20.

63. Yang Y, Lu QB, Liu MJ, et al. Epidemiological and clinical features of the 2019 novel coronavirus outbreak in China. Med Rxiv 2020. https://doi.org/10.1101/2020.02.10.20021675.

64. Liu Y, Gayle AA, Wilder-Smith A, et al. The reproductive number of COVID–19 is higher compared to SARS coronavirus. J Travel Med 2020;27(2):taaa021.

65. Arons MM, Hatfield KM, Reddy SC, et al. Presymptomatic SARS-CoV-2 infections and transmission in a skilled nursing facility. N Engl J Med 2020;382(22):2081–90.

Identification of Acute Coronary Syndrome in the Elderly

Michael McGarry, MD[a], Christina L. Shenvi, MD, PhD[b],*

KEYWORDS

- Acute coronary syndrome • Elderly • Geriatric • Chest pain • Atypical symptoms

KEY POINTS

- Consider acute coronary syndrome (ACS) in older patients who present with dyspnea, diaphoresis, syncope, nausea, vomiting, altered mental status, fatigue, or generalized weakness even if they do not have any chest pain.
- Have a low threshold to obtain an electrocardiogram and troponin level in elderly patients with symptoms of possible ACS even without chest pain.
- Once ACS is identified, treat patients with atypical symptoms just as aggressively as you would patients with active chest pain.
- Older adults with a high-risk non–ST-segment elevation myocardial infarction are more likely to have atypical symptoms than younger patients but may benefit more from early invasive therapy.
- Reframe the dichotomy of "typical" and "atypical" symptoms and, instead, consider the continuum and range of symptoms with which patients may present when having ACS.

RAPID FIRE: IDENTIFICATION OF ACUTE CORONARY SYNDROME IN THE OLDER ADULT

Case

A 77-year-old woman presented to the emergency department (ED) with a chief complaint of "allergic reaction." She had a past medical history of hypercholesterolemia and psoriatic arthritis. Per emergency medicine services (EMS) personnel, she had been sitting outside when she suddenly developed diaphoresis, nausea, and shortness of breath. She thought she had seen some ants around but denies any known bites. She denied urticaria or any skin itchiness. She was given intramuscular epinephrine and intravenous diphenhydramine and methylprednisolone by EMS and stated her nausea had improved.

[a] Department of Emergency Medicine, Northwest Medical Center, 2801 FL-7, Margate, FL 33063, USA; [b] Department of Emergency Medicine, University of North Carolina, 170 Manning Drive CB 7594, Chapel Hill, NC 27599, USA
* Corresponding author.
E-mail address: cshenvi@med.unc.edu
Twitter: @mike_mcgarry_ (M.M.); @clshenvi (C.L.S.)

Emerg Med Clin N Am 39 (2021) 339–346
https://doi.org/10.1016/j.emc.2020.12.003
0733-8627/21/© 2020 Elsevier Inc. All rights reserved.

At the time of evaluation, the patient reported that she was feeling well. She was in no acute distress and had a normal cardiopulmonary examination. She was placed on a cardiac monitor and monitored for four hours. As the physician was preparing the discharge instructions, as an afterthought, they ordered an electrocardiogram (ECG), which showed a normal sinus rhythm with inverted T waves in leads V1-V3. Laboratory tests were ordered. The physician was not sure if the T-wave inversions were new or old but wondered if the patient did have an anaphylactic response or if there was something else going on.

INTRODUCTION
The Problem

When older adults (aged 65 and over) experience acute coronary syndrome (ACS), they often present with what are considered "atypical" symptoms. Because their symptoms less often match the expected presentation of ACS, older patients can have delayed times to assessment, performance of an ECG, diagnosis, and definitive management. Unfortunately, studies in multiple different countries have shown that this group of patients is at the highest risk for having ACS and for complications from ACS.[1–4]

Definitions of Acute Coronary Syndrome

ACS includes a spectrum of presentations from unstable angina to non–ST-segment elevation myocardial infarction (NSTEMI) and ST-segment elevation myocardial infarction (STEMI) that occur when there is a mismatch between myocardial oxygen supply and demand.

- Unstable angina is defined as worsening symptoms (usually chest pain) with exertion, that are relieved by rest with no elevation of biomarkers.
- An NSTEMI occurs when there is evidence of subendocardial injury based on an elevated biomarker level without ECG findings of a transmural infarct.
- An STEMI occurs when there is transmural ischemia, as evidenced by ST-segment elevation on the ECG.

Epidemiology of Acute Coronary Syndrome

In the United States, the demographics of patients who are diagnosed with ACS are as follows:

- Average age of individuals diagnosed with ACS is 68 years.
- ACS is diagnosed in men and woman in a 3:2 ratio.
- The annual incidence of ACS in the United States is 780,000, of which 70% is due to NSTEMIs.[5]

Acute Coronary Syndrome Risk with Age

Age is a significant risk factor for ACS and an independent predictor of higher mortality.[2] It is estimated that 60% to 65% of STEMIs occur in patients aged 65 years or older, and 28% to 33% occur in patients aged 75 years or older. In addition, as many as 80% of all deaths related to myocardial infarction (MI) occur in persons 65 years and older.[6]

Older patients who present with NSTEMI[7] and STEMI[8] are less likely to present with "typical" chest pain symptoms. Sometimes, symptoms other than chest pain that can be present in a patient with ACS are termed "anginal-equivalent" symptoms. It is important to understand the range of ways in which ACS can present in the older population in order to diagnose and treat them more quickly and effectively.

PRESENTATION AND DIAGNOSIS

To diagnose ACS, clinicians must obtain a thorough history, ECG, and cardiac bio-markers, such as troponin level. Current guidelines recommend an ECG be performed within ten minutes of arrival to identify STEMI among patients presenting to the ED with chest pain.[9] However, many older adults who are ultimately found to have ACS do not present with chest pain as their primary concern, and so their ECG is often delayed.[7,8,10]

In a review of more than 430,000 patients with confirmed acute MI, one-third had no chest pain on presentation to the hospital, and those without chest pain were more often older, female, or diabetic.[11,12] Even in patients who are having an STEMI, the proportion of patients without chest pain increases significantly with age. Chest pain is present in more than 90% of patients having an STEMI who are under age 65, but in only 57% of patients over age 85 (**Fig. 1**).[8] Given this, traditional triage protocols may miss geriatric patients with ACS.

PATHOPHYSIOLOGY OF "ATYPICAL" SYMPTOMS

There are many potential reasons for the lack of chest pain in older adults presenting with ACS.[4] This population may have higher levels of endogenous opioids or increased opioid sensitivity that could blunt the sensation of chest pain.[4] In addition, they may have impaired peripheral or central pain sensation or neuropathy because of age-related changes or diabetes. Older patients may also have ischemic precondi-tioning, in which they have had many prior episodes of mild ischemia, which has desensitized them to the chest pain. Older patients also have a higher prevalence of multivessel disease and may have developed collateral flow. In addition, older patients may be *more* likely to experience dyspnea because of underlying lung disease and reduced pulmonary reserve.[4]

COMMON PRESENTATIONS OF ACUTE CORONARY SYNDROME IN OLDER ADULTS

Older adults who have confirmed ACS can present with a range of symptoms. Chest pain remains the most common chief complaint in patients with ACS. However, ACS

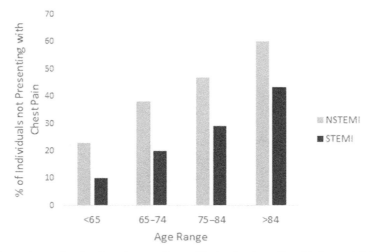

Fig. 1. Percentage of patients not presenting with chest pain as the chief complaint by age, with data from Refs.[6,7]

can present with a range of other symptoms and without chest pain. Among patients with ACS without a chief complaint of chest pain, the most common presenting symptom is dyspnea, present in about 50%, followed by diaphoresis (26%), nausea/vomiting (24%), and syncope (19%) (**Fig. 2**). Other possible symptoms include changes in mental status, "indigestion," and generalized weakness or fatigue.[13] It is important to identify these symptoms as potential manifestations of ACS, as patients with these symptoms experience a delay in diagnosis and definitive management, and higher morbidity and mortality.[13]

UTILITY OF TROPONIN IN PATIENTS WITH NONSPECIFIC SYMPTOMS

In recommending more liberal ECG or troponin assessments in older adults who lack chest pain, the authors are not necessarily suggesting that *all* older patients need both tests. In a 2019 retrospective study of 412 ED encounters by older adults, Wang and colleagues[14] found that among older patients with "nonspecific complaints" (NSC), there were low rates of ACS. They defined NSC as a chief complaint of "weak or weakness, dizzy or dizziness, fatigue, lethargy, altered mental status, light-headedness, medical problem, examination requested, failure to thrive, or multiple complaints.'" In their study, 20% of individuals tested had a positive troponin level, and overall, 1.2% were ultimately diagnosed with ACS. Although 1.2% is a relatively low number with ACS, the 20% who had a positive troponin level tended, as in other prior studies, to have higher mortalities.

The utility of a screening troponin test among patients with these NSC is likely low, but the true risks and benefits of testing have not been fully defined. However, among those with higher-risk symptoms, such as dyspnea, syncope, and the other symptoms listed in **Fig. 2**, the pretest probability of ACS is higher, and an ECG and troponin test may be helpful to assess for ACS while also performing a workup for other possible causes of the symptoms.

ELECTROCARDIOGRAPHIC INTERPRETATION IN OLDER ADULTS

To complicate matters further, ECG analysis can be more difficult in older adults. Older patients more often have chronic ECG findings or changes that can make diagnosis of the ischemic changes more challenging. For example, older adult patients are more likely to have a pacemaker, a bundle branch block, left ventricular hypertrophy, axis

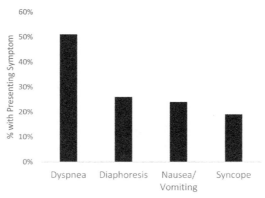

Fig. 2. Common presenting symptoms among older patients with ACS without chest pain as their chief complaint.[12]

deviation, premature ventricular contractions, premature atrial contractions, or prior MI findings, such as chronic inverted T waves or Q waves. Normal aging also frequently leads to first-degree atrioventricular blocks.[15,16]

OUTCOMES OF ACUTE CORONARY SYNDROME IN OLDER ADULTS WITHOUT CHEST PAIN

There are many significant differences in the rapidity of diagnosis and the outcomes between patients who have chest pain and those who do not at the time of presentation of ACS.[1,17] Of patients found to have an STEMI, those without chest pain who were transported by EMS received a prehospital ECG 72% of the time, compared with 87% of the time for those with chest pain. Patients who lack chest pain on presentation with ACS tend to have longer door-to-ECG times, and therefore, longer time to definitive management with percutaneous coronary intervention (PCI).[10]

For patients with an STEMI, those without chest pain receive fibrinolysis or PCI 37% of the time, compared with 67% of the time for those with chest pain. Patients without chest pain were also less likely to receive an aspirin within 24 hours and less likely to receive statins and beta-blockers at hospital discharge.[11]

Because of the delays in identification of MIs in patients without chest pain and their undertreatment, it is not surprising that mortality is higher in patients who lack chest pain. Among older women with an MI who present without chest pain, the mortality is 21%, compared with 13% for women with chest pain. For men, the mortality is 22% for those without chest pain and 7% for those with chest pain.[12]

REFRAMING "TYPICAL" SYMPTOMS

Much of the confusion and delay in diagnosis and management for older adults stems from the dogma that patients who have ACS will present with chest pain, and that if they are not having chest pain, the cause of their symptoms is likely nonischemic in nature. However, the data are contrary to this dogma and show that many older adults will present with ACS and have "atypical" symptoms.

Most physicians have a shared understanding of what "typical" ACS symptoms are. However, the individual interpretations of "atypical symptoms" are much broader, and there is poor consensus.[18] In addition, even among patients with chest pain, use of the terms "atypical" and "typical" chest pain can be misleading.

The description of "typical" symptoms of ischemic heart disease dates back to the 1700s when it was described as "a painful sensation in the breast accompanied by a strangling sensation, anxiety, and occasional radiation of pain to the left arm" that was worse with exertion and relieved by rest.[18,19] Subsequent early studies that defined typical symptoms of ACS were performed primarily in study populations of middle-aged men. Individuals in this younger male population do more often present with chest pain. As a result, those without chest pain were somewhat artificially dubbed "atypical." However, older adults are the very population who are more likely to have ACS, and who are more likely to lack "typical" chest pain symptoms.

Other investigators have also called for a retirement of the terms "typical" and "atypical" on the basis of their lack of specificity, particularly in women.[20] Therefore, the terms "typical" and "atypical" are misleading in the context of ACS and can lead to cognitive bias that could delay a patient's workup, diagnosis, and management. Instead of dichotomizing patients as having "typical" chest pain or not and treating them differently based on that, one should instead consider the diverse range of symptoms that can manifest in patients with ACS and be aware of the populations who may tend toward certain manifestations (dyspnea, diaphoresis, nausea) over others (chest pain).

SYSTEMATIC SOLUTIONS

Beyond reframing how individual physicians think about ACS, there are systematic solutions that can be implemented to prevent missing the diagnosis in older adults. ACS must be considered in older patients who present with dyspnea, diaphoresis, syncope, nausea, vomiting, altered mental status, fatigue, or generalized weakness. Clinicians should have a low threshold to obtain an ECG and troponin test in patients with these symptoms, but systems and protocols should also be developed to create safety nets to avoid missed or delayed diagnosis.

Long-term solutions to identification of older adults with ACS need to be systematic and easily implementable and not rely solely on clinician judgment. One option is to follow the prioritization rule developed and validated by Glickman and colleagues[9] to obtain an immediate ECG in the ED to identify STEMIs. They studied 3,575,178 ED patient visits to 107 EDs from 2007 to 2008. The prioritization rule found that those requiring an immediate ECG in the ED included age $\geq$30 years with chest pain, age $\geq$50 years with shortness of breath, altered mental status, upper extremity pain, syncope, or generalized weakness, and those with age $\geq$80 years with abdominal pain or nausea/vomiting in addition to the former symptoms. When the ECG prioritization rule was applied to a validation sample, it had a sensitivity of 91.9% (95% confidence interval [CI] 90.9%–92.8%) for STEMI and a negative predictive value of 99.98% (95% CI 99.98%–99.98%). ECG prioritization rule based on age and presenting symptoms in the ED is one simple, systematic method to better identify patients who are at high risk for STEMI. Similar criteria will need to be developed and validated for NSTEMIs.

Once ACS is identified, physicians should treat patients without "typical" symptoms just as aggressively as they would patients with active chest pain, taking into account individual goals of the patient and their baseline functional status.[2,21]

CASE REVISITED

Although the care team was not initially concerned for ACS in the patient who presented with purported anaphylaxis, after they noticed the T-wave inversions on the ECG, they send for a troponin test. However, when they thought more about it, they realized her symptoms of dyspnea, diaphoresis, and nausea could be signs of ACS rather than anaphylaxis, even though she never had chest pain. A troponin test is obtained, and the patient is kept on a cardiac monitor. The initial troponin level is 0.45 ng/mL (normal <0.034 ng/mL). The cardiologist is called because of concern for an NSTEMI. The patient is admitted and started on a heparin infusion, and serial troponin levels were obtained. The second troponin level three hours later is 0.83 ng/mL. She undergoes cardiac catheterization the next day, which shows 90% stenosis of the left anterior descending artery. She receives a drug-eluting stent and is discharged two days later.

This case illustrates the need for a high clinical suspicion for ACS in older adults. It also demonstrates the need for emergency physicians to advocate for the appropriate treatment of older adult patients with ACS, as delay in treatment or less aggressive treatment can cause increased morbidity and mortality. A systematic protocol to obtain an ECG among patients with dyspnea and recognizing dyspnea as a symptom of ACS may have expedited her diagnosis.

CLINICS CARE POINTS

- Acute coronary syndrome (ACS) occurs more frequently in older patients. However, with advancing age, patients are more likely to have symptoms other than chest pain as their presenting concern.
- Patients who have ACS but lack chest pain are at higher risk for delayed diagnosis and worse outcomes.
- It is important for clinicians to understand the spectrum of symptoms that can accompany ACS, particularly dyspnea, diaphoresis, nausea and vomiting, or syncope.
- Clinicians should have a low threshold for assessing for ACS with an EKG and troponin in older patients who have potential ACS symptoms, even if they do not have chest pain.

DISCLOSURE

The authors have nothing to disclose.

REFERENCES

1. Simms AD, Batin PD, Kurian J, et al. Acute coronary syndromes: an old age problem. J Geriatr Cardiol 2012;9(2):192–6.
2. Saunderson C, Brogan R, Simms A, et al. Acute coronary syndrome management in older adults: guidelines, temporal changes and challenges. Age Ageing 2014; 43(4):450–5.
3. Mirghani HO. Age related differences in acute coronary syndrome presentation and in hospital outcomes: a cross-sectional comparative study. Pan Afr Med J 2016;24. https://doi.org/10.11604/pamj.2016.24.337.8711.
4. Carro A, Kaski JC. Myocardial infarction in the elderly. Aging Dis 2011;2(2): 116–37.
5. Basit H, Malik A, Huecker MR. Non ST segment elevation (NSTEMI) myocardial infarction. Treasure Island, FL: StatPearls Publishing; 2020.
6. Yazdanyar A, Newman AB. The burden of cardiovascular disease in the elderly: morbidity, mortality, and costs. Clin Geriatr Med 2009;25(4):563–77.
7. Alexander KP, Newby LK, Cannon CP, et al. Acute coronary care in the elderly, part I: non-ST-segment-elevation acute coronary syndromes: a scientific statement for healthcare professionals from the American Heart Association Council on Clinical Cardiology: in collaboration with the Society of Geriatric Cardiology. Circulation 2007;115(19):2549–69.
8. Alexander KP, Newby LK, Armstrong PW, et al. Acute coronary care in the elderly, part II: ST-segment-elevation myocardial infarction: a scientific statement for healthcare professionals from the American Heart Association Council on Clinical Cardiology: in collaboration with the Society of Geriatric Cardiology. Circulation 2007;115(19):2570–89.
9. Glickman SW, Shofer FS, Wu MC, et al. Development and validation of a prioritization rule for obtaining an immediate 12-lead electrocardiogram in the emergency department to identify ST-elevation myocardial infarction. Am Heart J 2012;163(3):372–82.
10. Cannon AR, Lin L, Lytle B, et al. Use of prehospital 12-lead electrocardiography and treatment times among ST-elevation myocardial infarction patients with atypical symptoms. Acad Emerg Med 2014;21(8):892–8.

11. Canto JG, Shlipak MG, Rogers WJ, et al. Prevalence, clinical characteristics, and mortality among patients with myocardial infarction presenting without chest pain. J Am Med Assoc 2000;283(24):3223–9.

12. Canto JG, Rogers WJ, Goldberg RJ, et al. Association of age and sex with myocardial infarction symptom presentation and in-hospital mortality. JAMA 2012;307(8):813–22.

13. Brieger D, Eagle KA, Goodman SG, et al. Acute coronary syndromes without chest pain, an underdiagnosed and undertreated high-risk group: insights from the Global Registry of Acute Coronary Events. Chest 2004;126(2):461–9.

14. Wang AZ, Schaffer JT, Holt DB, et al. Troponin testing and coronary syndrome in geriatric patients with nonspecific complaints: are we overtesting? Acad Emerg Med 2020;27(1):6–14.

15. Khane RS, Surdi AD, Bhatkar RS. Changes in ECG pattern with advancing age. J Basic Clin Physiol Pharmacol 2011;22(4):97–101.

16. Wenger N. STEMI at elderly age. American College of Cardiology. 2016. Available at: https://www.acc.org/latest-in-cardiology/articles/2016/08/26/08/47/stemi-at-elderly-age. Accessed May 20, 2020.

17. Gale C, Cattle B, Woolston A, et al. Resolving inequalities in care? Reduced mortality in the elderly after acute coronary syndromes. The Myocardial Ischaemia National Audit Project 2003-2010. Eur Heart J 2012;33(5):630.

18. Swap CJ, Nagurney JT. Value and limitations of chest pain history in the evaluation of patients with suspected acute coronary syndromes. J Am Med Assoc 2005;294(20):2623–9.

19. Silverman ME. William Heberden and some account of a disorder of the breast. Clin Cardiol 1987;10(3):211–3.

20. DeVon HA, Mirzaei S, Zègre-Hemsey J. Typical and atypical symptoms of acute coronary syndrome: time to retire the terms? J Am Heart Assoc 2020;9(7): e015539.

21. Lattuca B, Kerneis M, Zeitouni M, et al. Elderly patients with ST-segment elevation myocardial infarction: a patient-centered approach. Drugs Aging 2019;36(6): 531–9.

Disaster Diagnoses in Geriatric Patients with Abdominal Pain

Ryan Spangler, MD*, Sara Manning, MD

KEYWORDS

- Geriatric • Abdominal pain • Biliary • Mesenteric ischemia

KEY POINTS

- Geriatric patients have increased morbidity and mortality compared with younger patients for most abdominal disorders.
- Geriatric patients show atypical signs and symptoms for many common abdominal conditions, contributing to misdiagnosis and worsened outcomes.
- Biliary disease is the most common surgical disease in older adults and often presents with complications.
- Acute mesenteric ischemia and abdominal aortic aneurysm are almost exclusively diseases of older adults and both carry very high mortalities.
- Potentially lethal conditions originating outside of the abdomen, including myocardial infarction, can present with abdominal pain in geriatric patients.

INTRODUCTION

Care of geriatric patients with abdominal pain can pose significant diagnostic and therapeutic challenges to emergency physicians. Older adults rarely present with classic signs, symptoms, and laboratory abnormalities. Incidence of life-threatening emergencies, including abdominal aortic aneurysm, mesenteric ischemia, perforated viscus, and other surgical emergencies, is high. This article explores the evaluation and management of several important causes of abdominal pain in geriatric patients, with an emphasis on high-risk presentations.

EPIDEMIOLOGY

Abdominal pain is among the most common presenting complaints in geriatric emergency department (ED) patients.[1] Altered physiology, comorbid conditions, medication side effects, and polypharmacy increase treatment difficulty and risk in this population. Despite widespread use of advanced imaging, diagnostic accuracy is

Department of Emergency Medicine, University of Maryland School of Medicine, 110 South Paca Street, 6th Floor, Suite 200, Baltimore, MD 21201, USA
* Corresponding author.
E-mail address: rspangler@som.umaryland.edu

Emerg Med Clin N Am 39 (2021) 347–360
https://doi.org/10.1016/j.emc.2021.01.011
0733-8627/21/© 2021 Elsevier Inc. All rights reserved.
emed.theclinics.com

reduced in patients more than 75 years old.[1] The need for surgery or other procedural intervention is high (25%–30%).[1,2] Many older adult patients require admission, and those who are discharged should be carefully selected, because the ED recidivism rate is about 10%.[1]

The risk of serious disorder and associated need for admission, morbidity, and mortality are all increased in older patients. In the past, morbidity rates for geriatric patients have been reported to be as high as 45%.[2] With improvements in the understanding of geriatric physiology and the availability of advanced imaging modalities and less invasive surgical techniques, mortalities have improved to approximately 5%.[1,3]

FEATURES OF COMMON CONDITIONS
Biliary and Gallstone Disease

Gallstone disease is a common surgical problem in the geriatric population. Biliary disease, most notably cholecystitis, is the most common abdominal surgical emergency in geriatric patients.[4] Older adult patients are at increased risk for complications, including emphysematous cholecystitis, perforation, and cholangitis (**Fig. 1**).[5,6] Physiologic factors, including atherosclerotic weakening of the gallbladder wall and age-related dilatation of the common bile duct, increase the risk for perforation and choledocholithiasis, respectively.[6,7]

Common symptoms such as nausea, vomiting, and fever are frequently lacking, often leading to delay in care or diagnosis, which contributes to the observed increase in complications.[8] In one series of older adults with acute cholecystitis, fever occurred in only 16% of cases.[9] Similarly, the Charcot triad of cholangitis (fever, jaundice, and right upper quadrant pain) is observed in only 20% to 45% of patients even in the setting of advanced disease.[10] Ultrasonography is the recommended imaging modality for suspected gallbladder disease; however, computed tomography (CT) may offer

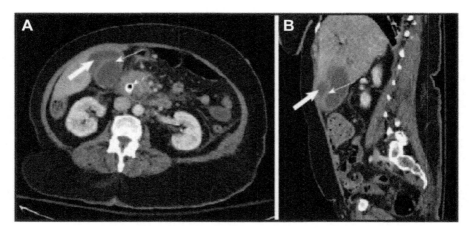

Fig. 1. Perforated gallbladder on computed tomography. (*A*) Transverse image showing fluid collection (*thick arrow*) adjacent to the gallbladder with thickened wall (*thin arrow*). Pancreatic stent placed because of coexisting malignancy also visible (*dashed arrow*). (*B*) Sagittal image showing fluid collection (*thick arrow*) anterior to gallbladder with thickened wall (*thin arrow*).

higher sensitivity, particularly for associated complications and alternative diagnoses.[11,12]

Older adult patients with confirmed acute cholecystitis should be referred for emergent surgical evaluation. Mounting evidence supports early surgical management of acute cholecystitis in geriatric patients because increased rates of morbidity and mortality have been observed with a delayed surgical approach.[13–15] Antibiotics should be administered in the setting of biliary disease with evidence of infection. The Infectious Diseases Society of America recommends single-agent cephalosporin coverage for most mild to moderate cases but recommends broader, dual-agent coverage for high-risk patients, including those of advanced age.[16]

Pancreatitis

Geriatric patients account for about one-third of cases of acute pancreatitis.[17] Compared with younger patients with acute pancreatitis, older patients develop severe disease more frequently and have higher rates of morbidity.[17] Advanced age does seem to increase mortality risk, particularly after age 80 years.[17–19] Gallstone disease remains an important cause of pancreatitis in the older adult population, but other causes, including medication-induced pancreatitis and ischemic pancreatitis, should also be carefully considered.[20,21] Diagnosis is made more difficult by the frequent absence of common symptoms. In one cohort of patients more than 65 years of age, abdominal pain was absent in almost 25% of patients and vomiting was absent in nearly 60%.[19] The aggressive early fluid resuscitation commonly prescribed to patients with acute pancreatitis may be less tolerated in geriatric patients because of their higher rates of comorbid cardiac disease.

Bowel Obstruction

Small bowel obstruction (SBO) increases in both incidence and associated mortality with advancing age.[22] Reported incidence ranges from around 30 to 40 cases per 100,000 in the 15-year to 44-year age group up to about 400 to 480 per 100,000 in patients more than 65 years old.[23] Large bowel obstructions (LBOs) are also more commonly encountered in the geriatric population.[24] The causes of bowel obstruction differ between the small and large bowel, with adhesions causing most SBOs and malignancy causing as many as 80% of LBOs (**Table 1**).[23,25] The symptoms of LBO can be more insidious in onset compared with SBO, although abdominal pain and decreased passage of stool and flatus are still common. Sigmoid volvulus occurs at

Table 1 Bowel obstruction causes[23,26]	
Small Bowel Obstruction[23]	**Large Bowel Obstruction**[26]
• Adhesions	• Malignancy
• Hernia	• Volvulus
• Malignancy	• Diverticulitis
• IBD	• Intussusception
• Stricture	• Hernia
	• IBD
	• Extrinsic compression
	• Fecal impaction

Causes listed by prevalence in descending order.
Abbreviation: IBD, inflammatory bowel disease.

a rate 3 to 4 times greater than cecal volvulus, likely a reflection of the chronic dilatation and redundancy observed in the sigmoid colons of geriatric patients.[26] Comorbidities associated with decreased gut motility are significant risk factors for the development of volvulus, with more than 60% of patients having comorbid neurologic or psychiatric conditions.[27] Complications of bowel obstruction can include ischemia, perforation, and intra-abdominal sepsis.

Although plain radiographs have poor sensitivity and specificity for SBO, they can offer rapid evidence of volvulus or free air.[23] CT offers the best diagnostic utility in the investigation of bowel obstruction in older adult patients, because CT can identify important features of an obstruction, including location, severity, presence of a predisposing lesion, and associated complications.

Evidence of bowel obstruction should prompt urgent surgical consultation. Although some bowel obstructions can be managed nonoperatively, nonoperative management is associated with a higher rate of recurrence.[23] Some cases of LBO, specifically volvulus, may be treated nonoperatively with endoscopic reduction and decompression with a rectal tube. Advanced age increases risk of mortality; however, some literature suggests that improvements in supportive care and surgical techniques are narrowing this gap.[22,23] Supportive care, including resuscitative fluids, analgesics, and antiemetics, should be administered. Placement of a nasogastric tube can be considered in the setting of severe symptoms from pain, distention, or intractable nausea; however, data regarding their impact on successful nonoperative management are limited.[28] Antibiotics covering gram-negative and anaerobic organisms should be administered to patients with obstructing diverticulitis or evidence of perforation or sepsis (**Table 2**).[16]

Appendicitis

Geriatric patients account for approximately 10% of appendicitis cases but a significantly greater proportion of deaths from the disease.[29] Complications including necrosis, gangrene, and (most commonly) perforation increase significantly after age 65 years.[29,30] The cause of this increased risk is likely multifactorial and includes physiologic changes such as vascular sclerosis and fibrotic narrowing of the appendix and fatty infiltration and weakening of the bowel wall.[31] In addition, older adult patients frequently have a delayed presentation from symptom onset compared with younger patients: 50 hours from symptom onset versus 31 hours in 1 large review.[32]

Presenting symptoms can be notably different in geriatric patients and include absence of fever, migratory pain, rebound tenderness, and nausea.[33,34] Right lower quadrant tenderness remains common and can be observed in more than 90% of geriatric patients.[33,34] Laboratory studies are of limited benefit because 20% to 25% of patients do not show increased white blood cell count or left shift.[33] Geriatric patients were poorly represented in the derivation of diagnostic scoring systems including the Alvarado and RIPASA scores.[35,36] The Alvarado score has been shown to perform poorly in a geriatric population; however, some have suggested that modification of traditional cutoffs may achieve adequate predictive values.[33,34] Further study is required to determine what, if any, utility these scores offer in the diagnosis of appendicitis in older adults.

The diagnosis of appendicitis is often aided by diagnostic imaging, and this is even more apparent in older adults. High rates of associated complications, underlying malignancy, and increased diagnostic uncertainty make imaging studies, particularly CT, a valuable diagnostic tool.[31]

Appendectomy remains the recommended treatment strategy for acute appendicitis; however, an approach including an initial trial of antibiotics for uncomplicated

Table 2
Common antibiotic regimens for complicated intra-abdominal infections

	Diagnosis	Mild Severity/Low Risk[a]	Moderate to Severe/High Risk[b]
Biliary	Cholecystitis	Ceftriaxone Cefazolin	Piperacillin/tazobactam, ciprofloxacin, meropenem, or cefepime
	Cholangitis	NA	Each in combination with metronidazole[c]
Extrabiliary	Appendicitis	Single agent: Cefoxitin Ertapenem Moxifloxacin Combination: Ceftriaxone, cefazolin, or ciprofloxacin Each in combination with metronidazole	Single agent: Piperacillin/tazobactam Meropenem Combination: Cefepime, ciprofloxacin, or meropenem Each in combination with metronidazole[d]
	Diverticulitis	Single Agent: Cefoxitin Ertapenem Moxifloxacin Combination: Ceftriaxone or ciprofloxacin Each in combination with metronidazole	
	Peritonitis	NA	

Abbreviation: NA, not available.
[a] Low risk: age less than 70 years, few medical comorbidities.
[b] High risk: advanced age, immunocompromise, health care–associated infections.
[c] May consider early oral therapy in select patients.
[d] Consider adding methicillin-resistant *Staphylococcus aureus* coverage with vancomycin for health care–associated infections.
Data from: Solomkin JS, Mazuski JE, Bradley JS, et al. Diagnosis and management of complicated intra-abdominal infection in adults and children: guidelines by the Surgical Infection Society and the Infectious Diseases Society of America. Clin Infect Dis. 2010;50(2):133-164. https://doi.org/10.1086/649554.

cases has shown some efficacy in the overall population.[31,37] This treatment strategy is not recommended in older adults because they have been poorly represented in antibiotic-first trials and show high rates of occult perforation and necrosis missed on CT imaging.[30,37] Antibiotics are strongly recommended in the setting of perforated appendicitis and preoperatively in uncomplicated cases (see **Table 2**).[16,31]

The World Society of Emergency Surgery recently produced guidelines for the diagnosis and treatment of appendicitis in older adult patients, which highlighted the overall lack of high-quality evidence in this population.[31]

Diverticulitis

Diverticulosis is the most common condition identified on routine colonoscopy.[38] The incidence of diverticulosis increases with age, affecting more than 70% of octogenarians.[38] The rate of development of diverticulitis in the setting of diverticulosis was long quoted in the 10% to 25% range; however, these figures predate routine screening colonoscopy and are thus likely overestimated.[39,40] A more recent study of more than 2000 veterans showed an incidence of diverticulitis of approximately 4%.[41]

In Western populations, more than 90% of cases affect the sigmoid and descending colon, producing the hallmark symptom of left lower quadrant pain.[42] The pain of diverticulitis is variable; it may be mild and intermittent or severe and constant. Other reported symptoms, including urinary symptoms, constipation, or diarrhea, can lead to misdiagnosis.[43] Markers of infection, including increased white blood cell count and fever, may be present; however, their absence should not be relied on to rule out disease.[42]

Although diverticulitis can be a clinical diagnosis, caution is warranted in geriatric patients. In a review of more than 400 geriatric patients who were ultimately diagnosed with diverticulitis, CT altered the pre-CT diagnosis in a significant proportion of patients.[44] Although diverticulitis is associated with a more aggressive presentation and higher recurrence rate in younger patients, older patients experience higher perioperative morbidity, prolonged hospitalization, and higher in-hospital mortality.[45]

A variety of treatments are available depending on disease severity and associated complications.[43] Uncomplicated cases have classically been treated with bowel rest and oral antibiotics. Evidence regarding the utility of antibiotics in the treatment of uncomplicated diverticulitis is evolving. At present, the available research suggests that antibiotic use does not reduce time to resolution, but it may reduce rates of recurrence and complications.[46] Antibiotic therapy alone may be used to treat mild to moderate diverticulitis, including patients with early complications such as a phlegmon. Treatment of more severe, complicated diverticulitis ranges from percutaneous drainage to staged resection. Antibiotics, both oral and intravenous preparations, should be selected to cover aerobic and anaerobic gram-negative bacteria (see **Table 2**).[16]

Mesenteric Ischemia

Older adult patients are more commonly affected by acute mesenteric ischemia (AMI), largely because of the concurrent and causative risk factors associated with AMI.[47] Despite advancements in treatment, the mortality from AMI remains as high at 40% to 50%.[47–49] The challenge of this cannot-miss diagnosis lies in its nonspecific presentation. Abdominal pain is common and is often described as pain out of proportion to the examination. Frequently leading to a misdiagnosis of gastroenteritis, symptoms commonly progress to include vomiting and/or diarrhea, although constipation has also been reported.[50] The duration of symptoms, as well as associated risk factors, are frequently tied to specific past medical comorbidities that the patient may carry.

Mesenteric ischemia is classified into 4 categories based on the cause of injury, with the categories exhibiting subtle differences in precipitating risk factors and clinical presentation (**Table 3**).[47,51–56] Regardless of cause, the pathologic result is significant bowel ischemia requiring urgent intervention to prevent permanent damage.

Laboratory evaluation for patients with AMI is helpful in assessing overall patient status and secondary injury, but no laboratory test is specific for the diagnosis of AMI.[57] Identification and correction of acid-base disturbance and electrolyte derangement can improve patient outcomes. Significant ischemia can lead to increased lactic acid level but a normal lactic acid level should not rule out the diagnosis; ideally, AMI will be diagnosed before irreversible bowel injury.[58] Importantly, diagnostic evaluation with imaging should be based on clinical suspicion rather than laboratory evaluation.

Computed tomographic angiography (CTA) is the preferred diagnostic tool to identify AMI as well as assess for complications and extent of disease.[58] CTA sensitivity is best for arterial disorders; however, multiphase imaging can improve diagnostic sensitivity for venous disease and should be specifically requested if venous thromboembolism is suspected. Ultrasonography with duplex imaging and magnetic resonance angiography can be used; however, patient illness, discomfort, time away from the

Table 3
Risk factors, presentation, and treatment of acute mesenteric ischemia

Category	Risk Factors	Presentation	Treatment
Thrombotic (40%)[56]	• Coronary artery disease • Hyperlipidemia • Diabetes • Hypertension[47]	• Prior history of food intolerance • Sudden worsening • Nausea/vomiting • Diarrhea • Pain out of proportion to examination[53]	• Heparin • Emergent revascularization or stenting
Embolic (25%)[56]	• Atrial fibrillation • Congestive heart failure • Endocarditis • Cardiac valvular dysfunction[52]	• Sudden onset • Severe pain • Nausea/vomiting • Diarrhea • Pain out of proportion to examination[53]	• Heparin • Emergent revascularization or stenting
Nonocclusive (25%)[56]	• Dialysis • Sepsis • Cardiogenic shock • Vasopressor use • Prolonged hypotension[51,54]	• Severe abdominal pain after hemodialysis • Critical illness with increasing lactic acid	• Treat underlying cause • Consider local vasodilator
Venous thrombosis (10%)[56]	• Hypercoagulability • Recent surgery • Malignancy • IBD	• Insidious • Severe abdominal pain • Younger population • Prior history of deep vein thrombosis or pulmonary embolism (20%)[55]	• Heparin • Long-term anticoagulation

department, and operator skill (for ultrasonography) often preclude their routine or recommended use. The diagnostic gold standard of catheter angiography has been largely supplanted by the less invasive and more widely available CTA. Catheter angiography is now mostly used to confirm and treat AMI.[58]

Definitive treatment of mesenteric ischemia is largely surgical; however, early medical intervention can improve outcomes. Once this diagnosis has been made, patients should be anticoagulated with heparin. Because many of these patients need open surgical intervention, longer-acting agents such as low-molecular-weight heparin should be avoided. Broad-spectrum antibiotics should be given because of the high incidence of bacterial translocation and risk of secondary infection (see **Table 2**).[16,58]

Peptic Ulcer Disease

Peptic ulcer disease (PUD) remains a frequent cause of hospitalization and mortality in older adult patients.[59] PUD is the most common cause of upper gastrointestinal (GI) bleeding in geriatric patients and carries a mortality up to 50-fold higher than that of younger populations.[60,61] *Helicobacter pylori* infection, found in 70% of geriatric patients with PUD, use of nonsteroidal antiinflammatory drugs, and smoking are important contributors to the development of bleeding ulcers.[62,63]

Typically, patients with PUD experience upper abdominal pain, pain with eating, nausea with or without vomiting, and food intolerance.[63] In contrast, as many as 50% of geriatric patients present with complications such as perforation or bleeding without any of the previously listed symptoms.[64] Even in the setting of perforated ulcer, a rigid abdomen is rarely present in older adults and cannot be relied on to rule out perforation.[64]

There is no emergency bedside diagnostic test to confirm or exclude PUD or a bleeding peptic ulcer; however, laboratory studies and an electrocardiogram (ECG) can aid in diagnosis and management. ECG in particular should always be obtained, because an acute myocardial infarction can present with abdominal pain, and myocardial injury can occur secondary to acute blood loss.[65]

Imaging for geriatric patients with suspected perforated PUD is always recommended. Upright chest radiograph can be diagnostic of a viscus perforation if free air is visualized. However, this finding occurs in only about 60% of cases; therefore absence of free air should not dissuade physicians from further imaging.[66] In geriatric patients, CT is useful for the diagnosis of occult perforation that would not be apparent on examination or radiograph.[67]

As with management of PUD and upper GI bleeding at any age, management of geriatric patients should focus on resuscitation and assessment for surgical emergencies. The benefits of proton pump inhibitors in the acute setting are debatable; however, their administration is generally recommended.[68] In patients that are at risk for variceal bleeding, administration of octreotide or a similar vasoactive agent is recommended, although poorly studied in the older population who may be at risk for increased side effects.[68] Antibiotics should be administered as early as possible for patients with perforation.

Most geriatric patients presenting with complicated PUD require admission. Gastroenterology should be consulted early in the case of an upper GI bleed. Endoscopy is the diagnostic and therapeutic test of choice for bleeding peptic ulcers. In the case of a suspected perforation, surgical consultation is necessary and should be obtained emergently. If the patient's symptoms are mild, well controlled, and there is no concern on examination or imaging for complicated disease, the patient may be discharged home with strict return precautions. Initiating proton pump inhibitor therapy is reasonable and avoidance of alcohol, nonsteroidal antiinflammatory drugs, and steroids is paramount to prevent further risk of bleeding and perforation.[59] Outpatient recommendations should include follow-up with primary care and gastroenterology for *H pylori* testing and treatment.

Abdominal Aortic Aneurysm

Abdominal aortic aneurysm (AAA) is largely a disease of older adults, with men experiencing the disease approximately 5 times more often than women.[69,70] Rupture of an AAA carries an extremely high mortality of 70% to 90%.[70] Alarmingly, the missed diagnosis rate remains high at about 42%.[71]

Although abdominal pain is a common presenting symptom, with 61% of patients reporting it, the classic triad of abdominal pain, hypotension, and pulsatile abdominal mass is present in fewer than half of patients with ruptured AAA.[71] Therefore, the presence of abdominal pain, back pain, syncope, or hypotension should prompt consideration of ruptured AAA. In addition, vascular compromise may cause lower extremity pain, numbness, or weakness.[72] Physical examination may reveal pulse deficits and atraumatic ecchymosis to the flank (Grey Turner sign), umbilical area (Cullen sign), or even the testicles (scrotal sign of Bryant).[73] Flank pain is a frequent complaint, often leading to a diagnosis of renal colic, the most frequent misdiagnosis in cases of ruptured AAA.[71] Transient symptoms or abnormal vital signs should raise alarm because a ruptured AAA can temporarily tamponade.

CTA can identify the size and location of an AAA, supply evidence of active bleeding, and provide guidance for operative intervention.[74] Non–contrast-enhanced CT

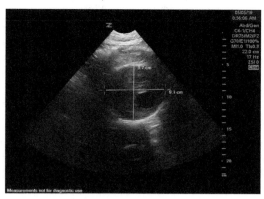

Fig. 2. POCUS showing large AAA with thrombus. (Image Courtesy of Dr. Leen Alblaihed, MBBS, MHA.)

remains highly sensitive for AAA as well as any retroperitoneal hematoma, but poorly visualizes active extravasation.[75] MRI may be used, but its practicality is limited by time, distance from the ED, and patient comfort and safety. Point-of-care ultrasonography (POCUS) has become the initial test of choice for most emergency physicians. Multiple studies have shown that POCUS performed by ED physicians requires little training and is both sensitive and specific for AAA (**Fig. 2**).[76,77] Although not sensitive for retroperitoneal bleeding, the presence of an AAA on POCUS in an unstable or clinically suspicious patient should prompt vascular surgery consultation with or without additional imaging.

Management of a ruptured AAA is surgical; once a rupture is identified, vascular surgery should be consulted emergently. In a hypotensive, bleeding patient, avoid over-resuscitation with crystalloids and aim to use a balanced administration of blood products to limit the impact on coagulopathy and improve mortality[78] Hypotensive patients that are otherwise stable with normal mental status may be allowed a degree of permissive hypotension (70–90 mm Hg systolic blood pressure) to limit bleeding and disruption of any clot formation.[74]

Box 1
Extra-abdominal causes of abdominal pain

- Drug ingestion (eg, NSAIDs, ethanol)
- Herpes zoster
- Metabolic acidosis
- Myocardial infarction
- Pneumonia
- Pulmonary embolus
- Pyelonephritis
- Urinary retention
- Urinary tract infection

Abbreviation: NSAIDs, nonsteroidal antiinflammatory drugs.

Extra-Abdominal Causes of Abdominal Pain

The atypical presentations of abdominal complaints in geriatric patients pose significant diagnostic challenges to emergency physicians. Their presentation is further complicated by the myriad of extra-abdominal causes of abdominal pain. Many of these causes can be life threatening and therefore require consideration in geriatric patients with abdominal pain (**Box 1**).

Myocardial infarction can present with abdominal pain or discomfort as the only symptom. The absence of chest pain in myocardial infarction is more common in geriatric women, patients with diabetes, and nonwhite patients.[79]

Disorders of the genitourinary tract, including urinary tract infections or pyelonephritis, are more common in older adults, particularly in nursing home populations.[80] Comorbid conditions such as benign prostatic hyperplasia and indwelling catheters often contribute to this increased prevalence in the geriatric population.

SUMMARY

Geriatric patients with abdominal disorders can show unusual patterns of symptoms, physical examination findings, and laboratory results, which can contribute to inaccurate or delayed diagnoses. Even when the correct diagnosis is made, older adult patients often have worse outcomes for a given condition compared with younger patients because of the geriatric patients' underlying comorbidities. Emergency physicians should remain cautious in their care of geriatric patients with abdominal pain and maintain a low threshold for advanced imaging and observation for serial examinations, and possibly repeat imaging.

ACKNOWLEDGMENTS

Deborah M. Stein, ELS, provided language editing of the article.

DISCLOSURE

The authors have nothing to disclose.

CLINICS CARE POINTS

- Charcot's triad of fever, jaundice and right upper quadrant pain is observed in as little as 20% of patients with acute cholangitis.[10]
- Geriatric patients with pancreatitis may require more judicious fluid resuscitation due to comorbid cardiac disease.
- Plain films offer poor sensitivity and specificity for small bowel obstruction but can provide quick evidence of volvulus or free air.[23]
- Right lower quadrant tenderness is still among the most common signs of appendicitis in the elderly, observed in >90% of cases.[36]
- Lab tests can be unreliable in geriatric patients and normal white blood cell counts or lactates cannot rule out important pathologies including appendicitis and mesenteric ischemia.[33,58]

REFERENCES

1. Lewis LM, Banet GA, Blanda M, et al. Etiology and clinical course of abdominal pain in senior patients: a prospective, multicenter study. J Gerontol A Biol Sci Med Sci 2005;60(8):1071–6.

2. Kizer KW, Vassar MJ. Emergency department diagnosis of abdominal disorders in the elderly. Am J Emerg Med 1998;16(4):357–62.

3. Marco CA, Schoenfeld CN, Keyl PM, et al. Abdominal pain in geriatric emergency patients: variables associated with adverse outcomes. Acad Emerg Med 1998; 5(12):1163–8.

4. Rosenthal RA, Andersen DK. Surgery in the elderly: observations on the pathophysiology and treatment of cholelithiasis. Exp Gerontol 1993;28(4–5):459–72.

5. Bedirli A, Sakrak O, Sözüer EM, et al. Factors effecting the complications in the natural history of acute cholecystitis. Hepatogastroenterology 2001;48(41): 1275–8.

6. Carrascosa MF, Salcines-Caviedes JR. Emphysematous cholecystitis. CMAJ 2012;184(1):E81.

7. Wilkins T, Agabin E, Varghese J, et al. Gallbladder dysfunction: cholecystitis, choledocholithiasis, cholangitis, and biliary dyskinesia. Prim Care 2017;44(4): 575–97.

8. Morrow DJ, Thompson J, Wilson SE. Acute cholecystitis in the elderly: a surgical emergency. Arch Surg 1978;113(10):1149–52.

9. Edlund G, Ljungdahl M. Acute cholecystitis in the elderly. Am J Surg 1990;159(4): 414–6.

10. Sharma BC, Kumar R, Agarwal N, et al. Endoscopic biliary drainage by nasobiliary drain or by stent placement in patients with acute cholangitis. Endoscopy 2005;37(5):439–43.

11. Yokoe M, Hata J, Takada T, et al. Tokyo Guidelines 2018: diagnostic criteria and severity grading of acute cholecystitis (with videos). J Hepatobiliary Pancreat Sci 2018;25(1):41–54.

12. Wertz JR, Lopez JM, Olson D, et al. Comparing the diagnostic accuracy of ultrasound and CT in evaluating acute cholecystitis. AJR Am J Roentgenol 2018; 211(2):W92–7.

13. Riall TS, Zhang D, Townsend CM, et al. Failure to perform cholecystectomy for acute cholecystitis in elderly patients is associated with increased morbidity, mortality, and cost. J Am Coll Surg 2010;210(5):668–77.

14. McKay A, Katz A, Lipschitz J. A population-based analysis of the morbidity and mortality of gallbladder surgery in the elderly. Surg Endosc 2013;27(7):2398–406.

15. Loozen CS, Van Ramshorst B, Van Santvoort HC, et al. Early cholecystectomy for acute cholecystitis in the elderly population: a systematic review and meta-analysis. Dig Surg 2017;34(5):371–9.

16. Solomkin JS, Mazuski JE, Bradley JS, et al. Diagnosis and management of complicated intra-abdominal infection in adults and children: guidelines by the Surgical Infection Society and the Infectious Diseases Society of America. Clin Infect Dis 2010;50(2):133–64.

17. Kara B, Olmez S, Yalcin MS, et al. Update on the effect of age on acute pancreatitis morbidity: a retrospective, single-center study. Prz Gastroenterol 2018; 13(3):223–7.

18. Moran RA, García-Rayado G, de la Iglesia-García D, et al. Influence of age, body mass index and comorbidity on major outcomes in acute pancreatitis, a prospective nation-wide multicentre study. United Eur Gastroenterol J 2018;6(10): 1508–18.

19. Quero G, Covino M, Ojetti V, et al. Acute pancreatitis in oldest old: a 10-year retrospective analysis of patients referred to the emergency department of a large tertiary hospital. Eur J Gastroenterol Hepatol 2020;32:159–65.

20. Gloor B, Ahmed Z, Uhl W, et al. Pancreatic disease in the elderly. Best Pract Res Clin Gastroenterol 2002;16(1):159–70.
21. Simons-Linares CR, Elkhouly MA, Salazar MJ. Drug-induced acute pancreatitis in adults: an update. Pancreas 2019;48(10):1263–73.
22. Scott FI, Osterman MT, Mahmoud NN, et al. Secular trends in small-bowel obstruction and adhesiolysis in the United States: 1988-2007. Am J Surg 2012; 204(3):315–20.
23. Springer JE, Bailey JG, Davis PJB, et al. Management and outcomes of small bowel obstruction in older adult patients: a prospective cohort study. Can J Surg 2014;57(6):379–84.
24. Pujahari AK. Decision making in bowel obstruction: a review. J Clin Diagn Res 2016;10(11):PE07–12.
25. Drozdz W, Budzyński P. Change in mechanical bowel obstruction demographic and etiological patterns during the past century: observations from one health care institution. Arch Surg 2012;147(2):175–80.
26. Jaffe T, Thompson WM. Large-bowel obstruction in the adult: classic radiographic and CT findings, etiology, and mimics. Radiology 2015;275(3):651–63.
27. Halabi WJ, Jafari MD, Kang CY, et al. Colonic volvulus in the United States: trends, outcomes, and predictors of mortality. Ann Surg 2014;259(2):293–301.
28. Paradis M. Towards evidence-based emergency medicine: Best BETs from the Manchester Royal Infirmary. BET 1: Is routine nasogastric decompression indicated in small bowel occlusion? Emerg Med J 2014;31(3):248–9.
29. Harbrecht BG, Franklin GA, Miller FB, et al. Acute appendicitis - not just for the young. Am J Surg 2011;202(3):286–90.
30. Dhillon NK, Barmparas G, Lin T, et al. Unexpected complicated appendicitis in the elderly diagnosed with acute appendicitis. Am J Surg 2019;218(6):1219–22.
31. Fugazzola P, Ceresoli M, Agnoletti V, et al. The SIFIPAC/WSES/SICG/SIMEU guidelines for diagnosis and treatment of acute appendicitis in the elderly (2019 edition). World J Emerg Surg 2020;15(1):1–15.
32. Segev L, Keidar A, Schrier I, et al. Acute appendicitis in the elderly in the twenty-first century. J Gastrointest Surg 2015;19(4):730–5.
33. Deiters A, Drozd A, Parikh P, et al. Use of the Alvarado score in elderly patients with complicated and uncomplicated appendicitis. Am Surg 2019;85(4):397–402.
34. Shchatsko A, Brown R, Reid T, et al. The utility of the Alvarado score in the diagnosis of acute appendicitis in the elderly. Am Surg 2017;83(7):793–8.
35. Alvarado A. A practical score for the early diagnosis of acute appendicitis. Ann Emerg Med 1986;15(5):557–64.
36. Chong CF, Adi MIW, Thien A, et al. Development of the RIPASA score: a new appendicitis scoring system for the diagnosis of acute appendicitis. Singapore Med J 2010;51(3):220–5.
37. Varadhan KK, Neal KR, Lobo DN. Safety and efficacy of antibiotics compared with appendicectomy for treatment of uncomplicated acute appendicitis: meta-analysis of randomised controlled trials. BMJ 2012;344(7855):1–15.
38. Everhart JE, Ruhl CE. Burden of digestive diseases in the United States part II: lower gastrointestinal diseases. Gastroenterology 2009;136(3):741–54.
39. Parks TG. Natural history of diverticular disease of the colon. Clin Gastroenterol 1975;4(1):53–69.
40. Hughes LE. Postmortem survey of diverticular disease of the colon. I. Diverticulosis and diverticulitis. Gut 1969;10(5):336–44.

41. Shahedi K, Fuller G, Bolus R, et al. Long-term risk of acute diverticulitis among patients with incidental diverticulosis found during colonoscopy. Clin Gastroenterol Hepatol 2013;11(12):1609–13.
42. Horesh N, Shwaartz C, Amiel I, et al. Diverticulitis: does age matter? J Dig Dis 2016;17(5):313–8.
43. Feuerstein JD, Falchuk KR. Diverticulosis and diverticulitis. Mayo Clin Proc 2016; 91(8):1094–104.
44. Gardner CS, Jaffe TA, Nelson RC. Impact of CT in elderly patients presenting to the emergency department with acute abdominal pain. Abdom Imaging 2015; 40(7):2877–82.
45. Razik R, Nguyen GC. Diverticular disease: changing epidemiology and management. Drugs Aging 2015;32(5):349–60.
46. Strate LL, Peery AF, Neumann I. American Gastroenterological Association Institute technical review on the management of acute diverticulitis. Gastroenterology 2015;149(7):1950–76.e12.
47. Kärkkäinen JM, Acosta S. Acute mesenteric ischemia (part I) – incidence, etiologies, and how to improve early diagnosis. Best Pract Res Clin Gastroenterol 2017;31(1):15–25.
48. Kassahun WT, Schulz T, Richter O, et al. Unchanged high mortality rates from acute occlusive intestinal ischemia: six year review. Langenbecks Arch Surg 2008;393(2):163–71.
49. Zettervall SL, Lo RC, Soden PA, et al. Trends in treatment and mortality for mesenteric ischemia in the United States from 2000 to 2012. Ann Vasc Surg 2017; 42(March):111–9.
50. Mastoraki A. Mesenteric ischemia: pathogenesis and challenging diagnostic and therapeutic modalities. World J Gastrointest Pathophysiol 2016;7(1):125.
51. Acosta S. Epidemiology of mesenteric vascular disease: clinical implications. Semin Vasc Surg 2010;23(1):4–8.
52. Liao G, Chen S, Cao H, et al. Review: acute superior mesenteric artery embolism: a vascular emergency cannot be ignored by physicians. Medicine (Baltimore) 2019;98(6):e14446.
53. Kärkkäinen JM. Acute mesenteric ischemia in elderly patients. Expert Rev Gastroenterol Hepatol 2016;10(9):985–8.
54. John AS, Tuerff SD, Kerstein MD. Nonocclusive mesenteric infarction in hemodialysis patients. J Am Coll Surg 2000;190(1):84–8.
55. Acosta S, Alhadad A, Svensson P, et al. Epidemiology, risk and prognostic factors in mesenteric venous thrombosis. Br J Surg 2008;95(10):1245–51.
56. Lehtimäki TT, Kärkkäinen JM, Saari P, et al. Detecting acute mesenteric ischemia in CT of the acute abdomen is dependent on clinical suspicion: review of 95 consecutive patients. Eur J Radiol 2015;84(12):2444–53.
57. Memet O, Zhang L, Shen J. Serological biomarkers for acute mesenteric ischemia. Ann Transl Med 2019;7(16):394.
58. Clair DG, Beach JM. Mesenteric ischemia. N Engl J Med 2016;374(10):959–68.
59. Pilotto A, Franceschi M, Maggi S, et al. Optimal management of peptic ulcer disease in the elderly. Drugs Aging 2010;27(7):545–58.
60. Ahmed A, Stanley AJ. Acute upper gastrointestinal bleeding in the elderly: aetiology, diagnosis and treatment. Drugs Aging 2012;29(12):933–40.
61. Thorsen K, Søreide JA, Kvaløy JT, et al. Epidemiology of perforated peptic ulcer: age- and gender-adjusted analysis of incidence and mortality. World J Gastroenterol 2013;19(3):347–54.

62. Pilotto A, Malfertheiner P. Review article: an approach to Helicobacter pylori infection in the elderly. Aliment Pharmacol Ther 2002;16(4):683–91.
63. Chung KT, Shelat VG. Perforated peptic ulcer - an update. World J Gastrointest Surg 2017;9(1):1–12.
64. Khaghan N, Holt PR. Peptic disease in elderly patients. Can J Gastroenterol 2000;14(11):922–8.
65. Bellotto F, Fagiuoli S, Pavei A, et al. Anemia and ischemia: myocardial injury in patients with gastrointestinal bleeding. Am J Med 2005;118(5):548–51.
66. Anbalakan K, Chua D, Pandya GJ, et al. Five year experience in management of perforated peptic ulcer and validation of common mortality risk prediction models - are existing models sufficient? A retrospective cohort study. Int J Surg 2015;14:38–44.
67. Pinto A, Scaglione M, Romano L, et al. Helical computed tomography diagnosis of gastrointestinal perforation in the elderly. Emerg Radiol 2000;7(5):259–62.
68. Stanley AJ, Laine L. Management of acute upper gastrointestinal bleeding. BMJ 2019;364:l536.
69. Lederle FA, Johnson GR, Wilson SE, et al. The aneurysm detection and management study screening program: validation cohort and final results. Aneurysm Detection and Management Veterans Affairs Cooperative Study Investigators. Arch Intern Med 2000;160(10):1425–30.
70. Karthikesalingam A, Holt PJ, Vidal-Diez A, et al. Mortality from ruptured abdominal aortic aneurysms: clinical lessons from a comparison of outcomes in England and the USA. Lancet 2014;383(9921):963–9.
71. Azhar B, Patel SR, Holt PJE, et al. Misdiagnosis of ruptured abdominal aortic aneurysm: systematic review and meta-analysis. J Endovasc Ther 2014;21(4):568–75.
72. Kamano S, Yonezawa I, Arai Y, et al. Acute abdominal aortic aneurysm rupture presenting as transient paralysis of the lower legs: a case report. J Emerg Med 2005;29(1):53–5.
73. Ratzan RM, Donaldson MC, Foster JH, et al. The blue scrotum sign of Bryant: a diagnostic clue to ruptured abdominal aortic aneurysm. J Emerg Med 1987;5(4):323–9.
74. Chaikof EL, Dalman RL, Eskandari MK, et al. The Society for Vascular Surgery practice guidelines on the care of patients with an abdominal aortic aneurysm. J Vasc Surg 2018;67(1):2–77.e2.
75. Siegel CL, Cohan RH. CT of abdominal aortic aneurysms. AJR Am J Roentgenol 1994;163(1):17–29.
76. Rubano E, Mehta N, Caputo W, et al. Systematic review: emergency department bedside ultrasonography for diagnosing suspected abdominal aortic aneurysm. Acad Emerg Med 2013;20(2):128–38.
77. Kuhn M, Bonnin RLL, Davey MJ, et al. Emergency department ultrasound scanning for abdominal aortic aneurysm: accessible, accurate, and advantageous. Ann Emerg Med 2000;36(3):219–23.
78. Kawatani Y, Nakamura Y, Kurobe H, et al. Correlations of perioperative coagulopathy, fluid infusion and blood transfusions with survival prognosis in endovascular aortic repair for ruptured abdominal aortic aneurysm. World J Emerg Surg 2016;11(1):1–6.
79. Canto JG, Shlipak MG, Rogers WJ, et al. Prevalence, clinical characteristics, and mortality among patients with myocardial infarction presenting without chest pain. J Am Med Assoc 2000;283(24):3223–9.
80. Foxman B. Epidemiology of urinary tract infections: incidence, morbidity, and economic costs. Am J Med 2002;113(Suppl 18):5S–13S.

Genitourinary Emergencies in Older Adults

Nicole Soria, MD[a,b,1], Danya Khoujah, MBBS, MEHP[c,d,]*

KEYWORDS

- Urinary tract infections • Urinary incontinence • Pelvic organ prolapse • Scrotal pain
- Urologic trauma • Varicoceles

KEY POINTS

- Asymptomatic bacteriuria in older adults is common. It is frequently misdiagnosed and inappropriately treated.
- Urinary tract infections in geriatric patients are more likely to be complicated, caused by a multidrug-resistant organism, and require a longer course of treatment.
- Urinary incontinence has a broad differential; emergent conditions include urinary tract infections, spinal cord pathology, and delirium.
- Abuse of older adults is under-recognized, whether in the form of neglect, physical abuse, or sexual abuse.
- Microscopic hematuria should not be dismissed and should always be referred for outpatient follow-up.

INTRODUCTION

Older adults comprise 15% of the US population and are expected to reach 21% in 2040.[1] With this population growth comes a more pronounced use of emergency care,[2] necessitating a thorough understanding of the unique considerations of this age group. Many genitourinary (GU) complaints, such as retention, incontinence, pelvic organ prolapse, and urinary tract infections (UTIs), are more likely to occur in older adults.[3–5] However, older adults may be less likely to seek care for GU complaints,[6] and when they do, they are less likely to receive evidence-based care.[7] Older adults' emergency department (ED) visits may further be complicated by acute or chronic

[a] Emergency Medicine, US Acute Care Solutions, Mercy Health West Hospital, Cincinnati, OH, USA; [b] Geriatric Division, Department of Family & Community Medicine, University of Cincinnati, Cincinnati, Ohio, USA; [c] Emergency Medicine, MedStar Franklin Square Medical Center, 9000 Franklin Square Dr, Baltimore, MD 21237, USA; [d] Department of Emergency Medicine, University of Maryland School of Medicine, 110 S Paca St, 6th Floor, Suite 200, Baltimore, MD 21201, USA
[1] Present address: 30 East Central Parkway #502, Cincinnati, OH.
* Corresponding author. PSC 473 Box 487, FPO, AP 96349.
E-mail address: dkhoujah@gmail.com
Twitter: @npsi86 (N.S.); @DanyaKhoujah (D.K.)

Emerg Med Clin N Am 39 (2021) 361–378
https://doi.org/10.1016/j.emc.2021.01.003
0733-8627/21/© 2021 Elsevier Inc. All rights reserved.

emed.theclinics.com

cognitive impairments limiting the ability to obtain an adequate history, shame or embarrassment related to the sensitive nature of GU complaints as well as challenges associated with the fast-paced nature of EDs themselves. Moreover, several life-threatening conditions may masquerade as benign genital complaints, as summarized in **Box 1**.

BACKGROUND
Pertinent History

Sexual history
Clinician questions should avoid assumptions of heterosexuality or abstinence when discussing a geriatric patient's sexual behavior[8]; lesbian, gay, bisexual, and transgender people make up 5% to 10% of the population overall[9] and 25% of patients in their 80s are sexually active.[10] One approach to start the conversation with the patient may be to ask, "Are you currently satisfied with your sexual activity?" Follow-up questions regarding gender identity, sexual orientation, number of partners, frequency and type of activity, penile implants, hormone replacement, and medications can ensue. Lesbian, gay, bisexual, and transgender older adults are less likely to divulge their sexual history to health care providers for fear of discrimination and refusal of care,[11] especially given that they grew up in a time when their behavior was considered pathologic.

Medications
Polypharmacy is common among older adults[12] and may contribute to acute urologic complaints. Older adults presenting to the ED should have their medications reviewed (prescribed, over the counter, and recreational) for iatrogenic causes of their presentation,[13] specifically for medications with peripheral alpha-1 blockers and anticholinergic properties.[14] Medications used to treat menopausal symptoms or erectile dysfunction may not be thought of as "medications" and should be specifically inquired about as well.

Mistreatment and abuse
Older adults should be screened for elder abuse, especially those with cognitive or physical impairment. The most common type of mistreatment is neglect, such as improper toileting, poor hygiene, and delay in seeking care, and should raise a red flag for further inquiry.

Pertinent Physical Examination

Evaluating a patient with a GU complaint should include abdominal palpation to detect a distended bladder as well as abdominal masses and chaperoned genital and rectal examinations. All patients with irritative voiding symptoms should be offered a genital examination, because they may not recognize the presence of genital culprit for their symptoms or be too embarrassed to disclose it to the physician. Fecal impaction,

---

Box 1
Life-threatening conditions presenting as urogenital complaints

Emphysematous pyelonephritis

Incarcerated hernia

Necrotizing fasciitis (Fournier's gangrene)

Renal infarction

Testicular torsion

prostate enlargement or tenderness, perineal sensation, and abnormal sphincter tone should be elicited on rectal examination.[15] Positioning a patient in a manner that allows adequate GU examination and visualization of the perineum, such as the lithotomy position, may be logistically challenging and uncomfortable for older adult patients and require the assistance of other health care team members. Patients suspected to have a hernia or pelvic organ prolapse should be examined while standing, if possible. A neurologic examination is essential to identify spinal cord abnormalities and peripheral neuropathy.[16] Signs of physical or sexual abuse may be uncovered while performing a physical examination and should be addressed immediately. Logistical difficulties should not deter the physician from performing a thorough examination.

URINARY TRACT PATHOLOGY
Acute Kidney Injury

Older adults are susceptible to acute kidney injury (AKI) given that renal blood flow decreases by 10% every decade after the age of 50, especially in patients with hypertension and chronic heart disease.[17] When compared with those without AKI, patients with AKI are more likely to be older, have underlying chronic kidney disease, progress to end-stage renal disease, and have increased mortality, especially in the setting of sepsis or heart failure.[18,19]

Older adults with renal failure are more likely than younger adults to present with vague concerns and report symptoms of weakness, dizziness, or feeling tired and generally unwell.[20] Questions regarding urine color and output, uremic symptoms (such as nausea, vomiting, and headache), and fluid overload are important. Physical examination ranges from unremarkable to signs of dyspnea with rales, disorientation, and an ill appearance.

Serum creatinine is the most commonly used laboratory value to estimate kidney function.[21] However, the levels can be confounded by volume overload, low body weight, and a decrease in production during acute illness, particularly in older adults.[22] Calculating the creatinine clearance by taking into account the patient's weight and age is a more reliable estimate for renal function than serum creatinine alone.[9]

An investigation of the cause of the AKI requires consideration of prerenal (hypovolemia), renal (intrinsic renal injury), and postrenal (obstruction at any level along the urinary tract) etiologies, which may occur concurrently or independently. For example, AKI in the setting of sepsis may be due to exposure to nephrotoxic drugs, diminished renal flow secondary to inflammation from sepsis, hypovolemia, or underlying renal disease.[19]

The managing the underlying cause of AKI improves symptoms and may resolve the injury. Treatment for AKI in older adults does not generally differ from that in younger patients, with some exceptions. Comorbidities such as diastolic heart failure require frequent reassessment during fluid resuscitation to avoid fluid overload. Ethical considerations and shared decision making are necessary before starting a life-altering treatment such as dialysis.[23]

Hematuria

Hematuria may be visible (gross) or seen only on urinalysis (microscopic); the latter is commonly found incidentally during an evaluation for other complaints. A confirmation of the origin of any hematuria may require a physical examination and potentially a straight catheterization, because many patients reporting hematuria actually have a vaginal or rectal source of their bleeding. The timing of bleeding relevant to urination can give clues regarding its potential urinary source, as outlined in **Fig. 1**.

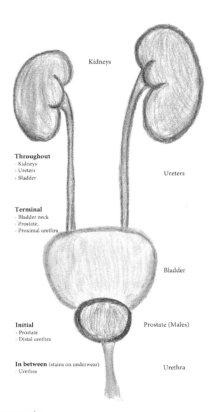

Kidneys

Throughout
- Kidneys
- Ureters
- Bladder

Ureters

Terminal
- Bladder neck
- Prostate,
- Proximal urethra

Bladder

Initial
- Prostate
- Distal urethra

Prostate (Males)

In between (stains on underwear)
- Urethra

Urethra

Fig. 1. The timing of hematuria.

Infection and anticoagulation are common causes of gross hematuria in older adults.[24] With advancing age, more worrisome etiologies should be considered, such as aortic dissection with extension into the renal vasculature, renal vein thrombosis, urinary tract tumors, or acute tubular necrosis. Myoglobinuria resulting from rhabdomyolysis should be considered in the differential of "blood in the urine" as well.

The etiology of the bleeding determines disposition and treatment. Benign prostatic hyperplasia (BPH) causing significant bleeding and hemodynamic instability is an indication for emergent intervention such as transurethral resection of the prostate.[20,25] Asymptomatic microscopic hematuria is commonly due to BPH or urologic malignancy.[24] Older adults, particularly current or former smokers, have a high risk of malignancy and should follow up with urology.[26]

Urinary Retention

Acute urinary retention (AUR) is the inability to voluntarily void and can lead to infection, hydronephrosis, and renal failure.[27] Comorbidities and polypharmacy can alter the presentation in older adults; AUR is often associated with fecal impaction, delirium, and constitutional symptoms.[16] AUR affects up to 10% of men in their 70s and one-third of men in their 80s.[28] BPH is the most common cause of AUR in older males and age is the greatest risk factor for BPH. Obstructive symptoms such as frequency, nocturia, and dribbling of urine affect 25% of men by age 60 years and 45% by age 85.[25] However, it is prudent to avoid anchoring on BPH in older men and consider other causes of AUR such as acute prostatitis, especially in the presence of additional symptoms such as fever.

There are few published data addressing occurrence rates and treatment of AUR in women.[29] The most common causes of AUR in women are detrusor underactivity, obstruction (such as bladder masses and pelvic organ prolapse), or iatrogenic (gynecologic surgery).[30] Causes of AUR in both sexes are summarized in **Box 2**. A list of medications causing retention is in **Box 3**.

Draining a distended bladder provides pain relief and should be done immediately unless contraindications exist, such as a recent urologic procedure.[28] Rapid emptying of an enlarged bladder has been reported to cause a vagal response, resulting in temporary hypotension and/or hematuria; however, studies show neither is common nor clinically significant.[31,32] When a precipitating cause of AUR can be identified, such as infection, constipation, or medication, it should be rectified and a spontaneous voiding trial performed. The optimal timing for a voiding trial is unclear[16]; it is reasonable to attempt spontaneous voiding while in the ED and discharge the patient with an indwelling catheter if voiding fails. Men with BPH may be started on alpha blockers in the ED; alpha blockers before removal of the catheter increase the success rate of voiding.[28,33] In contrast, there are few data for the benefit of alpha blockers in treating female urinary retention.[34] Alpha blockers may cause hypotension and are best taken at bedtime.[28] Follow-up in three days improves outcomes and reduces complications.[28]

The postvoid residual (PVR) is the amount of urine retained in the bladder after a voluntary void and can be an objective measure of urinary retention. Clinically significant PVR volume is unclear; it is highly dependent on the clinical context and may range from 100 to 500 mL.[27] Asymptomatic individuals should be followed up in the primary care setting for the development of symptoms, especially those without prior history of elevated PVR volumes. Symptomatic patients with an elevated PVR or those with obstructive complications require an urgent urology referral.[35] Hospitalization is indicated when AUR precipitates or exacerbates comorbid medical conditions or is associated with acute renal failure, urosepsis, malignancy, or spinal cord compression.

Urinary Incontinence

Discerning the acuity of urinary incontinence is necessary, because 20% of older adults in the community have some element of urinary incontinence at baseline, a percentage that increases to 75% in residents of long-term care facilities.[36] There are

---

Box 2
Causes of AUR in males and females

Bladder cancer or stones

Infection

Medication side effects

Neurogenic bladder secondary to chronic diseases (eg, diabetes, peripheral neuropathy)

Spinal compression

Trauma (bladder, hip, pelvis, or urethra)

Urethral stricture

Data from: Serlin DC, Heidelbaugh JJ, Stoffel JT. Urinary Retention in Adults: Evaluation and Initial Management. *Am Fam Physician*. 2018;98(8):496-503.

Box 3
Medications causing urinary retention

Anticholinergics

Antidepressants

Antihistamines

Antiparkinsonian agents

Antipsychotics

Muscle relaxants

Nonsteroidal anti-inflammatory drugs

Over-the-counter cold medications

Sympathomimetics

Data from: American Geriatrics Society 2019 Updated AGS Beers Criteria® for Potentially Inappropriate Medication Use in Older Adults. *J Am Geriatr Soc.* 2019;67(4):674-694; Curtis LA, Dolan TS, Cespedes RD. Acute Urinary Retention and Urinary Incontinence. *Emerg Med Clin North Am.* 2001;19(3):591-620.

---

different types of incontinence and more than one type may coexist (**Table 1**). Urge incontinence is more common in the older population. However, stress and mixed incontinence have similar frequencies in younger and older women.[3] The differential diagnosis of acute incontinence is broad, encompassing GU, neurologic, and pharmacologic causes.[6,37] A helpful mnemonic for the differential of acute incontinence is DIAPERS, summarized in **Table 2**.[38] The disposition and management depend on the underlying etiology.

URINARY TRACT INFECTIONS

Older adults are more likely than their younger counterparts to have a UTI, have a more complicated course, and require a longer course of antibiotics.[5] In addition to frailty,

Table 1
Different types of urinary incontinence

Type	Definition	Cause
Urgency incontinence	Involuntary urinary loss with a sensation of urgency	Idiopathic; systemic neurologic condition
Stress incontinence	Involuntary urinary loss with activities that increase intra-abdominal pressure (eg, exertion, sneezing, coughing)	Abnormal urethral closure; repetitive increase in intra-abdominal pressure.
Mixed incontinence	A combination of urgency and stress incontinence	Any of the causes above
Overflow incontinence	Incomplete urinary bladder emptying from detrusor underactivity or areflexia	Systemic neurologic conditions; urethral obstruction

Data from: Nitti VW, Blaivas JG. Urinary incontinence: Epidemiology, pathophysiology, evaluation, and management overview. In: Wein AJ, Kavoussi LR, Novick AC, Partin AW, Peters CA, eds. Campbell's Urology, ed 9. Philadelphia: WB Saunders Co; 2007: 2046; and Lukacz ES, Santiago-Lastra Y, Albo ME, Brubaker L. Urinary incontinence in women. *JAMA.* 2017;318(16):1592.

Table 2
Differential diagnosis of acute urinary incontinence: the DIAPERS mnemonic

	Causes of Acute Urinary Incontinence
D	Delirium Dementia Diabetes (neurogenic bladder, hyperglycemia)
I	Infection (UTI) Inflammation
A	Atrophic vaginitis
P	Pharmacology (eg, anticholinergics, alpha agonists, calcium channel blockers)
E	Excessive urine output (eg, excessive intake, diuretics)
R	Restricted mobility
S	Stool impaction Sacral nerve root pathology

Abbreviation: UTI, urinary tract infection.

Adapted from: Lukacz ES, Santiago-Lastra Y, Albo ME, Brubaker L. Urinary incontinence in women. *JAMA.* 2017;318(16):1592; and Resnick NM. Initial evaluation of the incontinent patient. *J Am Geriatr Soc.* 1990;38(3):311-316.

many factors may predispose older adults to a worsened outcome and are summarized in **Table 3**.

Clinical Presentation

Similar to their younger counterparts, UTIs in older adults can affect any location along the urinary tract. Older adults are less likely to have flank pain with pyelonephritis and may present with gastrointestinal or pulmonary symptoms.[39] As with all infections,

Table 3	
Factors predisposing older adults to complicated UTIs[48,56]	
Risk Factor	**Example**
Anatomic and structural abnormalities	Urinary tract calculi Urinary tract tumor (including prostate) Extraurinary tumors compression ureters or bladder Urethral stricture Pelvic floor prolapse (eg, uterine prolapse, cystocele) Benign prostatic hypertrophy
Functional abnormalities	Urinary retention Urinary incontinence Neurogenic bladder Postmenopausal estrogen deficiency
Instrumentation and foreign bodies	Urethral catheterization (including Foley catheter placement) Cystoscopy Transurethral surgery Stent placement Lysis of calculi Penile implant
Systemic factors	Immunocompromise Renal transplant Single kidney

older adults are less likely to have a fever or leukocytosis, even in the presence of bacteremia.[40] Older adults are more likely to have chronic GU symptoms and the acuity of presenting symptoms must be clarified.[25,36] Eliciting symptoms can be challenging in residents of long-term care facilities, especially those with catheters.[41,42] Consensus-based recommendations on clinical presentations suggestive of a UTI in this population are presented in **Table 4**.[41] These criteria have not been validated in the ED and should not substitute for the clinician's judgment.

Emphysematous pyelonephritis
Severe necrotizing infection of the kidney owing to gas-forming pathogens is more likely to occur in diabetics, especially in the presence of an obstruction, and carries a high morbidity and mortality.[43]

Urinary tract infection in males
As infection ascends through the male GU tract, urethritis can progress to epididymitis, orchitis, or prostatitis (**Table 5**). Identifying the presence of prostatitis is important because this diagnosis requires longer antibiotic treatment and may present with systemic complications.[44] Patients with prostatitis may present with perineal or rectal pain with or without urinary symptoms as well as constitutional symptoms, such as fever and malaise, or AUR.[44] A digital rectal examination may reveal exquisite prostate tenderness. Prostatic massage in a patient with acute bacterial prostatitis may precipitate bacteremia and/or shock and is best avoided in immunocompromised or ill-appearing individuals.[45] A prostate abscess should be suspected in patients who remain febrile despite being on antibiotics for 36 hours or more.[46]

Causes

UTIs in older adults are most likely due to a urinary pathogen, although sexually transmitted infections and noninfectious etiologies should be considered as well. Mumps and other systemic viral infections such as rubella, coxsackievirus, varicella, echovirus, and cytomegalovirus should be considered in patients with orchitis.[47]

Diagnosis

Urine macroanalysis, microscopy, and culture
Obtaining a noncontaminated voided urine sample may be logistically challenging in older adults, particularly those with underlying incontinence or cognitive impairment. A single intermittent catheter can be used to obtain a sterile sample.[45] Indwelling catheters should be placed only in cases of acute outlet obstruction or critical illness to monitor urinary output.[13] Acute bacterial prostatitis is diagnosed using midstream urine with or without expressed prostate secretions.[45]

Table 4 Symptoms suggestive of a UTI in residents of long-term care facilities[41,42]	
No Indwelling Urinary Catheter	**Indwelling Urinary Catheter in Place**[a]
New or worsening urgency	New or worsening fever
Frequency	Rigors
Suprapubic pain	Altered mental state
Frank hematuria	General malaise
Costovertebral angle tenderness	Lethargy
Urinary incontinence	New costovertebral angle tenderness

[a] In the absence of another cause.

Table 5
Male genital infections[44,47,55]

Disorder	Epididymitis	Orchitis	Acute Bacterial Prostatitis
History	Gradual onset of pain with radiation to lower abdomen, UTI symptoms	Rare in isolation. Usually progression of epididymitis with acute pain of 1 testis, which may spread to include whole scrotum	Symptoms of UTI and obstructed voiding. Systemic symptoms: fever, chills, malaise
Physical examination	Localized tenderness over the epididymis, pain relief with testicular elevation	Testicular swelling and tenderness	Prostate tenderness on rectal examination may be the only finding

Urine macroanalysis (dipstick testing) is used initially to screen for UTIs and microscopic urine evaluation is frequently the next step. Both tests have variable sensitivity and specificity for UTI in the general population (as detailed in **Table 6**).[48,49] The usefulness and accuracy of dipsticks and microscopy seems to be comparable in older adults.[50]

Table 6
Sensitivity and specificity of urinalysis and urine microscopy for a positive urine culture

Population	Test	Element	Sensitivity (%)	Specificity (%)
General population	Urine dipstick (macroanalysis)	Positive leukocyte esterase	77	59–96
		Positive nitrite*	81	95–98
		Positive leukocyte esterase and nitrite	35–84	98–100
Concomitant renal stone	Urine microscopy	WBCs >5/hpf	86	79
		WBCs >20/hpf	68	93
Catheter-associated UTI	Urine dipstick	Positive leukocyte esterase	87.5	72.0
		Positive nitrite*	25	100
	Urine microscopy	WBCs >5/hpf	73.3	90.0

Abbreviations: hpf, high-power field; WBC, white blood cells.

*Falsely negative in non–nitrate-reducing organisms (*S saprophyticus, Pseudomonas,* and enterococci).

Data From: Abrahamian FM, Krishnadasan A, Mower WR, Moran GJ, Talan DA. Association of pyuria and clinical characteristics with the presence of urinary tract infection among patients with acute nephrolithiasis. Ann Emerg Med. 2013;62(5):526-533; and Lane DR, Takhar SS. Diagnosis and Management of Urinary Tract Infection and Pyelonephritis. Emerg Med Clin North Am. 2011;29(3):539-552; and Lee SP, Vasilopoulosb T, Gallagher TJ, Vasilopoulos T, Gallagher TJ. Sensitivity and specificity of urinalysis samples in critically ill patients. Anaesthesiol Intensive Ther. 2017;49(3):204-209; and Rehmani R. Accuracy of urine dipstick to predict urinary tract infections in an emergency department. J Ayub Med Coll Abbottabad 2004;16(1):4–7; and Tambyah PA, Maki DG. The relationship between pyuria and infection in patients with indwelling urinary catheters: a prospective study of 761 patients. Arch Intern Med. 2000;160(5):673-677.

Urine cultures should be sent on all older adults except those with simple cystitis.[5,51] The definition of a UTI on urine culture depends on the method of collection; a lower threshold is required in catheterized samples than in spontaneously voided ones.[45] Recurrent UTIs secondary to mixed enteric bacteria in straight-catheterized samples should raise suspicion of an enteric urinary fistula.[45]

Imaging

Emergency medicine physicians should maintain a low threshold of imaging in ill-appearing older adults and those with multiple comorbidities to assess for the presence of a complication, such as renal stones, renal or perinephric or prostate abscess, or emphysematous pyelonephritis, and for an alternate non-GU diagnosis, such as cholecystitis or appendicitis.[44]

Management

Antibiotics

All UTIs in older adults must be managed as complicated except for cystitis in a community-dwelling older female with no predisposing factors.[48,52] Antibiotic choice depends on the location of the infection, kidney function, local antibiogram, and available prior culture results. Simple cystitis requires antibiotics that concentrate well in the urine. Infection of the renal or prostate parenchyma requires a longer course of antibiotics with adequate serum levels. Creatinine clearance must be calculated for patients given renally excreted antibiotics, such as nitrofurantoin and piperacillin–tazobactam. Nitrofurantoin can be given in patients with cystitis and a creatinine clearance of 30 mL/min or greater,[14] despite prior reports recommending its avoidance in patients with creatinine clearance of less than 60 mL/min.[53] Fluoroquinolones are the first-line treatment for pyelonephritis and prostatitis in general,[44,51] but should be avoided if possible in older adults given the high risk of complications.[14,54] A more appropriate alternative is a third-generation cephalosporin or piperacillin–tazobactam.[44,51] Trimethoprim–sulfamethoxazole may be used if susceptibility data are known.

Patients with epididymitis who do not require inpatient admission should follow up with a physician within 72 hours.[55] The treatment of prostatitis is similar to other UTIs with a longer antibiotic course of up to 4 weeks.[44] A low threshold should be maintained for intravenous antibiotics and admission, especially in patients with predisposing factors, complications, or unreliable follow-up.

Intervention

Obstruction at any level along the urinary tract should be relieved as soon as possible, whether using a Foley catheter, suprapubic catheter, or percutaneous nephrostomy tube. Renal abscesses of more than 3 to 5 cm, perinephric abscesses of more than 3 cm, or any abscess in a hemodynamically unstable patient should be drained, whether percutaneously or surgically, as early as possible.[56] Patients with emphysematous pyelonephritis may require a nephrectomy in severe cases. Fungus balls associated with candidal UTIs require surgical intervention.[57]

Special Populations

Asymptomatic Bacteriuria

Asymptomatic bacteriuria (ASB) is the presence of 10^5 or more colony-forming units/mL of one or more species of bacteria in the absence of specific GU signs or symptoms attributable to UTI, irrespective of the presence of pyuria.[58] Bacteriuria is common in older adults (**Table 7**) and should not be treated because treatment leads to unnecessary antibiotic use with a resulting increased antibiotic resistance,

Table 7
Prevalence of ASB in specific populations

Population		Bacteriuria (%)
Older adults in the community	Female	10.8–16.0
	Male	3.6–19.0
Older adults in long-term care facilities	Female	25–50
	Male	15–50
Urinary catheter	Intermittent catheterization	1–3
	Indwelling catheter Short term (<30 d)	3–5/day catheter
	Long term (≥30 d)	100

Data from: Nicolle LE, Gupta K, Bradley SF, et al. Clinical Practice Guideline for the Management of Asymptomatic Bacteriuria: 2019 Update by the Infectious Diseases Society of America. *Clin Infect Dis*. March 2019; and Tambyah PA, Maki DG. Catheter-associated urinary tract infection is rarely symptomatic. Arch Intern Med 2000;160:678–87.

Clostridioides difficile infections, and adverse drug events.[58,59] Overtreating ASB is common; one-third of so-called UTIs diagnosed and treated in older adults are in fact ASB.[7] The common practice of treating older adults presenting with a fall or delirium for a UTI in the absence of GU symptoms is not recommended.[58] Bacteriuric patients who are hemodynamically unstable or febrile without specific GU symptoms should receive broad antibiotic coverage for both urinary and nonurinary source,[58] because premature closure on the diagnosis of UTI can lead to anchoring bias and missing serious diagnoses. Asymptomatic candiduria should not be treated in non-neutropenic individuals.[57]

Indwelling catheters
ASB in patients with indwelling catheters is common and should not be treated.[42,45,58] Sampling the urine from indwelling catheters is strongly discouraged. If necessary, specimens must be taken from a newly inserted device.[45] In patients with a UTI, discontinue the catheter completely if possible. If not, replace the catheter to hasten recovery and prevent recurrence.[42] Patients with catheter-associated UTIs are more likely to have *Pseudomonas* and *Proteus*. Patients with asymptomatic candiduria should have their indwelling catheters discontinued if possible and require no further treatment.[57]

Sexually transmitted infections
On par with their younger counterparts, UTIs in older adults may be caused by sexually transmitted infections. An assumption of sexual abstinence, monogamy, or heterosexuality in older patients may lead to missed diagnoses, especially given that older adults may not use condoms because pregnancy is not an issue.

FEMALE GENITAL PATHOLOGY
Vulvovaginitis

With advancing age, estrogen and progesterone decrease, resulting in atrophy of the estrogen-responsive tissue, tissue friability, and decreased healing. Vulvar irritation and vaginitis may occur separately or coexist (vulvovaginitis). Atrophic vaginitis, as part of the GU syndrome of menopause, is a common culprit. Exposure to chemical irritants may cause inflammation as well. Bacterial vaginosis may occur given increased vaginal pH in older women. Candida is less common, and usually occurs in the setting of incontinence, poorly controlled diabetes, immunosuppression, or estrogen therapy.[60] Local treatments may be preferred over systemic for both conditions to decrease polypharmacy.[60] Desquamation reaction, a self-limiting asymptomatic white discharge, results from replacement of uterine prolapse or estrogen therapy. The discharge has scant white blood cells, is filled with epithelial cells, and does not require treatment.[60] Sexually transmitted infections should be considered as part of the differential for vulvovaginal complaints. Thick, malodorous discharge may be a sign of endometrial cancer necessitating further outpatient workup.[60]

Vesicovaginal (vagina and bladder) and enterovaginal (vagina and rectum) fistulas should be considered in all older adults reporting vaginal discharge. Fistulae may result from cancer, radiation treatment, or surgery and should be investigated. Patients with a mass in the Bartholin's gland area should be referred to a specialist to rule out cancer and not assumed to be a benign "Bartholin's cyst."[60]

Vaginal Bleeding

Vaginal bleeding in postmenopausal women should be considered a sign of cancer until proven otherwise. Ten percent of cases are caused by endometrial cancer[61] and the rest are mostly caused by endometrial atrophy.[62] Local or systemic estrogen use can cause vaginal bleeding as well.[63] A thorough examination should evaluate for other causes of bleeding, such as vulvar pathology, rectal bleeding, and hematuria. Patients should be examined for signs of trauma and vascular malformations. As with all bleeding complaints, the patient should be assessed for systemic coagulopathy or a bleeding tendency and systemic illness. If the bleeding is not life threatening, the patient can be referred for outpatient ultrasound examination and gynecologic follow-up for a possible hysteroscopy.

Pelvic Organ Prolapse

Pelvic organ prolapse is more common in women above the age of 70.[3] Pelvic organ prolapse is usually multifactorial, resulting from pelvic injury (such as pregnancy, delivery, surgery, and radiation) and age-related weakening of connective tissue.[15] Patients may present with symptoms of urinary incontinence, difficulty with voiding and/or defecation, or sexual dysfunction; these patients require referral to a gynecologist for a pessary, pelvic floor muscle training, estrogen therapy, and/or surgery.[15] Measuring a PVR volume assesses for chronic urinary retention that, if present, would require follow-up as well.[15] Patients whose only symptoms are a vaginal bulge and vaginal or pelvic pressure do not require any specific treatment by a specialist.[15,64]

MALE EXTERNAL GENITAL PATHOLOGY
Infectious and Inflammatory Disorders

Balanitis and balanoposthitis

Balanitis is inflammation of the glans of the penis; balanoposthitis includes inflammation of the foreskin (the glans and the prepuce). These conditions are usually localized processes that rarely present with systemic symptoms and are diagnosed clinically. The most common cause is a candida infection, which can be treated topically with antifungal (azole) creams, although severe cases require oral treatment. Risk factors for the development of balanitis include diabetes, uncircumcised or immunocompromised patients, poor hygiene, use of certain drugs (salicylates, sulfonamides, tetracyclines), and chemical irritants (soap, spermicides, lotion). Older patients with penile skin changes such as discoloration and scarring should be referred for further evaluation for the possibility of carcinoma in situ or squamous cell cancer.[65]

Phimosis and paraphimosis

Phimosis is defined as the inability to retract the foreskin over the glans penis. Although typically nonemergent, it may cause obstructive uropathy requiring a renal ultrasound examination to evaluate for a distended bladder and hydronephrosis.

Paraphimosis is the inability to reduce the retracted foreskin back over the glans penis and is a urologic emergency owing to the concern for necrosis of the glans secondary to arterial compromise and constriction of lymphatic and venous drainage. Urgent reduction is indicated, either manually or surgically. Applying ice to the penis may decrease edema, which will increase the success of reduction.[66] A gauze soaked with a mixture of 50% dextrose solution and 2% lidocaine jelly, which is then held in place with a condom catheter for 1 hour may decrease edema as well.[67]

Scrotal cellulitis and Fournier's gangrene

Fournier's gangrene, a life-threatening necrotizing emergency that can be deceptively subtle in presentation, presents similarly to scrotal cellulitis with erythema and swelling. Older adults are at increased risk owing to their decreased immunity. High-risk individuals are those with a history of diabetes, malignancy, chronic steroid use, human immunodeficiency virus, or alcohol abuse.[68] Suspicion for Fournier's gangrene should prompt further imaging with a computed tomography scan, broad-spectrum antibiotics, and emergent surgical consultation for definitive management.[69]

Male Genitourinary Cancer

Male GU cancer is not usually diagnosed in the ED. However, two important scenarios that must be kept in mind are: (1) prostate cancer presenting with back pain owing to spinal metastasis and (2) retroperitoneal space cancer presenting with a varicocele.

Prostate cancer and back pain

Prostate cancer is the most common solid organ cancer found in males in the United States and the cause of 30% of cases of bony metastases of unknown primary site.[70] Metastases to the spine can result in pathologic fractures and metastatic spinal cord compression, the latter developing in 5.5% of patients with prostate cancer.[71] Older adults with new or worsening low back pain should be evaluated for potential metastases, even in the absence of neurologic deficits.[72] Any patient with cancer with new back pain should be considered to have spinal metastasis until proven otherwise.[73,74]

Patients with suspected spinal metastasis should receive an MRI with and without intravenous contrast of the entire spine,[75] because spinal metastasis will involve multiple sites in up to 38% of patients.[76] Moreover, sensory deficits and mechanical pain may be present 2 to 4 vertebral levels away from the actual lesion.[76,77] Noncontrast MRI may be considered if there is low suspicion of epidural or intraspinal disease. If MRI is contraindicated or unavailable then computed tomography imaging may be helpful.

Testicular varicocele and retroperitoneal cancer

A testicular varicocele is an abnormal enlargement of the veins in the pampiniform plexus that affects 15% of men, with incidence increasing with age.[78] Sudden onset of right sided varicocele in an older adult should prompt further investigation with a computed tomography scan or retroperitoneal ultrasound examination looking for retroperitoneal space pathology, such as renal cell carcinoma.[78]

Trauma

Isolated external GU trauma is relatively uncommon in older adults.[79] Injuries in older adults usually occur in males after a fall with direct trauma to genitals against furniture, bathroom fixtures, or climbing fixtures (such as stairs or stepstools).[79] In the setting of testicular trauma, the physical examination helps to distinguish between a simple testicular contusion and testicular rupture or penetrating injury through the dartos fascia. The latter diagnoses are true urologic emergencies requiring surgical exploration.[80] The treatment for external GU trauma does not vary by age and injuries limited to the external genitalia are managed on an outpatient basis. A voiding trial before discharge is prudent.

CLINICS CARE POINTS

- ASB is frequently misdiagnosed and treated. A "positive" urinalysis does not mean the patient has a UTI.
- UTIs in geriatric patients are more likely to be complicated and caused by a multidrug-resistant organism. Choose the appropriate antibiotic for a longer course of treatment.
- Emergent differential for urinary incontinence includes UTIs, spinal cord pathology, and delirium.
- Have a high index of suspicion for elder abuse, whether in the form of neglect, physical abuse, or sexual abuse.
- Microscopic hematuria should always be referred for outpatient follow-up.
- A thorough medication list review may provide important clues for the etiology of GU complaints.

DISCLOSURE

The authors have nothing to disclose.

REFERENCES

1. Administration for community living. 2018 Profile of older Americans. 2018. Available at: https://acl.gov/sites/default/files/Aging and Disability in America/2018OlderAmericansProfile.pdf. Accessed June 20, 2020.
2. Pines JM, Mullins PM, Cooper JK, et al. National trends in emergency department use, care patterns, and quality of care of older adults in the United States. J Am Geriatr Soc 2013;61(1):12–7.
3. Luber KM, Boero S, Choe JY. The demographics of pelvic floor disorders: current observations and future projections. Am J Obstet Gynecol 2001;184(7): 1496–503.
4. Jacobsen SJ, Jacobson DJ, Girman CJ, et al. Natural history of prostatism: risk factors for acute urinary retention. J Urol 1997;158(2):481–7.
5. Liang SY. Sepsis and Other Infectious Disease Emergencies in the Elderly. Emerg Med Clin North Am 2016;34(3):501–22.
6. ACOG Practice Bulletin No. 155: urinary incontinence in women. Obstet Gynecol 2015;126(5):e66–81.
7. Woodford HJ, George J. Diagnosis and management of urinary tract infection in hospitalized older people. J Am Geriatr Soc 2009;57(1):107–14.
8. American Geriatrics Society Ethics Committee. American Geriatrics Society care of lesbian, gay, bisexual, and transgender older adults position statement. J Am Geriatr Soc 2015;63(3):423–6.
9. American Geriatrics Society. In: Harper GM, Lyons WL, Potter JF, editors. Geriatric review syllabus (GRS): a core curriculum in geriatric medicine. 10th edition. American Geriatrics Society; 2009.

10. Wilson MMG. Sexually transmitted diseases. Clin Geriatr Med 2003;19(3):637–55.
11. When Health Care Isn't Caring. Legal's Survey of Discrimination against LGBT People and People Living with HIV. New York, NY, . Lambda. Available at: www.lambdalegal.org/health-care-report.
12. Jörgensen T, Johansson S, Kennerfalk A, et al. Prescription drug use, diagnoses, and healthcare utilization among the elderly. Ann Pharmacother 2001;35(9): 1004–9.
13. American College of Emergency Physicians; American Geriatrics Society. Emergency Nurses Association; Society for Academic Emergency Medicine; Geriatric Emergency Department Guidelines Task Force. Geriatric emergency department guidelines. Ann Emerg Med 2014;63(5):e7–25.
14. American Geriatrics Society 2019 Updated AGS Beers Criteria® for Potentially Inappropriate Medication Use in Older Adults. J Am Geriatr Soc 2019;67(4): 674–94.
15. Bales G, Chung D, Ballert K. Pelvic organ prolapse in older adults. In: Griebling TL, editor. Geriatric urology. New York: Springer New York; 2014. p. 181–206.
16. Thorne MB, Geraci SA. Acute urinary retention in elderly men. Am J Med 2009; 122(9):815–9.
17. Wiggins J, Patel SR. Changes in kidney function. Hazzards Geriatr Med Gerontol 2009;6(8):10–3.
18. Selby NM, Kolhe NV, McIntyre CW, et al. Defining the cause of death in hospitalised patients with acute kidney injury. PLoS One 2012;7(11):1–7.
19. Anderson S, Eldadah B, Halter JB, et al. Acute kidney injury in older adults. J Am Soc Nephrol 2011;22(1):28–38.
20. Nagaratnam N, Nagaratnam K, Cheuk G. Geriatric diseases: evaluation and management. Cham (Switzerland): Springer; 2018.
21. Gaibi T, Ghatak-Roy A. Approach to acute kidney injuries in the emergency department. Emerg Med Clin North Am 2019;37(4):661–77.
22. Raman M, Middleton RJ, Kalra PA, et al. Estimating renal function in old people: an in-depth review. Int Urol Nephrol 2017;49(11):1979–88.
23. Del Vecchio L, Locatelli F. Ethical Issues in the elderly with renal disease. Clin Geriatr Med 2009;25(3):543–53.
24. Willis GC, Tewelde SZ. The approach to the patient with hematuria. Emerg Med Clin North Am 2019;37(4):755–69.
25. AUA Guideline on Management of Benign Prostatic Hyperplasia (2003). Chapter 1: diagnosis and treatment recommendations. J Urol 2003;170(2):530–47.
26. Gonzalez AN, Lipsky MJ, Li G, et al. The prevalence of bladder cancer during cystoscopy for asymptomatic microscopic hematuria. Urology 2019;126:34–8.
27. Kaplan SA, Wein AJ, Staskin DR, et al. Urinary retention and post-void residual urine in men: separating truth from tradition. J Urol 2008;180(1):47–54.
28. Marshall JR, Haber J, Josephson EB. An evidence-based approach to emergency department management of acute urinary retention. Emerg Med Pract 2014;16(1):1–20 [quiz: 21].
29. Klarskov P, Andersen JT, Asmussen CF, et al. Acute urinary retention in women: a prospective study of 18 consecutive cases. Scand J Urol Nephrol 1987;21(1): 29–31.
30. Malik RD, Cohn JA, Bales GT. Urinary retention in elderly women: diagnosis & management. Curr Urol Rep 2014;15(11):454.

31. Boettcher S, Brandt AS, Roth S, et al. Urinary retention: benefit of gradual bladder decompression - myth or truth? A randomized controlled trial. Urol Int 2013;91(2): 140–4.

32. Etafy MH, Saleh FH, Ortiz-Vanderdys C, et al. Rapid versus gradual bladder decompression in acute urinary retention. Urol Ann 2017;9(4):339–42.

33. Fisher E, Subramonian K, Omar MI. The role of alpha blockers prior to removal of urethral catheter for acute urinary retention in men. Cochrane Database Syst Rev 2014;2014(6):CD006744.

34. Nitti VW. Is there a role for alpha-blockers for the treatment of voiding dysfunction unrelated to benign prostatic hyperplasia? Rev Urol 2005;7(Suppl 4):S49–55.

35. Taylor JA, Kuchel GA. Detrusor underactivity: clinical features and pathogenesis of an underdiagnosed geriatric condition. J Am Geriatr Soc 2006;54(12): 1920–32.

36. Adelmann PK. Prevalence and detection of urinary incontinence among older Medicaid recipients. J Health Care Poor Underserved 2004;15(1):99–112.

37. Lukacz ES, Santiago-Lastra Y, Albo ME, et al. Urinary incontinence in women: a review. JAMA 2017;318(16):1592–604.

38. Resnick NM. Initial evaluation of the incontinent patient. J Am Geriatr Soc 1990; 38(3):311–6.

39. Roberts JA. Management of pyelonephritis and upper urinary tract infections. Urol Clin North Am 1999;26(4):753–63.

40. Caterino JM. Evaluation and management of geriatric infections in the emergency department. Emerg Med Clin North Am 2008;26(2):319–43.

41. Loeb M, Bentley DW, Bradley S, et al. Development of minimum criteria for the initiation of antibiotics in residents of long-term-care facilities: results of a consensus conference. Infect Control Hosp Epidemiol 2001;22(2):120–4.

42. Hooton TM, Bradley SF, Cardenas DD, et al. Diagnosis, Prevention, and Treatment of Catheter-Associated Urinary Tract Infection in Adults: 2009 International Clinical Practice Guidelines from the Infectious Diseases Society of America. Clin Infect Dis 2010;50(5):625–63.

43. Huang JJ, Tseng CC. Emphysematous pyelonephritis: clinicoradiological classification, management, prognosis, and pathogenesis. Arch Intern Med 2000; 160(6):797–805.

44. Lipsky BA, Byren I, Hoey CT. Treatment of bacterial prostatitis. Clin Infect Dis 2010;50(12):1641–52.

45. Miller JM, Binnicker MJ, Campbell S, et al. A guide to utilization of the microbiology laboratory for diagnosis of infectious diseases: 2018 update by the Infectious Diseases Society of America and the American Society for Microbiologya. Clin Infect Dis 2018;67(6):e1–94.

46. Nickel JC. Recommendations for the evaluation of patients with prostatitis. World J Urol 2003;21(2):75–81.

47. Azmat CE, Vaitla P. Orchitis. In: StatPearls. Treasure Island (FL): StatPearls Publishing; November 4, 2020.

48. Beveridge LA, Beveridge LA, Davey PG, et al. Optimal management of urinary tract infections in older people. Clin Interv Aging 2011;6:173–80.

49. Cortes-Penfield NW, Trautner BW, Jump RLP. Urinary tract infection and asymptomatic bacteriuria in older adults. Infect Dis Clin North Am 2017;31(4):673–88.

50. Sundvall P-D, Gunnarsson RK. Evaluation of dipstick analysis among elderly residents to detect bacteriuria: a cross-sectional study in 32 nursing homes. BMC Geriatr 2009;9(1):32.

51. Gupta K, Hooton TM, Naber KG, et al. International Clinical Practice Guidelines for the Treatment of Acute Uncomplicated Cystitis and Pyelonephritis in Women: a 2010 update by the Infectious Diseases Society of America and the European Society for Microbiology and Infectious Diseases. Clin Infect Dis 2011;52(5): e103–20.
52. Nicolle LE. Urinary tract infections in the elderly. Clin Geriatr Med 2009;25(3): 423–36.
53. American Geriatrics Society updated beers criteria for potentially inappropriate medication use in older adults. J Am Geriatr Soc 2012;60(4):616–31.
54. Stahlmann R, Lode H. Safety considerations of fluoroquinolones in the elderly: an update. Drugs Aging 2010;27(3):193–209.
55. Epididymitis - 2015 STD treatment guidelines. Centers for Disease Control and Prevention; 2015. Available at: https://www.cdc.gov/std/tg2015/epididymitis. htm. Accessed July 23, 2020.
56. Dubbs SB, Sommerkamp SK. Evaluation and management of urinary tract infection in the emergency department. Emerg Med Clin North Am 2019;37(4):707–23.
57. Pappas PG, Kauffman CA, Andes DR, et al. Clinical Practice Guideline for the Management of Candidiasis: 2016 Update by the Infectious Diseases Society of America. Clin Infect Di 2015;62(4):e1–50.
58. Nicolle LE, Gupta K, Bradley SF, et al. Clinical Practice Guideline for the Management of Asymptomatic Bacteriuria: 2019 Update by the Infectious Diseases Society of America. Clin Infect Dis 2019;68(10):e83–110.
59. American Geriatrics Society Identifies Five Things That Healthcare Providers and Patients Should Question. J Am Geriatr Soc 2013;61(4):622–31.
60. Miller KL, Griebling TL. Gynecologic disorders. In: Halter JB, Ouslander JG, Studenski S, et al, editors. Hazzard's geriatric medicine and gerontology. 7th edition. New York: McGraw-Hill; 2017; p. 629–46.
61. Karlsson B, Granberg S, Hellberg P, et al. Comparative study of transvaginal sonography and hysteroscopy for the detection of pathologic endometrial lesions in women with postmenopausal bleeding. J Ultrasound Med 1994;13(10):757–62.
62. Reinhold C, Khalili I. Postmenopausal bleeding: value of imaging. Radiol Clin North Am 2002;40(3):527–62.
63. Krause M, Wheeler TL 2nd, Snyder TE, et al. Local effects of vaginally administered estrogen therapy: a review. J Pelvic Med Surg 2009;15(3):105–14.
64. Pelvic Organ Prolapse. Obstet Gynecol 2019;134(5):e126–42.
65. Buechner SA. Common skin disorders of the penis. BJU Int 2002;90(5):498–506.
66. Jones MP, Mekuria K. Genitourinary Procedures. Emerg Med Clin North Am 2019; 37(4):811–9.
67. Fu J, Watts M, Coralic Z. Trick of the trade: paraphimosis - pour some sugar on me. ALiEM Academic Life in Emergency Medicine. Available at: https://www. aliem.com/trick-trade-management-paraphimosis/.
68. Yilmazlar T, Işik Ö, Öztürk E, et al. Fournier's gangrene: review of 120 patients and predictors of mortality. Turkish J Trauma Emerg Surg 2014;20(5):333–7.
69. Levenson RB, Singh AK, Novelline RA. Fournier gangrene: role of imaging. Radiographics 2008;28(2):519–28.
70. Cross W, Prescott S. The prostate. In: Fillit H, Rockwood K, Young JB. Brocklehurst's textbook of geriatric medicine and gerontology. 2010. Amsterdam, Netherlands: Elsevier; p. 689–701.
71. Mak KS, Lee LK, Mak RH, et al. Incidence and treatment patterns in hospitalizations for malignant spinal cord compression in the United States, 1998-2006. Int J Radiat Oncol Biol Phys 2011;80(3):824–31.

72. Loblaw DA, Perry J, Chambers A, et al. Systematic review of the diagnosis and management of malignant extradural spinal cord compression: the Cancer Care Ontario Practice Guidelines initiative ' s neuro-oncology disease site group. J Clin Oncol 2020;23(9):2028–37.
73. Helweg-Larsen S, Laursen H. Clinical and autopsy findings in spinal cord compression due to metastatic disease. Eur J Neurol 1998;5:587–92.
74. Viets-upchurch J, Silvestre J, Rice TW, et al. Metastatic spinal cord compression: a review. Emergency Medicine. 2014 January;46(1):10
75. Patel ND, Broderick DF, Burns J, et al. ACR Appropriateness Criteria Low Back Pain. J Am Coll Radiol 2016;13(9):1069–78.
76. Lu C, Gonzalez RG, Jolesz FA, et al. Suspected spinal cord compression in cancer patients: a multidisciplinary risk assessment. J Support Oncol 2005;3(4): 305–12.
77. Wong D, Fornasier V, MacNab I. Spinal metastases: the obvious, the occult, and the impostors. Spine (Phila Pa 1976) 1990;15:1–4.
78. Beddy P, Geoghegan T, Browne RF, et al. Testicular varicoceles. Clin Radiol 2005; 60(12):1248–55.
79. Bagga HS, Tasian GE, Fisher PB, et al. Product related adult genitourinary injuries treated at emergency departments in the United States from 2002 to 2010. J Urol 2013;189(4):1362–8.
80. Bourke MM, Silverberg JZ. Acute Scrotal Emergencies. Emerg Med Clin North Am 2019;37(4):593–610.

Infections in Older Adults

Mary Morgan Scott, MD[a], Stephen Y. Liang, MD, MPHS[b],*

KEYWORDS

- Infections • Pneumonia • Urinary tract infection • Gastrointestinal infections
- Skin and soft tissue infections • Elderly • Emergency department
- Antimicrobial stewardship

KEY POINTS

- Older patients with infection can present atypically (altered mental status, lack of fever).
- Symptoms of chronic conditions common in the elderly can mimic infectious symptoms.
- Diagnosis should be made considering all patient factors, including history, risk factors, presentation, and objective data.
- Asymptomatic bacteriuria is common in the elderly and should not be treated with antibiotics.
- Unnecessary use of antibiotics contributes to increased morbidity and emergence of drug-resistant pathogens.

INTRODUCTION

The world's population is aging. A 2015 report estimates that, by 2050, the world's population aged 65 years and older will have increased by almost 150%.[1] In the United States, it is estimated that, by 2035, the elderly will account for more than one-fifth of the population.[2] As the number of elders in the United States increases, so will the number presenting to US emergency departments (EDs). In 2009 to 2010, elders accounted for 15% of all ED visits. The rate of ED visits increased with age, 511 per 1000 persons aged 65 years and older compared with 832 per 1000 persons aged 85 and older.[3]

A substantial number of ED visits and hospitalizations in the elderly are related to infectious diseases (IDs). In 2012 alone, US elders had more than 3 million visits to the ED for IDs, representing 13.5% of all geriatric ED visits that year. This number was more than the rates of both myocardial infarction and congestive heart failure combined. Lower respiratory tract infections, urinary tract infections (UTIs), and septicemia accounted for most ID-related ED visits.[4] ID-related hospitalization rates are consistently higher in the geriatric population and have steadily increased over the

[a] Department of Medicine, Washington University School of Medicine, 660 S. Euclid Avenue, Campus Box 8066, St. Louis, MO 63110, USA; [b] Divisions of Emergency Medicine and Infectious Diseases, Washington University School of Medicine, 4523 Clayton Avenue, Campus Box 8051, St Louis, MO 63110, USA
* Corresponding author.
E-mail address: syliang@wustl.edu

Emerg Med Clin N Am 39 (2021) 379–394
https://doi.org/10.1016/j.emc.2021.01.004   emed.theclinics.com
0733-8627/21/© 2021 Elsevier Inc. All rights reserved.

past 2 decades.[5,6] The nation's elderly tend to have longer and more costly hospitalizations for IDs compared with younger patients.[6,7]

Considering the anticipated steady increase in the elderly population, their consistent and increasing use of EDs and hospitals, and the significant burden of IDs on these visits, emergency physicians must be prepared to effectively evaluate and treat elderly patients presenting with possible infection. This requirement can be especially challenging because elderly patients frequently present atypically.

AGING AND THE ATYPICAL PRESENTATION

A loss of integrity in physical barriers (such as skin), decreased effectiveness of both the innate and adaptive immune systems, and disease-induced and iatrogenic immunosuppression all put elders at greater risk of contracting and ineffectively fighting infections. The mucociliary apparatus and cough/gag reflex help prevent unwanted material from entering the lower respiratory tract. Both are impaired in the aging population. In addition to natural barrier breakdown, iatrogenic perturbation with implanted medical devices such as cardiac pacemakers and defibrillators, heart valves, prosthetic joints, and indwelling urinary catheters can serve as a nidus of infection.

The aging immune system places elders in a chronic state of immunosuppression, called immunosenescence. Both the adaptive and innate immune systems decline in efficacy with age. The bone marrow produces fewer naive B cells ready to react to new antigens.[8] Thymic involution by the fifth decade leaves elders with reduced numbers of available naive T cells, and a breakdown of T-cell homeostasis by the seventh decade results in a dramatically decreased repertoire of T cells.[9] The T cells that remain tend to have defects that inhibit their ability to effectively proliferate in response to antigen activation and contribute to decreased protective antibody response following vaccination.[10,11] Older dendritic cells have been shown to activate B cells 70% less effectively than in younger people.[12] Neutrophils, macrophages, and natural killer cells all take a similar hit in functionality.[13–15]

Unsurprisingly, elders with infections tend to present differently than their younger counterparts. Nonspecific symptoms commonly seen in the elderly include confusion, generalized malaise/fatigue, failure to thrive, difficulty ambulating with frequent falls, weight loss, and urinary incontinence, none of which are specific to an infectious cause. Presence of dementia and polypharmacy can make history-taking difficult and/or unreliable. In addition, the tendency of patients to associate some symptoms with normal aging can lead to delays in presentation and underrepresentation of symptoms.

Atypical presentation has been associated with increased mortality in the elderly.[16] In a recent study of patients aged 65 years or older, altered mental status and malaise/fatigue did not predict diagnosis of bacterial infection; however, fever greater than 38.0°C was largely predictive.[17] The presence of fever is a helpful benchmark, but fever is absent or blunted in up to a third of elderly patients with an acute infection.[18] In addition, elders tend to have lower baseline temperatures, suggesting that a normal febrile response in elders may not reach traditional fever cutoffs,[19,20] and development of fever can be delayed by as much as 12 hours.[21]

PNEUMONIA AND INFLUENZA
Incidence and Mortality

Pneumonia and influenza remain the leading causes of infectious death in the older population.[22] One in 20 people aged 85 years or older have a new episode of community-acquired pneumonia (CAP) every year.[23] Those aged 65 years and older account for more than 90% of influenza-related mortality in the United States every year.[24] Age-related changes in lung function and comorbid conditions increase risk of pneumonia (**Table 1**) and reduce the elder's ability to successfully recover from respiratory infections, often making these events a trigger of further functional decline.

Presentation

Atypical presentation of pneumonia is common in elders. The classic triad of fever, dyspnea, and productive cough may be absent in more than 40% of elders with pneumonia.[25,26] Instead, they may present with delirium or other acute change in mental status, generalized fatigue, decreased functional status, urinary incontinence, and falls.[27,28] Older adults with pneumonia tend to report fewer symptoms than their younger counterparts, and a change in mental status is often the sole indication of an acute decline caused by infection. Incidence of tachypnea has been shown to increase with age and may indicate an underlying pulmonary process in an otherwise atypical presentation.[25]

Diagnosis

All patients presenting to the ED with suspicion of pneumonia should receive a chest radiograph. Clinical features and examination findings alone are notoriously inaccurate in diagnosing pneumonia.[29,30] If the initial chest radiograph is negative but clinical suspicion remains high, a chest computed tomography (CT) scan can be considered.[31] The 2007 Infectious Diseases Society of America (IDSA)/American Thoracic Society (ATS) guidelines suggest empiric initiation of antibiotics and repeat chest radiograph in 24 to 48 hours.[32] Further recommendations regarding diagnostic testing depend on the severity and treatment setting. Per 2019 IDSA/ATS guidelines, pneumococcal and *Legionella* antigen testing can be considered in patients with severe CAP (**Box 1**). Blood and sputum cultures should be obtained in patients with severe CAP and in those empirically treated for methicillin-resistant *Staphylococcus aureus* (MRSA) or *Pseudomonas aeruginosa*. Influenza testing should be done if in season. Procalcitonin measurements are not recommended by the IDSA to help determine whether or not to initiate antibiotics.[33]

Several prognostic tools, such as the Pneumonia Severity Index and the CURB-65 (**C**onfusion; **U**remia, blood urea nitrogen >7 mmol/L or 20 mg/dL; **R**espiratory rate ≥30 breaths per minutes; **B**lood pressure, systolic <90 mmHg or diastolic ≤60 mmHg; **A**ge ≥**65** years) criteria have been used for decades as decision aids to determine which patients with CAP can be safely managed as outpatients.[34,35] However, recent studies have suggested these tools may not be as accurate in older individuals, citing inappropriate emphasis on age and the lack of assessment of comorbidities such as

Table 1	
Risk factors for pneumonia and aspiration	
Risk Factors for Pneumonia	**Risk Factors for Aspiration**
Tobacco use	Impaired cough reflex
Lung cancer	Impaired mucociliary apparatus
Chronic obstructive pulmonary disease	Impaired swallowing mechanism
Asthma	
Dementia	
Stroke	

functional status.[36,37] Emergency physicians should use these tools with caution and ultimately rely on their own best clinical judgment when deciding whether a patient needs hospitalization. The 2007 IDSA/ATS CAP severity criteria can also be used to determine level of care (see **Box 1**).

Management

Antibiotic management of CAP is summarized in **Table 2**. Fluoroquinolones should be used with caution in the elderly because they can increase the risk of life-threatening side effects, including aortic dissection and aortic aneurysm rupture.[38,39] They should be reserved for situations when other treatment options are prohibited. Macrolides as monotherapy should also be used cautiously because of high resistance patterns in some areas.

If the patient has risk factors for MRSA or *Pseudomonas* (previous infection with these organisms or recent intravenous [IV] antibiotics), coverage for these organisms should be added to the regimen. Cultures should be obtained (eg, nasal MRSA polymerase chain reaction [PCR]) and, if negative, additional coverage should be discontinued. Risk factors such as residence in a nursing home, recent hospitalization, and chronic dialysis that defined the health care–associated pneumonia classification in previous guidelines have been abandoned because they do not consistently identify individuals at higher risk for antibiotic-resistant pathogens.[40] Current guidelines do not recommend routinely adding anaerobic coverage for suspected aspiration pneumonia unless there is suspicion for lung abscess or empyema.[33,41,42] Evidence suggests timely administration of empiric antibiotics (within 4–8 hours of arrival to the hospital) results in reduced mortality.[43,44] Patients with pneumonia who test positive for influenza should be given antiviral therapy regardless of timing of symptom onset.[33]

Box 1
Criteria for diagnosis of severe community-acquired pneumonia

2007 IDSA/ATS criteria for diagnosis of severe CAP
    Defined as presence of either 1 major or 3 or more minor criteria

Minor criteria
    Respiratory rate $\geq$30 breaths/min
    Pao_2/Fio_2 ratio $\leq$ 250
    Multilobar infiltrates
    Confusions/disorientation
    Uremia (blood urea nitrogen level $\geq$20 mg/dL)
    Leukopenia[a] (white blood cell count <4000 cells/μL)
    Thrombocytopenia (platelet count <100,000/μL)
    Hypothermia (core temperature <36°C)
    Hypotension requiring aggressive fluid resuscitation

Major criteria
    Septic shock with need for vasopressors
    Respiratory failure requiring mechanical ventilation

[a]Caused by infection alone (ie, not chemotherapy induced).

Adapted from Mandell LA, Wunderink RG, Anzueto A, et al. Infectious Diseases Society of America/American Thoracic Society consensus guidelines on the management of community-acquired pneumonia in adults. Clin Infect Dis Off Publ Infect Dis Soc Am. 2007;44 Suppl 2:S27-72.

Table 2
Management of community-acquired pneumonia

	Treatment	Duration
Outpatient without comorbidities	Monotherapy with amoxicillin, doxycycline, or a macrolide	At least 5 d and should not be discontinued until the patient is afebrile for at least 48 h and clinically improving
Outpatient with comorbidities[a]	(1) Amoxicillin/clavulanate, (2) cephalosporin plus macrolide or doxycycline, or (3) monotherapy with a respiratory fluoroquinolone (levofloxacin or moxifloxacin)	Patients initially started on intravenous antibiotics may transition to equivalent oral therapy when they are clinically improving, hemodynamically stable, and can tolerate oral medications
Inpatient	(1) Combination therapy with a beta-lactam (ampicillin-sulbactam, cefotaxime, ceftriaxone) and a macrolide (azithromycin or clarithromycin) or (2) monotherapy with a respiratory fluoroquinolone	

[a] Comorbidities such as chronic cardiac, pulmonary, hepatic, or renal disease; diabetes; alcoholism; malignancy; or asplenia.

Data from Metlay JP, Waterer GW, Long AC, et al. Diagnosis and Treatment of Adults with Community-acquired Pneumonia. An Official Clinical Practice Guideline of the American Thoracic Society and Infectious Diseases Society of America. Am J Respir Crit Care Med. 2019;200(7):e45-e67.

Elders tend to have extended recovery times, and many do not return to their previous functional status. Given the extensive burden these infections can have on the geriatric population, routine pneumococcal and influenza vaccination is warranted.

URINARY TRACT INFECTION
Prevalence and Risk Factors

The incidence of UTI is second only to respiratory infections in adults more than 65 years old. It is the most common infection diagnosed in nursing home residents.[45–47] UTI is more common in women, but the incidence in men increases with age.[48] Functional disability and neurogenic bladder resulting from stroke, Alzheimer's and Parkinson's disease, as well as bladder outlet obstruction from prostatic hypertrophy in men contribute to urinary retention and allow microorganisms to colonize and proliferate. Urinary incontinence, urogynecologic surgery, and chronic indwelling urinary catheters promote bacterial seeding of the urinary tract.

Diagnosis and Asymptomatic Bacteriuria

Diagnostic criteria for UTI and asymptomatic bacteriuria (ASB) are defined in **Table 3**.[49] ASB is common in the geriatric population.[50,51] In people living in long-term care facilities, the prevalence of ASB may be as high as 50% in women and 35% in men.[52] Current IDSA guidelines recommend against treating ASB in the geriatric population because this has not been shown to improve outcomes.[53]

Distinguishing between ASB and true UTI is challenging in older patients. Many elders regularly experience urinary incontinence, increased frequency or urgency,

Table 3
Definition of urinary tract infection based on symptoms and urinalysis

Term	Definition
Pyuria	>10 WBC/mm^3 per HPF
Bacteriuria	Urinary pathogen of $\geq 10^5$ CFU/mL
Laboratory-confirmed UTI	Pyuria (>10 WBC/mm^3/HPF) plus bacteriuria ($\geq 10^5$ CFU/mL)
Asymptomatic bacteriuria	Bacteriuria in the absence of genitourinary signs or symptoms
Symptomatic UTI	Bacteriuria in the presence of genitourinary symptoms (ie, dysuria, suprapubic pain or tenderness, frequency, or urgency)
Uncomplicated UTI	Genitourinary symptoms (ie, dysuria, suprapubic pain or tenderness, frequency, or urgency) with evidence of pyuria plus bacteriuria in a structurally normal urinary tract
Complicated UTI	UTI occurring in a patient with evidence that infection extends beyond the bladder

Abbreviations: CFU, colony-forming units; HPF, high-power field; WBC, white blood cells.
Adapted from Rowe TA, Juthani-Mehta M. Diagnosis and Management of Urinary Tract Infection in Older Adults. Infect Dis Clin North Am. 2014;28(1):75-89.

dysuria, and pelvic pain even when infection is not present. More than half of women aged 80 years and older experience urinary incontinence, with a third experiencing it several times a week.[54] These symptoms can reflect other conditions often seen in the elderly, such as bladder and pelvic floor dysfunction, atrophic vaginitis in women, and prostatic hypertrophy and chronic prostatitis in men. Patients with neurogenic bladder and UTI tend to present with back pain, increased spasticity, and urinary incontinence.[55]

Vague presentations are clouded by shortcomings of the urinalysis (UA) or dipstick (**Table 4**). Proper collection technique is paramount to ensure reliability. Even when

Table 4
Limitations of urinalysis or dipstick

Dipstick Finding	Suggests	Limitation
Positive leukocyte esterase	Pyuria	False-positive with contamination, concurrent trichomoniasis, use of medication, or consumption of food that colors the urine red
Positive nitrite	Presence of nitrate-reducing bacteria (Enterobacteriaceae)	Absent with non–nitrate-reducing bacteria (*Staphylococcus saprophyticus* and *Enterococcus*)

Data from Gupta K, Hooton TM, Naber KG, et al. International Clinical Practice Guidelines for the Treatment of Acute Uncomplicated Cystitis and Pyelonephritis in Women: A 2010 Update by the Infectious Diseases Society of America and the European Society for Microbiology and Infectious Diseases. Clin Infect Dis. 2011;52(5):e103-e120; and Oplinger M, Andrews CO. Nitrofurantoin contraindication in patients with a creatinine clearance below 60 mL/min: looking for the evidence. Ann Pharmacother. 2013;47(1):106-111.

the clinical presentation and UA suggest a UTI, culture data may take several days to result. In 1 study, 43% of elderly patients diagnosed with UTI in the ED ended up having a negative culture, and 95% of those were inappropriately treated with antibiotics.[56]

Clinicians should be wary when accepting UTI as the explanation for a patient's vague constellation of symptoms. Other disease processes may be overlooked at the sight of a positive UA. In a nonseptic patient, UA should only be sent when there is a clinical suspicion for UTI.

Management

Escherichia coli is the most common pathogen isolated from urine cultures in older adults. Other commonly isolated organisms include *Klebsiella*, *Proteus*, and *Enterococcus* spp. *Klebsiella* and *Proteus* spp are seen most frequently in nursing home residents.[57,58] The prevalence of multidrug-resistant organisms (MDROs) is higher in long-term care residents but is growing in community populations as well. The higher incidence of MDROs in nursing home residents is attributed in part to more frequent and inappropriate use of antibiotics.

According to the 2010 IDSA guidelines, preferred antibiotics for treatment of uncomplicated UTI include:

- Nitrofurantoin monohydrate/macrocrystals (100 mg twice a day for 5 days) or
- Trimethoprim-sulfamethoxazole (160/800 mg twice a day for 3 days)

Fosfomycin (3 g, single dose) is an alternative but has been shown to have inferior efficacy compared with other regimens. Beta-lactams such as amoxicillin-clavulanate, cefdinir, cefaclor, and cefpodoxime-proxetil are appropriate alternatives when other regimens cannot be used. Fluoroquinolones should be avoided. Antibiotics with local resistance prevalence greater than 20% should only be used if urine culture with antimicrobial sensitivities is available.[59]

Nitrofurantoin use may be limited in older individuals with impaired renal function. However, data have shown that it is safe and effective to treat acute UTI in patients with creatinine clearance greater than 30 mL/min.[60,61] In patients with history of UTI caused by MDROs, initial treatment should be selected with previous resistance patterns in mind. In all cases, antibiotics should be tailored to susceptibility data if available from urine culture.

GASTROINTESTINAL INFECTIONS

Gastrointestinal infections in the elderly are common, and the effects of such are often underappreciated. Elders are at greater risk for severe dehydration in the setting of diarrheal illness because of decreased thirst perception, which places elders at greater risk for complications such as malnutrition, electrolyte abnormalities, and orthostatic hypotension resulting in falls.[62]

Clostridiodes difficile

C difficile is the most common cause of acute bacterial diarrhea in nursing homes, skilled nursing facilities, and hospitals.[63] Its incidence has doubled over recent years, with rates higher in patients aged 65 years and older.[64] It is primarily related to the use of antibiotics. Presentation typically involves acute onset of watery diarrhea, abdominal pain, and leukocytosis, but can be as severe as fulminant colitis with sepsis, intestinal perforation, and death.[62]

Antibiotics most frequently associated with *C difficile* infection include clindamycin, fluoroquinolones, and to a lesser extent third-generation cephalosporins; however, any antibiotic has the potential to cause infection.[65–67] Longer exposure and exposure to multiple antibiotics increase risk.[68] The use of proton pump inhibitors, diuretics, and nonsteroidal antiinflammatory medications, which are frequently used in older adults, has also been associated with increased risk.[69–71]

A liquid stool sample should be sent for nucleic acid amplification testing (NAAT) or enzyme immunoassay (EIA). NAAT is generally preferred to EIA for its higher specificity, but NAAT does not test for active *C difficile* toxin and therefore is positive even in asymptomatic carriers. Repeat testing is of no clinical utility if performed within 7 days.[72–74]

In addition to discontinuing the responsible antibiotic agent, the IDSA recommends the following regimens for treatment of initial *C difficile* infection:

- Vancomycin 125 mg by mouth 4 times daily for 10 days, or
- Fidaxomicin 200 mg by mouth twice daily for 10 days

Metronidazole is no longer recommended as first-line therapy and should only be used if the agents discussed earlier are not available. For patients with recurrent infections, options include using a vancomycin taper or using fidaxomicin if vancomycin was used for the initial episode. For frequent recurrent episodes, the addition of rifaximin or fecal transplant can be considered.[74]

Other Gastrointestinal Infections

Other common causes of acute infectious diarrhea in older patients include viral and bacterial gastroenteritis and foodborne illness. *Salmonella*, *Shigella*, and *Campylobacter jejuni* are frequent causes of bacterial diarrhea in elders.[62] Older patients with these infections may present atypically. In 1 study of patients with *Campylobacter*, only 18% of those greater than 75 years old had bloody diarrhea, compared with 92% of those in the age cohort 5 to 24 years old. Similar findings were reported in those with *Salmonella*.[75] *Salmonella* is the most commonly identified pathogen in nursing home outbreaks of bacterial gastroenteritis, accounting for 52% of outbreaks and 81% of deaths.[76]

Maintaining adequate hydration (either enteral or parenteral) is the most important intervention in older patients with diarrheal illness. Empiric antibiotic therapy is not recommended except when presentation is consistent with *Shigella* or in patients who have recently traveled internationally with temperatures greater than 38.5°C and/or signs of sepsis. When indicated, empiric therapy should include either ciprofloxacin or azithromycin. Antibiotics should not be used in patients infected with toxin-producing bacteria.

SKIN AND SOFT TISSUE INFECTIONS

The skin serves as a crucial barrier to prevent entrance of pathogens into the human body. Aging skin is dry and thin, making it susceptible to tears and abrasions that provide convenient portals of entry for pathogens. Common skin infections in the elderly population include bacterial infections (cellulitis, erysipelas, necrotizing fasciitis) and herpes zoster.

Cellulitis and Erysipelas

Cellulitis and erysipelas are usually caused by gram-positive bacteria, and they can often be distinguished clinically. Erysipelas is a superficial infection of the dermis with a rash that tends to be sharply demarcated. Cellulitis involves the deeper subcutaneous tissues and is more ill-defined. Both tend to occur more often in the lower extremities of older patients. Differential diagnoses to exclude include chronic venous stasis and venous thromboembolism. Venous stasis changes are usually bilateral, whereas infection is more likely to present unilaterally.[77] Blood cultures should be obtained in patients with malignancy, underlying immunosuppression, and those with systemic symptoms (ie, hypotension and high fever). Skin swabs and biopsy cultures are usually of low yield and are not recommended but can be considered in the at-risk populations described above.

For uncomplicated cellulitis and erysipelas, IDSA guidelines recommend covering for streptococci and MSSA (**Table 5**).[78] MRSA coverage is usually not necessary unless the patient has risk factors such as penetrating trauma, especially from IV drug use. IV antibiotics should be reserved for more severe infections requiring hospitalization and for patients who are immunocompromised or have signs of systemic inflammatory response.

Necrotizing Soft Tissue Infections

Necrotizing fasciitis (NF) is a severe deep soft tissue infection traversing muscle fascia and subcutaneous fat. It can present similarly to cellulitis. Distinguishing characteristics include (1) pain out of proportion to presentation; (2) hard, wooden feel of the subcutaneous tissue when palpated; (3) signs of systemic toxicity; (4) failure to respond to initial antibiotics; and (5) palpable crepitus or evidence of skin necrosis.[78] NF is a clinical diagnosis, and imaging studies such as CT or MRI are of limited utility. Many times,

Table 5			
Treatment of skin and soft tissue infections in older adults			
Infection	**Pathogen**	**Antimicrobial**	**Duration**
Cellulitis/ erysipelas	*Streptococcus, S aureus (uncommon in erysipelas)*	**Covering streptococci and MSSA** IV: cefazolin PO: amoxicillin, amoxicillin-clavulanate, cephalexin, clindamycin **Covering MRSA:** IV: vancomycin, daptomycin, linezolid PO: doxycycline, clindamycin, TMP-SMX **Covering MRSA and streptococci:** PO: clindamycin alone or doxycycline/TMP-SMX + beta-lactam	5 d, can be extended if no improvement
Necrotizing fasciitis	*Streptococcus, Staphylococcus, Vibrio vulnificus*	Polymicrobial: MRSA coverage + (1) piperacillin-tazobactam, (2) carbapenem, (3) ceftriaxone + metronidazole, or (4) fluroquinolone + metronidazole. Clindamycin should be added for antitoxin effect	Should be continued until no further debridement and afebrile 48–72 h
Herpes zoster	Varicella zoster virus	Acyclovir 800 mg 5 times daily or valacyclovir 1000 mg TID or famciclovir 500 mg TID	7 d

Abbreviations: MSSA, methicillin-sensitive *S aureus*; PO, orally; TID, 3 times daily; TMP-SMX, trimethoprim-sulfamethoxazole.

Data from Stevens DL, Bisno AL, Chambers HF, et al. Practice Guidelines for the Diagnosis and Management of Skin and Soft Tissue Infections: 2014 Update by the Infectious Diseases Society of America. Clin Infect Dis. 2014;59(2):e10-e52.

diagnosis and subsequent urgent surgical treatment of NF is delayed in the elderly when vague complaints are thought to be explained by other infectious causes.[79,80] NF should remain on the differential in geriatric patients until symptoms are reliably explained by other causes and the patient is improving clinically.

Initial management involves surgical debridement and broad-spectrum antibiotics. The most commonly identified pathogens include *Streptococcus pyogenes*, *S aureus*, and *Vibrio vulnificus*. Causative bacteria may be identified via blood cultures or tissue cultures obtained in the operating room. Patients at risk for polymicrobial infection include those with perianal abscesses or surgical procedures involving the bowel, decubitus ulcers, IV drug users, and those with perivaginal infections.[78] **Table 5** outlines suggested initial antibiotic regimens. Antibiotics should be narrowed based on culture data and continued until there is no need for further debridement and the patient is clinically improving and afebrile for 48 to 72 hours.

Herpes Zoster

Herpes zoster (shingles) is caused by the reactivation of latent varicella zoster virus. Patients may experience pain in a dermatomal distribution for 1 to 3 days before the vesicular skin eruption. The rash is described as clusters of vesicles on an erythematous base that evolve into pustules and eventually crust over. Patients are contagious until all lesions have turned into crusted plaques. Treatment with antivirals (see **Table 5**) is important to shorten duration of illness and for the prevention of postherpetic neuralgia, which is especially common in the elderly, occurring in approximately 50% of patients aged 60 years and older.[81] Treatment initiation more than 72 hours after onset of lesions is of unclear utility unless there are new lesions still forming.[82] Patients with ophthalmic zoster or disseminated zoster should be treated with IV acyclovir.[83] Patients with Ramsey-Hunt syndrome respond better when treated with both an antiviral agent and prednisone (1 mg/kg for 5 days).[84] Vaccination with recombinant zoster vaccine is indicated in immunocompetent patients aged 50 years and older. Those with a history of herpes zoster should also receive vaccination. Timing of vaccination after infection is not clearly defined but is generally recommended after the acute phase of infection has resolved or within 1 year.[85]

ANTIMICROBIAL STEWARDSHIP

Emerging antimicrobial resistance now poses a serious threat to public health. According to the Centers for Disease Control and Prevention (CDC), the most urgent threats currently are *Candida auris*, *Clostridioides difficile*, carbapenem-resistant Enterobacteriaceae and *Acinetobacter*, and drug-resistant *Neisseria gonorrhoeae*.[86] Every year, 2.8 million people are infected with an antibiotic-resistant infection, and more than 35,000 people die.[87] Aggressive application of antimicrobial stewardship is crucial because the rate of emerging resistance currently far outpaces the development of new antimicrobials.[88,89]

The goal of antimicrobial stewardship is to treat infection with minimal toxicity to the patient and minimal contribution to development of resistance. The 4 Ds of antimicrobial stewardship, initially described by Joseph and Rodvold,[90] are (1) right **drug**, (2) right **dose**, (3) **deescalation** to pathogen-directed therapy, and (4) right **duration** of therapy (**Table 6**). Some institutions have added a fifth D for right **diagnosis**, which emphasizes the need to prevent unnecessary use of antibiotics.

By carefully assessing every patient and making decisions using these principles, clinicians can contribute to the safe and effective use of antimicrobials and ensure

Table 6	
Five Ds of antimicrobial stewardship	
Right diagnosis	Rule out noninfectious causes and treat with antimicrobials appropriate for the suspected infection
Right drug	Choose a drug or drugs that cover clinically suspected microbes, taking into account local resistance patterns
Right dose	Make sure each antimicrobial is dosed appropriately for infection source and patient factors such as weight and renal function
Deescalation	As soon as possible, narrow coverage to pathogens isolated in culture. Discontinue expanded coverage for patients without risk factors for drug resistance
Right duration	Make sure antimicrobials have a stop date consistent with established recommendations. Ensure patients take all medication as prescribed

medicine stays on the winning side of the battle against antimicrobial resistance. When in doubt regarding any of the principles discussed earlier, consultation with an infectious disease specialist is encouraged. Referencing local antibiograms is also recommended to aid in understanding of local resistance patterns and provide direction in antibiotic prescribing tailored to the specific geographic region and patient population.

SUMMARY

Infections in older patients can prove diagnostically challenging. Age-related factors affecting the immune system in elderly individuals contribute to nonspecific presentations. Other age-related factors and chronic conditions cloud the picture with symptoms that may or may not point to an infectious diagnosis. Delay in administration of antimicrobials can lead to poor outcomes; however, unnecessary administration of antimicrobials can lead to increased morbidity in older patients and contribute to the emergence of MDROs. When evaluating an older patient for infection in the ED, careful clinical assessment and consideration of patient history and risk factors are critical. Objective data should be interpreted with these factors in mind. When necessary, antimicrobials should be chosen that are appropriate for the diagnosis and deescalated as soon as possible.

CLINICS CARE POINTS

- Older patients with infection can present atypically (altered mental status, lack of fever).
- Symptoms of chronic conditions common in the elderly can mimic infectious symptoms.
- Diagnosis should be made considering all patient factors, including history, risk factors, presentation, and objective data.
- Asymptomatic bacteriuria is common in the elderly and should not be treated with antibiotics.
- Unnecessary use of antibiotics contributes to increased morbidity and emergence of drug-resistant pathogens.

DISCLOSURE

MMS and SYL have no conflicts of interest to disclose. SYL received support through the Foundation for Barnes-Jewish Hospital and the Washington University Institute of

Clinical and Translational Sciences which is, in part, supported by the NIH/National Center for Advancing Translational Sciences (NCATS), Clinical and Translational Science Award (CTSA) program (UL1TR002345).

REFERENCES

1. He W, Kowal P. An aging world. 2015. Available at: https://www.academia.edu/30886740/An_Aging_World_2015. Accessed June 29, 2020.
2. Bureau UC. National population projections tables: main series. The United States census bureau. 2017. Available at: https://www.census.gov/data/tables/2017/demo/popproj/2017-summary-tables.html. Accessed May 17, 2020.
3. Albert M. Emergency department visits by persons aged 65 and over: United States, 2009–2010. NCHS Data Brief 2013;(130):8.
4. Goto T, Yoshida K, Tsugawa Y, et al. Infectious disease-related emergency department visits of elderly adults in the United States, 2011-2012. J Am Geriatr Soc 2016;64(1):31–6.
5. Kennedy JL, Haberling DL, Huang CC, et al. Infectious disease hospitalizations: United States, 2001 to 2014. Chest 2019;156(2):255–68.
6. Christensen KLY, Holman RC, Steiner CA, et al. Infectious disease hospitalizations in the United States. Clin Infect Dis 2009;49(7):1025–35.
7. Curns AT, Steiner CA, Sejvar JJ, et al. Hospital charges attributable to a primary diagnosis of infectious diseases in older adults in the United States, 1998 to 2004. J Am Geriatr Soc 2008;56(6):969–75.
8. Cancro MP. B cells and aging: gauging the interplay of generative, selective, and homeostatic events. Immunol Rev 2005;205:48–59.
9. Goronzy JJ, Weyand CM. T cell development and receptor diversity during aging. Curr Opin Immunol 2005;17(5):468–75.
10. Fagnoni FF, Vescovini R, Passeri G, et al. Shortage of circulating naive CD8(+) T cells provides new insights on immunodeficiency in aging. Blood 2000;95(9):2860–8.
11. Saurwein-Teissl M, Lung TL, Marx F, et al. Lack of antibody production following immunization in old age: association with CD8(+)CD28(-) T cell clonal expansions and an imbalance in the production of Th1 and Th2 cytokines. J Immunol 2002;168(11):5893–9.
12. Aydar Y, Balogh P, Tew JG, et al. Age-related depression of FDC accessory functions and CD21 ligand-mediated repair of co-stimulation. Eur J Immunol 2002;32(10):2817–26.
13. Borrego F, Alonso MC, Galiani MD, et al. NK phenotypic markers and IL2 response in NK cells from elderly people. Exp Gerontol 1999;34(2):253–65.
14. Wenisch C, Patruta S, Daxböck F, et al. Effect of age on human neutrophil function. J Leukoc Biol 2000;67(1):40–5.
15. Jorge L, Antonio C. Effect of aging on macrophage function. Exp Gerontol 2002;37(12):1325–31.
16. Hyernard C, Breining A, Duc S, et al. Atypical presentation of bacteremia in older patients is a risk factor for death. Am J Med 2019;132(11):1344–52.e1.
17. Caterino JM, Kline DM, Leininger R, et al. Nonspecific symptoms lack diagnostic accuracy for infection in older patients in the emergency department. J Am Geriatr Soc 2019;67(3):484–92.
18. Norman DC. Fever in the elderly. Clin Infect Dis 2000;31(1):148–51.
19. Downton JH, Andrews K, Puxty JA. "Silent" pyrexia in the elderly. Age Ageing 1987. https://doi.org/10.1093/ageing/16.1.41.

20. Sloane PD, Kistler C, Mitchell CM, et al. Role of body temperature in diagnosing bacterial infection in nursing home residents. J Am Geriatr Soc 2014. https://doi.org/10.1111/jgs.12596.
21. McAlpine CH, Martin BJ, Lennox IM, et al. Pyrexia in infection in the elderly. Age Ageing 1986. https://doi.org/10.1093/ageing/15.4.230.
22. Heron M. Deaths: leading causes for 2017. Natl Vital Stat Rep 2019;68(6):1–77.
23. Jackson ML, Neuzil KM, Thompson WW, et al. The burden of community-acquired pneumonia in seniors: results of a population-based study. Clin Infect Dis 2004;39(11):1642–50.
24. Thompson WW, Shay DK, Weintraub E, et al. Mortality associated with influenza and respiratory syncytial virus in the United States. JAMA 2003;289(2):179–86.
25. Metlay JP, Schulz R, Li YH, et al. Influence of age on symptoms at presentation in patients with community-acquired pneumonia. Arch Intern Med 1997;157(13):1453–9.
26. Janssens J-P, Krause K-H. Pneumonia in the very old. Lancet Infect Dis 2004;4(2):112–24.
27. Marrie TJ. Community-acquired pneumonia in the elderly. Clin Infect Dis 2000;31(4):1066–78.
28. Faverio P, Aliberti S, Bellelli G, et al. The management of community-acquired pneumonia in the elderly. Eur J Intern Med 2014;25(4):312–9.
29. Metlay JP, Kapoor WN, Fine MJ. Does this patient have community-acquired pneumonia? Diagnosing pneumonia by history and physical examination. JAMA 1997;278(17):1440–5.
30. Moore M, Stuart B, Little P, et al. Predictors of pneumonia in lower respiratory tract infections: 3C prospective cough complication cohort study. Eur Respir J 2017;50(5). https://doi.org/10.1183/13993003.00434-2017.
31. Syrjälä H, Broas M, Suramo I, et al. High-resolution computed tomography for the diagnosis of community-acquired pneumonia. Clin Infect Dis 1998;27(2):358–63.
32. Mandell LA, Wunderink RG, Anzueto A, et al. Infectious diseases society of America/American thoracic Society consensus guidelines on the management of community-acquired pneumonia in adults. Clin Infect Dis 2007;44(Suppl 2):S27–72.
33. Metlay JP, Waterer GW, Long AC, et al. Diagnosis and treatment of adults with community-acquired pneumonia. An official clinical practice guideline of the American thoracic society and infectious diseases society of America. Am J Respir Crit Care Med 2019;200(7):e45–67.
34. Lim WS, van der Eerden MM, Laing R, et al. Defining community acquired pneumonia severity on presentation to hospital: an international derivation and validation study. Thorax 2003;58(5):377–82.
35. Fine MJ, Auble TE, Yealy DM, et al. A prediction rule to identify low-risk patients with community-acquired pneumonia. N Engl J Med 1997;336(4):243–50.
36. Parsonage M, Nathwani D, Davey P, et al. Evaluation of the performance of CURB-65 with increasing age. Clin Microbiol Infect 2009;15(9):858–64.
37. Chen J-H, Chang S-S, Liu JJ, et al. Comparison of clinical characteristics and performance of pneumonia severity score and CURB-65 among younger adults, elderly and very old subjects. Thorax 2010;65(11):971–7.
38. Zhang Y-Q, Zou S-L, Zhao H, et al. Ceftriaxone combination therapy versus respiratory fluoroquinolone monotherapy for community-acquired pneumonia: a meta-analysis. Am J Emerg Med 2018;36(10):1759–65.
39. Research C for DE. FDA warns about increased risk of ruptures or tears in the aorta blood vessel with fluoroquinolone antibiotics in certain patients. FDA 2019.

Available at: https://www.fda.gov/drugs/drug-safety-and-availability/fda-warns-about-increased-risk-ruptures-or-tears-aorta-blood-vessel-fluoroquinolone-antibiotics. Accessed July 26, 2020.

40. Chalmers JD, Rother C, Salih W, et al. Healthcare-associated pneumonia does not accurately identify potentially resistant pathogens: a systematic review and meta-analysis. Clin Infect Dis 2014;58(3):330–9.

41. El-Solh AA, Pietrantoni C, Bhat A, et al. Microbiology of severe aspiration pneumonia in institutionalized elderly. Am J Respir Crit Care Med 2003;167(12):1650–4.

42. Marik PE, Careau P. The role of anaerobes in patients with ventilator-associated pneumonia and aspiration pneumonia: a prospective study. Chest 1999;115(1):178–83.

43. Houck PM, Bratzler DW, Nsa W, et al. Timing of antibiotic administration and outcomes for Medicare patients hospitalized with community-acquired pneumonia. Arch Intern Med 2004;164(6):637–44.

44. Lee JS, Giesler DL, Gellad WF, et al. Antibiotic therapy for adults hospitalized with community-acquired pneumonia: a systematic review. JAMA 2016;315(6):593–602.

45. Rowe TA, Juthani-Mehta M. Urinary tract infection in older adults. Aging Health 2013;9(5). https://doi.org/10.2217/ahe.13.38.

46. Curns AT, Holman RC, Sejvar JJ, et al. Infectious disease hospitalizations among older adults in the United States from 1990 through 2002. Arch Intern Med 2005;165(21):2514–20.

47. Tsan L, Langberg R, Davis C, et al. Nursing home-associated infections in department of veterans affairs community living centers. Am J Infect Control 2010;38(6):461–6.

48. Beyer I, Mergam A, Benoit F, et al. Management of urinary tract infections in the elderly. Z Gerontol Geriatr 2001;34(2):153–7.

49. Rowe TA, Juthani-Mehta M. Diagnosis and management of urinary tract infection in older adults. Infect Dis Clin North Am 2014;28(1):75–89.

50. Nicolle LE. Asymptomatic bacteriuria in the elderly. Infect Dis Clin North Am 1997;11(3):647–62.

51. Rodhe N, Löfgren S, Matussek A, et al. Asymptomatic bacteriuria in the elderly: high prevalence and high turnover of strains. Scand J Infect Dis 2008;40(10):804–10.

52. Hedin K, Petersson C, Widebäck K, et al. Asymptomatic bacteriuria in a population of elderly in municipal institutional care. Scand J Prim Health Care 2002;20(3):166–8.

53. Nicolle LE, Gupta K, Bradley SF, et al. Clinical practice guideline for the management of asymptomatic bacteriuria: 2019 update by the infectious diseases society of America. Clin Infect Dis 2019. https://doi.org/10.1093/cid/ciy1121.

54. Melville JL, Katon W, Delaney K, et al. Urinary incontinence in US women: a population-based study. Arch Intern Med 2005;165(5):537–42.

55. Jahromi MS, Mure A, Gomez CS. UTIs in patients with neurogenic bladder. Curr Urol Rep 2014;15(9):433.

56. Gordon LB, Waxman MJ, Ragsdale L, et al. Overtreatment of presumed urinary tract infection in older women presenting to the emergency department. J Am Geriatr Soc 2013;61(5):788–92.

57. Marques LPJ, Flores JT, Barros Junior O de O, et al. Epidemiological and clinical aspects of urinary tract infection in community-dwelling elderly women. Braz J Infect Dis 2012;16(5):436–41.

58. Hu KK, Boyko EJ, Scholes D, et al. Risk factors for urinary tract infections in post-menopausal women. Arch Intern Med 2004;164(9):989–93.

59. Gupta K, Hooton TM, Naber KG, et al. International clinical practice guidelines for the treatment of acute uncomplicated cystitis and pyelonephritis in women: a 2010 update by the infectious diseases society of America and the European society for microbiology and infectious diseases. Clin Infect Dis 2011;52(5): e103–20.

60. Oplinger M, Andrews CO. Nitrofurantoin contraindication in patients with a creatinine clearance below 60 mL/min: looking for the evidence. Ann Pharmacother 2013;47(1):106–11.

61. Cunha BA, Cunha CB, Lam B, et al. Nitrofurantoin safety and effectiveness in treating acute uncomplicated cystitis (AUC) in hospitalized adults with renal insufficiency: antibiotic stewardship implications. Eur J Clin Microbiol Infect Dis 2017;36(7):1213–6.

62. Trinh C, Prabhakar K. Diarrheal diseases in the elderly. Clin Geriatr Med 2007; 23(4):833–856, vii.

63. Simor AE, Bradley SF, Strausbaugh LJ, et al. Clostridium difficile in long-term-care facilities for the elderly. Infect Control Hosp Epidemiol 2002;23(11):696–703.

64. McDonald LC, Owings M, Jernigan DB. Clostridium difficile infection in patients discharged from US short-stay hospitals, 1996-2003. Emerg Infect Dis 2006; 12(3):409–15.

65. Unger JL, Penka WE, Lyford C. Clindamycin-associated colitis. Am J Dig Dis 1975;20(3):214–22.

66. Yip C, Loeb M, Salama S, et al. Quinolone use as a risk factor for nosocomial Clostridium difficile-associated diarrhea. Infect Control Hosp Epidemiol 2001; 22(9):572–5.

67. Muto CA, Pokrywka M, Shutt K, et al. A large outbreak of Clostridium difficile-associated disease with an unexpected proportion of deaths and colectomies at a teaching hospital following increased fluoroquinolone use. Infect Control Hosp Epidemiol 2005;26(3):273–80.

68. Pépin J, Saheb N, Coulombe M-A, et al. Emergence of fluoroquinolones as the predominant risk factor for Clostridium difficile-associated diarrhea: a cohort study during an epidemic in Quebec. Clin Infect Dis 2005;41(9):1254–60.

69. Brown E, Talbot GH, Axelrod P, et al. Risk factors for Clostridium difficile toxin-associated diarrhea. Infect Control Hosp Epidemiol 1990;11(6):283–90.

70. Dial S, Alrasadi K, Manoukian C, et al. Risk of Clostridium difficile diarrhea among hospital inpatients prescribed proton pump inhibitors: cohort and case-control studies. CMAJ 2004;171(1):33–8.

71. Dial S, Delaney JaC, Barkun AN, et al. Use of gastric acid-suppressive agents and the risk of community-acquired Clostridium difficile-associated disease. JAMA 2005;294(23):2989–95.

72. Miller JM, Binnicker MJ, Campbell S, et al. A guide to utilization of the microbiology laboratory for diagnosis of infectious diseases: 2018 update by the infectious diseases society of America and the American society for microbiology. Clin Infect Dis 2018;67(6):e1–94.

73. Deshpande A, Pasupuleti V, Patel P, et al. Repeat stool testing to diagnose Clostridium difficile infection using enzyme immunoassay does not increase diagnostic yield. Clin Gastroenterol Hepatol 2011;9(8):665–9.e1.

74. McDonald LC, Gerding DN, Johnson S, et al. Clinical practice guidelines for clostridium difficile infection in adults and children: 2017 update by the infectious

diseases society of America (IDSA) and society for healthcare epidemiology of America (SHEA). Clin Infect Dis 2018;66(7):e1–48.

75. White AE, Ciampa N, Chen Y, et al. Characteristics of campylobacter and salmonella infections and acute gastroenteritis in older adults in Australia, Canada, and the United States. Clin Infect Dis 2019;69(9):1545–52.

76. Levine WC, Smart JF, Archer DL, et al. Foodborne disease outbreaks in nursing homes, 1975 through 1987. JAMA 1991;266(15):2105–9.

77. Scheinfeld N. Infections in the elderly. Dermatol Online J 2005;11(3). Available at: https://escholarship.org/uc/item/9x6912pv. Accessed June 17, 2020.

78. Stevens DL, Bisno AL, Chambers HF, et al. Practice guidelines for the diagnosis and management of skin and soft tissue infections: 2014 update by the infectious diseases society of America. Clin Infect Dis 2014;59(2):e10–52.

79. Cheah KL, Surrun SK. Necrotising fasciitis in the elderly: a double delay. Proc Singapore Healthc 2010;19(1):73–7. https://doi.org/10.1177/201010581001900111.

80. Yu C-M, Huang W-C, Tung K-Y, et al. Necrotizing fasciitis risk factors in elderly taiwan patients. Int J Gerontol 2011;5(1):41–4.

81. Raeder CK, Hayney MS. Immunology of varicella immunization in the elderly. Ann Pharmacother 2000;34(2):228–34.

82. Cohen JI, Brunell PA, Straus SE, et al. Recent advances in varicella-zoster virus infection. Ann Intern Med 1999;130(11):922–32.

83. Laube S. Skin infections and ageing. Ageing Res Rev 2004;3(1):69–89.

84. Coulson S, Croxson GR, Adams R, et al. Prognostic factors in herpes zoster oticus (ramsay hunt syndrome). Otol Neurotol 2011;32(6):1025–30.

85. Dooling KL, Guo A, Patel M, et al. Recommendations of the advisory committee on immunization practices for use of herpes zoster vaccines. MMWR Morb Mortal Wkly Rep 2018;67(3):103–8.

86. CDC. Antibiotic-resistant Germs: new threats. centers for disease control and prevention. 2020. Available at: https://www.cdc.gov/drugresistance/biggest-threats.html. Accessed June 27, 2020.

87. CDC. Antibiotic resistance threatens everyone. Centers for disease control and prevention. 2020. Available at: https://www.cdc.gov/drugresistance/index.html. Accessed June 27, 2020.

88. Barriere SL. Clinical, economic and societal impact of antibiotic resistance. Expert Opin Pharmacother 2015;16(2):151–3.

89. Doron S, Davidson LE. Antimicrobial Stewardship. Mayo Clin Proc 2011;86(11):1113–23.

90. Joseph J, Rodvold KA. The role of carbapenems in the treatment of severe nosocomial respiratory tract infections. Expert Opin Pharmacother 2008;9(4):561–75.

Rapid Fire
Polypharmacy in the Geriatric Patient

Ashley N. Martinelli, PharmD, BCCCP

KEYWORDS

• Polypharmacy • Geriatric • Medication safety

KEY POINTS

- Geriatric patients are at increased risk for falls owing to prescription medications and polypharmacy.
- Several tools are available to highlight high-risk medications in the geriatric pharmacy.
- Patients with polypharmacy or high-risk medications should be screened for opportunities to remove potentially inappropriate medications, select alternative agents, or adjust doses to improve safety.

CASE

Pertinent history: a 70-year-old woman presents for evaluation of a witnessed fall while walking across her living room. Per the spouse, she had no head trauma or loss of consciousness and did not trip on any objects before the fall. Over the past week, she has been suffering from muscle spasm and pain in her lower back for which she was seen in the emergency department. Her spouse noted that she has been less active and more fatigued than usual over the past 2 days.

Past medical history: hypertension, hyperlipidemia, hypothyroidism, chronic kidney disease.

Surgical history: tubal ligation, hernia repair.

Medications: lisinopril 5 mg/d, metoprolol tartrate 25 mg twice daily, atorvastatin 20 mg/d, ezetimibe 10 mg/d, levothyroxine 88 μg daily, tramadol 50 mg every 6 hours as needed for pain, diazepam 10 mg every 8 hours as needed for muscle spasms.

Family history: breast cancer in mother; diabetes and hypertension in sister and father.

S history: drinks 1 to 2 alcoholic beverages per week socially, no tobacco or illicit substance use.

Pertinent physical examination: Height: 60 inches; weight: 50 kg; temperature: 36.7C; blood pressure: 128/80 mm Hg; heart rate 85 beats per minutes; respiratory rate 16 breaths per minute; oxygen saturation on room air 98%.

Emergency Medicine, Department of Pharmacy, University of Maryland Medical Center, 22 South Greene Street, Room WGL 136, Baltimore, MD 21201, USA
E-mail address: Ashley.martinelli@umm.edu
Twitter: @RxMartinelli (A.N.M.)

Emerg Med Clin N Am 39 (2021) 395–404
https://doi.org/10.1016/j.emc.2021.01.001
0733-8627/21/© 2021 Elsevier Inc. All rights reserved.

General: slow to respond to questions, fatigued, alert and oriented ×3.

Head, eyes, ears, nose, and throat: pupils equal, round, and reactive to light, mucous membranes slightly dry.

Neck: full range of motion, no pain or tenderness.

Cardiovascular: regular rhythm, no murmurs, rubs, or gallops; all pulses equal.

Pulmonary: clear lungs, no wheezing, rales, or rhonchi.

Abdominal: soft, nontender, nondistended, slow bowel sounds.

Neurologic: 5/5 strength and normal sensation in all 4 extremities, tenderness noted on the lumbar spine.

Musculoskeletal: full range of motion, no edema, no deformities of the extremities.

Skin: small abrasion and bruising to left shin.

Diagnostic testing: A workup for the fall was initiated.

WBC	10.4 K/mcL
Hgb	10.6 g/dL
Hct	40.1%
Plt	260 K/mcL
Na	140 mmol/L
K	4.2 mmol/L
Cl	108 mmol/L
CO_2	23 mmol/L
Glucose	98 mg/dL
BUN	18 mg/dL
Creatinine	1.5 mg/dL
Lactate	1.2 mmol/L
Troponin	<0.02 ng/mL
Ammonia	12 mmol/L
aPTT	25 s
PT	1.1
INR	14.7 s

Abbreviations: aPTT, activated partial thromboplastin time; BUN, blood urea nitrogen; Cl, chloride; CO_2, bicarbonate; Hct, hematocrit; Hgb, hemoglobin; INR, international normalized ratio; K, potassium; Na, sodium; Plt, platelet count; PT, prothrombin time; WBC, white blood cells.

Electrocardiogram: normal sinus rhythm, no signs of ischemia or ectopy.

Chest radiograph: normal.

Head computed tomography scan: no acute intracranial abnormalities.

Lumbar spine computed tomography scan: degenerative changes of the lumbar spine, no fracture or dislocation.

Clinical Course

A workup was promptly initiated for her fall, including basic laboratory assessments, coagulation tests, electrocardiogram, and imaging with a chest radiograph and a computed tomography scan of the head and lumbar spine. The only abnormality was her renal function with a calculated creatinine clearance of 28 mL/min, which is consistent with her chronic kidney disease. She had no acute abnormalities on imaging.

Upon further questioning, she recently injured her back while working in her garden. She "did not want an opioid medication" so the emergency department physician started her on tramadol for pain in addition to diazepam for muscle spasms. She had been taking these medications around the clock as prescribed for the past 3 days.

LEARNING POINTS

- As patients age, they experience changes in their pharmacokinetic and pharmacodynamic responses to medications. This change can increase a patient's overall sensitivity and the risk of adverse events. Dose adjustments or alternative agent selection may be necessary to mitigate the risk.
- Polypharmacy is commonly defined as the use of five or more medications at a time and taking more medications than clinically appropriate for the patient's underlying clinical condition.[1]
- Overall prescription numbers have increased by more than 85% in the past two decades disproportionately to the 21% increase in overall US population. The number of patients with polypharmacy also increased from 12.8% to 39.0% during the same time frame. In patients greater than 65 years old, 40% take five to nine medications per day and 18% take more than ten.[2–4]
- This increase in medication use can be problematic owing to drug–drug interactions, the potential for adverse drug events, added cost, and, most important, increased hospitalization and mortality.[5,6]
- Several tools are available to help avoid inappropriate medications therapy and polypharmacy in the geriatric patient.

Physiology and Pathophysiology

With advancing age, patients experience several changes with respect to pharmacokinetics and pharmacodynamics that generally cause medications to be more potent and have a longer duration of action than predicted compared with their younger counterparts.[7] (**Table 1**).

Renal insufficiency

Chronic kidney disease is prevalent in 15% (37 million people) of the US adult population and is more common in persons aged 65 or older.[9] Many medications with renal clearance require adjustment for chronic kidney disease to prevent adverse events and/or accumulation of the medication.

Creatinine clearance as calculated by the Cockcroft-Gault equation is the gold standard for assessing renal function as it relates to medication safety. Most package insert dose adjustments are based on this formula.[10] Most medications cleared by the kidneys do not require dose adjustment until the creatinine clearance is less than 60 mL/min. Each medication should be checked with a reliable drug reference as the cutoffs vary.

Cockcroft-Gault equation for creatinine clearance:
 Creatinine clearance = [((140 − age) × ideal body weight)/(72 × SCr)] × 0.85 if female, where SCr is the serum creatinine.

Hepatic insufficiency

Less frequently, medications are adjusted based on the presence of hepatic insufficiency; however, there is not a similar standardized scoring tool on which to base the adjustments. For those patients, it is generally recommended to use a medication that does not undergo hepatic metabolism or start with the lowest dose and decrease the dosing frequency when possible.

Table 1
Effects of aging on medication response[7,8]

Pharmacokinetic/ Pharmacodynamic Change	Effect on Medications	Medication Examples
Decreased muscle mass and circulating plasma proteins	Highly protein-bound medications may have increased serum concentrations.	Verapamil, haloperidol, propranolol
Increased total body fat	Lipophilic medications may have lower plasma concentrations and prolonged duration of effect.	Diazepam, midazolam, lorazepam
Decreased water concentration	Hydrophilic medications may have increased plasma concentrations and effect.	Lithium, digoxin
Decreased renal function	Decreased clearance of medication eliminated by the kidneys.	Sulfamethoxazole-trimethoprim, ciprofloxacin, apixaban, rivaroxaban, enoxaparin, tramadol, gabapentin, famotidine
Decreased hepatic CYP enzyme capacity and lower hepatic blood flow	Reduced clearance of medication metabolized by CYP enzymes or cleared by the liver including first pass metabolism. Decreased conversion of prodrugs.	Propranolol, verapamil, theophylline, risperidone, carbamazepine

Geriatric patients in clinical trials

Historically, geriatric patients have had limited enrollment in clinical trials, which is remarkable given the prevalence of medications usage in this demographic. Because of this circumstance, there is limited information on medication dosing in this patient population. A recent analysis of medications reviewed by the Federal Drug Administration for authorization demonstrated a remarkable lack of pharmacokinetic data in geriatric patients before 1979. This lack has improved in recent years with approximately 75% of new medications from 2010 to 2018 reporting this information.[11] Detailed geriatric safety information has remained unchanged throughout this same time period for approximately 45% of medications. Although the data may be limited, it is advisable to review prescribing information for specific geriatric considerations.

In the absence of geriatric-specific data:

- Determine if the patient has renal or hepatic insufficiency.
- If so, assess for renal and hepatic dose recommendations in package inserts.
- Follow the general rule of "start low, go slow" when initiating new medications while regularly titrating to the desired clinical effect.[12]

Making the Diagnosis

Given that adverse drug events lead to many emergency department visits within the geriatric population, it is important to keep medication causes on the differential diagnosis. In addition to assessing for organ dysfunction and required dose adjustments, there are several resources that highlight inappropriate medications for the geriatric patient and can be used to screen medication lists for high-risk medications (**Boxes 1** and **2**).

A medication adverse event can contribute to or be the sole cause of worsening of a chronic condition, fatigue, falls, or altered mental status. Specific attention should be paid to medications that can increase adverse central nervous system effects and falls, such as anticholinergic medications, opioids, benzodiazepines, antidepressants, and antipsychotics.[13] A more comprehensive list is presented in **Box 2**.

Patients presenting for evaluation after a fall should also be assessed for the presence of anticoagulant or antiplatelet agents on their home medication list. While these medications do not increase the risk for falls, they increase the risk for bleeding events, even after minor falls or injuries.

Pain Management in Older Adults

Although the list of high-risk medications to review as found in Box 2 is extensive, the purpose of this case is to illustrate the challenges with pain management in the geriatric patient, because it can be complex owing to their increased sensitivity to medication effects. It is important to have an ongoing risks and benefits discussion with patients and their families.

Opioids are not recommended as first-line therapy for mild pain in older adults and should only be considered in moderate to severe pain or for mild pain when acetaminophen and non-steroidal anti-inflammatory drugs (NSAIDs) have been ineffective or are contraindicated.[14] Opioids such as morphine, hydromorphone, and tramadol are cleared by the kidneys, thus any reductions in renal function can prolong the effect of these medications. It is generally recommended to start opioids at a lower dose in older patients, 25% to 50% of the usual starting dose in their younger counterparts.[15]

Tramadol is often thought to be a safer alternative to opioid medications.[16] This is not the case and prescribing tramadol should be done with as much care as prescribing an opioid. With simultaneous opioid agonist and serotonin HT and norepinephrine reuptake inhibition activities, tramadol has a unique mechanism of action. It is a prodrug that is metabolized by the CYP enzymes and genetic polymorphisms can lead to differences in both the analgesic effect and adverse events. Dose adjustments and/or alternative agent selection are required for patients with severe hepatic disease or renal dysfunction.[17] Although not limited to the geriatric patient, tramadol also lowers the seizure threshold, has the potential to cause serotonin syndrome, carries a risk of hyponatremia and development of syndrome of inappropriate antidiuretic hormone, and rarely has been linked to hypoglycemia thus making it a potentially unsafe medication to use in the geriatric patient.[13]

Benzodiazepines are commonly used for the treatment of anxiety, but are sometimes prescribed for patients with low back pain or muscle spasms. They are considered potentially inappropriate medications owing to their risk of cognitive impairment,

---

Box 1
Resources for geriatric medication recommendations

- American Geriatric Society Beers Criteria for Potentially Inappropriate Medication Use in Older Adults[13]
- Screening Tool of Older People's Prescriptions (STOPP) and Screening Tool to Alert to Right Treatment (START) Criteria[14]

Box 2
High-risk medications in older adults[2,13,14]

Anticoagulants

Antiplatelet medications

Antihyperglycemics

Anticholinergic medications (diphenhydramine, tricyclic antidepressants)

Antipsychotics

Benzodiazepines

Cardiac medications (digoxin, amiodarone, beta-blockers, calcium channel blockers)

Diuretics

Immunosuppressant medications including chemotherapy

Opioid medications

Sleep aids

---

delirium, falls, fractures, and motor vehicle crashes in geriatric patients and should be avoided in combination with an opioid medication owing to the risk of additive adverse events.[13,14] Recent data have demonstrated that diazepam was not better than placebo for back pain when added to an NSAID.[18] Additionally, skeletal muscle relaxants have questionable benefit in these patients with back pain and are often not recommended in geriatric patients owing to the increased anticholinergic effects such as sedation, and increased risk of fractures.[13,19]

When selecting alternative agents, many consider the risk to benefit ratio of oral NSAIDs and acetaminophen as these are readily available in the community and easily accessible. NSAIDs have the potential to increase blood pressure (by approximately 5 mm Hg), increase adverse cardiovascular events, and increase the risk of gastrointestinal bleeding.[20] The risk of gastrointestinal bleeding increases with duration of use (approximately 1% with three to six months of use, 2%–4% with up to a year of use).[13] Finally, although renal adverse events are less common, the American Geriatric Society recommends avoiding NSAID use in patients with stage IV and V chronic kidney disease.[13] In the absence of the aforementioned risk factors, short courses of low-dose NSAID therapy may be beneficial. In addition, topical preparations may be used because they have minimal adverse events and can be directly applied to intact skin.[21]

Acetaminophen is a safe analgesic option for most geriatric patients. The daily maximum dose should not exceed 4000 mg when used under the direction of a clinician, but the over-the-counter preparations are labeled with a lower maximum dose of approximately 3000 mg to decrease the risk of hepatotoxicity. Although contraindicated in patients with severe liver failure, lower doses are recommended in patients with mild to moderate liver disease and in patients with routine alcohol use.[22] With clear instructions, acetaminophen can be safely used as a first-line treatment for mild to moderate pain (**Box 3**).

Geriatric Medication Safety in the Emergency Department

All patients should have their medication lists reviewed during their emergency department visit. Patients with high-risk medications or who are on more than five medications at home should have special attention by the medical team and/or pharmacist.[2] The addition of a clinical pharmacist in the emergency department has been demonstrated to decrease medication errors and adverse drug events, improve compliance

---

Box 3
Geriatric general pain management recommendations

- Use nonpharmacologic options such as heat, ice, and/or physical therapy.
- First-line pharmacologic options include acetaminophen or NSAIDs.
- Add low-dose opioids only for moderate to severe pain or if acetaminophen or NSAIDs are ineffective or contraindicated
- Dose reduce opioids by 25% to 50% of the typically adult starting dose and titrate slowly.
- Avoid tramadol, especially for patients with renal or hepatic dysfunction.
- Avoid benzodiazepines and skeletal muscle relaxants.
- Have a risks and benefits discussion with patients and families; for example, "Treating pain in older adults can be tricky because side effects are more common. I don't want you to be in pain but I also don't want to prescribe a medication that increases your chance of a fall."
- For all pain management prescriptions, include clear instructions such as: Take 1 tablet by mouth every 4 hours as needed for back pain, use for no more than 5 days.

---

with clinical practice guidelines, decrease emergency department and hospital read-missions, and provide education for the medical and nursing team. Emergency department clinical pharmacists should be considered as essential team members in both urban and rural settings.[23]

After identifying medication safety concerns in the emergency department patient as a team, it is important to develop a plan to make the substitutions. Some of the therapeutic substitutions are easier to make than others. Changing a patient's maintenance antipsychotic or antihypertensive regimen while in the emergency department may pose a difficult problem owing to extreme care coordination and may require an inpatient admission or close outpatient follow-up with the prescribing clinician. Whenever possible, consider if adjustments to the medication regimen are required and determine the most appropriate treatment team to complete the transition. A summary of optimal medication management for older adults is summarized in **Box 4**.

Box 4
Geriatric medication management in the emergency department[2]

1. All geriatric patients presenting to the emergency department should have their medication list reviewed.

2. The updated medication list should be screened by the medical team for patients with:
   a. Polypharmacy (>5 medications)
   b. Presence of any high-risk medications

3. Patients requiring hospitalization with either polypharmacy or high-risk medications would ideally be referred to a multidisciplinary team including a pharmacist with the goal of reducing polypharmacy and minimizing drug–drug interactions and high-risk medications.

4. Patients eligible for discharge with polypharmacy or high-risk medications would ideally be reviewed by a pharmacist for potential medication modifications in addition to referral to the patient's primary care provider for long-term management.

CASE CONCLUSION

After reviewing all of the laboratory and imaging results, it was determined that the most likely cause of the patient's fatigue and subsequent fall was medication related; that is, sedation owing to the combination of tramadol and diazepam and the likely accumulation of tramadol in a patient with a decrease creatinine clearance. She was observed in the emergency department for several hours, completed an ambulatory assessment, and was counseled by the pharmacist and team to avoid taking the diazepam and tramadol owing to their drug–drug interaction, her renal function, and her age. For her acute pain management, she was instructed to take acetaminophen 650 mg every 6 hours as needed until she followed up with her primary care physician. A summary of the visit was also sent to the primary care physician's office for continuity of care.

DISCUSSION

With the increasing geriatric population, the frequency of falls and drug–drug interactions owing to polypharmacy is increasing. All geriatric patients should have their medication list reviewed with screening specifically for polypharmacy and high-risk medications. When polypharmacy or high-risk medications are identified, determine if switching to a different agent or other adjustments are required; however, this process may require a discussion with the prescribing physician or coordination with a primary care practitioner, depending on the offending medication category. Regardless of age, limit the coprescribing of opioids with benzodiazepines because they can have additive effects on sedation. Additionally, tramadol has a wide range of side effects that does not make it a safe alternative to opioid medications and renal function must be calculated because decreased clearance will also increase sedative effects. Finally, consider the implementation of a pharmacist in the emergency department and a service focused on obtaining high-quality medication histories, ideally performed or managed by pharmacy personnel, to provide accurate medication information in the hectic environment of the emergency department.

CLINICS CARE POINTS

- Geriatric falls and drug-drug interactions due to polypharmacy are common.
- Utilize established tools to screen home medication lists for polypharmacy and high-risk medications.
- Consider implementing pharmacy services in the emergency department to perform high-quality medication histories.

DISCLOSURE

The author has nothing to disclose.

REFERENCES

1. Masnoon N, Shakib S, Kalisch-Ellett, et al. What is polypharmacy? A systematic review of definitions. BMC Geriatr 2017;17:230.
2. American College of Emergency Physicians; American Geriatrics Society. Emergency Nurses Association; Society for Academic Emergency Medicine; Geriatric

Emergency Department Guidelines Task Force. Geriatric emergency department guidelines. Ann Emerg Med 2014;63(5):e7–25.

3. Ellenbogen MI, Wang P, Overton HN, et al. Frequency and predictors of polypharmacy in US Medicare patients: a cross-sectional analysis at the patient and physician levels. Drugs Aging 2020;37:57–65.

4. Carr T. Too Many Meds? America's love affair with prescription medication [Internet]. Consumer reports. Available at: https://www.consumerreports.org/prescription-drugs/too-many-medsamericas-love-afair-with-prescription-medication/. Accessed June 23, 2020.

5. Jensen GL, Friedmann JM, Coleman CD, et al. Screening for hospitalization and nutritional risks among community-dwelling older persons. Am J Clin Nutr 2001; 74(2):201–5. 6.

6. Richardson K, Ananou A, Lafortune L, et al. Variation over time in the association between polypharmacy and mortality in the older population. Drugs Aging 2011; 28(7):547–60.

7. Chau DL, Walker V, Pai L, et al. Opiates and the elderly: use and side effects. Clin Interv Aging 2008;3(2):273–8.

8. ElDesoky ES. Pharmacokinetic-pharmacodynamic crisis in the elderly. Am J Ther 2007;14:488–98.

9. Centers for Disease Control and Prevention. Chronic kidney disease in the United States, 2019. Atlanta (GA): US Department of Health and Human Services, Centers for Disease Control and Prevention; 2019.

10. Cockcroft DW, Gault MH. Prediction of creatinine clearance from serum creatinine. Nephron 1976;16(1):31–41.

11. Ruiter R, Burggraaf J, Rissmann R. Under-representation of elderly in clinical trials: an analysis of the initial approval documents in the Food and Drug Administration database. Br J Clin Pharmacol 2019;85(4):838–44.

12. Tan JL, Eastment JG, Poudel A, et al. Age-related changes in hepatic function: an update on implications for drug therapy. Drugs Aging 2015;32:999–1008.

13. American Geriatrics Society 2019 Updated AGS Beers Criteria® for Potentially Inappropriate Medication Use in Older Adults. J Am Geriatr Soc 2019;67(4): 674–94.

14. O'Mahony D, O'Sullivan D, Byrne S, et al. STOPP/START criteria for potentially inappropriate prescribing in older people: version 2. Age Ageing 2015;44(2): 213–8.

15. Clark PM. Pharmacologic pain management on the elderly cancer patient. Presented at the 26th Congress of the Oncology Nursing Society; San Diego, CA. 2001, May 17–20, 2001.

16. Miotto K, Cho AK, Mohamed K, et al. Trends in tramadol: pharmacology, metabolism, and misuse. Anesth Analg 2017;124(1):44–51.

17. Product information: ULTRAM® oral tablets, tramadol HCl oral tablets. Titusville (NJ): Janssen Pharmaceuticals Inc (per FDA); 2019.

18. Friedman BW, Irizarry E, Solorzano C, et al. Diazepam is no better than placebo when added to naproxen for acute low back pain. Ann Emerg Med 2017;70(2): 169–76.

19. Friedman BW, Irizarry E, Solorzano C, et al. A randomized, placebo-controlled trial of ibuprofen plus metaxalone, tizanidine, or baclofen for acute low back pain. Ann Emerg Med 2019;74(4):512–20.

20. Wongrakpanich S, Wongrakpanich A, Melhado K, et al. A comprehensive review of non-steroidal anti-inflammatory drug use in the elderly. Aging Dis 2018;9(1): 143–50.

21. Derry S, Moore R, Gaskell H, et al. Topical NSAIDs for acute musculoskeletal pain in adults. Cochrane Database Syst Rev 2015;(6):CD007402.

22. Product Information: TYLENOL(R) oral, acetaminophen oral. Skillman (NJ): McNeil Consumer Healthcare; 2010.

23. Rahman Morgan S, Acquisto NM, Coralic Z, et al. Clinical pharmacy services in the emergency department. Am J Emerg Med 2018;36(10):1727–32.

Elder Abuse—A Guide to Diagnosis and Management in the Emergency Department

Nicole Cimino-Fiallos, MD[a],*, Tony Rosen, MD, MPH[b]

KEYWORDS

- Elder abuse • Elder abuse neglect • Elder abuse mandatory reporting
- Elder mistreatment • Elder abuse emergency department

KEY POINTS

- Emergency physicians should consider elder abuse and neglect when evaluating older adults in the emergency department (ED), because these conditions are both common and dangerous.
- The utilization of elder abuse screening tools in the ED can increase the detection of elder mistreatment.
- ED clinicians are mandatory reporters of suspected elder abuse in most US states. In addition to reporting suspected mistreatment, an ED physician should ensure a patient's safety and utilize a multidisciplinary team if available to develop a treatment plan for vulnerable older adults.

BACKGROUND

Emergency medicine clinicians are trained to identify and treat life-threatening medical conditions. Although elder abuse is difficult to diagnose and challenging to treat and prevent, physicians must be trained to address this morbid and potentially mortal condition. Elder mistreatment is defined as action or negligence against an older adult that causes harm or risk of harm committed by a person in a relationship with an expectation of trust or when an older person is targeted based on age or disability.[1] Several different types of maltreatment exist[2] (**Table 1**), and each poses different diagnostic and treatment hurdles to physicians. Approximately 10% of Americans over the age of 65 experience some form of mistreatment.[3]

Most older adults live at home, with approximately 95% of older people living either independently or with their spouses, children, or other relatives, rather than in institutions.[3] Therefore, the home is where most elder abuse occurs. As older adults age in

---

[a] Department of Emergency Medicine, Meritus Medical Center, 11116 Medical Campus Road, Hagerstown, MD 21742, USA; [b] Department of Emergency Medicine, Weill Cornell Medical College, New York-Presbyterian Hospital, 525 East 68th Street, New York, NY 10065, USA
* Corresponding author.
E-mail address: nfiallos105@gmail.com

Emerg Med Clin N Am 39 (2021) 405–417
https://doi.org/10.1016/j.emc.2021.01.009
0733-8627/21/© 2021 Elsevier Inc. All rights reserved.

emed.theclinics.com

Table 1
Types of elder abuse

Type	Definition	Examples
Physical abuse	Intentional use of physical force that may result in bodily injury, physical pain, or impairment	• Slapping, hitting, kicking, pushing, pulling hair • Use of physical restraints, force-feeding • Burning, use of household objects as weapons, use of firearms and knives
Sexual abuse	Any type of sexual contact with an elderly person that is nonconsensual or sexual contact with any person incapable of giving consent	• Sexual assault or battery, such as rape, sodomy, coerced nudity, and sexually explicit photographing • Unwanted touching, verbal sexual advances • Indecent exposure
Neglect	Refusal or failure to fulfill any part of a person's obligations or duties to an elder, which may result in harm—may be intentional or unintentional	• Withholding of food, water, clothing, shelter, medications • Failure to ensure elder's personal hygiene or to provide physical aids, including walker, cane, glasses, hearing aids, dentures • Failure to ensure elder's personal safety and/or appropriate medical follow-up
Emotional/psychological abuse	Intentional infliction of anguish, pain, or distress through verbal or nonverbal acts	• Verbal berating, harassment, or intimidation • Threats of punishment or deprivation • Treating the older person like an infant • Isolating the older person from others
Abandonment	Desertion of an elderly person by an individual who has assumed responsibility for providing care for an elder or by a person with physical custody	• The desertion of an elder at a hospital, a nursing facility, or other similar institution

(continued on next page)

Table 1 (*continued*)		
Type	**Definition**	**Examples**
Financial/material exploitation	Illegal or improper use of an older adult's money, property, or assets	• Stealing money or belongings • Cashing an older adult's checks without permission and/or forging his or her signature • Coercing an older adult into signing contracts, changing a will, or assigning durable power of attorney against his or her wishes or when the older adult does not possess the mental capacity to do so
Self-neglect	Behavior of an older adult that threatens his/her own health or safety—excluding when an older adult who understands the consequences of his or her actions makes a conscious and voluntary decision to engage in acts that threaten his/her health or safety	• Refusal or failure of an older adult to provide him or herself with basic necessities, such as food, water, shelter, medications, and appropriate personal hygiene • Disregard for maintenance of safe home environment and/or hoarding

Data from NCEA - Types of Abuse. Available at https://ncea.acl.gov/Suspect-Abuse/Abuse-Types. aspx. Accessed Aug 24, 2020.

place, the increased dependency on others for care that occurs for some puts them at higher risk for abuse. Victims of elder abuse most commonly are female and older than age 74.[4,5] Some studies also suggest victims of abuse are more likely to have mental health disorders.[6] Cognitive impairment also increases a person's risk for abuse, with older adults diagnosed with dementia approximately 5 times as likely to experience abuse than those without this diagnosis.[7,8] Social isolation also increases risk dramatically whereas a strong social support system is protective against elder abuse.[4]

Elder abuse is perpetrated most commonly by someone close to the victim, frequently a male spouse or adult child.[3] Mental illness, substance abuse, and financial dependency on the victim make someone more likely to commit abuse.[4]

Although a small percentage (4.5%) of older adults live in nursing facilities,[9] many will at some point in their lives (35%).[10] A paucity of data exists to describe the prevalence of abuse in long-term care facilities, but experts believe and studies suggest it may be higher than in the community.[11] There are two types of abuse that exist in nursing facilities: staff-to-resident abuse and resident-to-resident abuse. In resident-to-resident abuse, two forms of mistreatment are occurring simultaneously—the abuse itself and neglect by staff members who are not supervising effectively to prevent these events.

Despite popular perception, resident-to-resident abuse actually may be more prevalent than staff-to-resident abuse at nursing facility.[12] This may be, due to the number of nursing residents with cognitive impairments, such as dementia and related behavioral disturbances. Page and colleagues[13] report a 20.2% 1-month prevalence of resident-to-resident elder mistreatment. Although most cases of elder abuse revolve around the perpetrator's intent, in these cases, the abuser frequently is confused and both the victim and the abuser may suffer harm from the encounter.[14]

OUTCOMES OF ABUSE

The effects of elder abuse are far-reaching. Older adults who suffer from abuse have worse outcomes from preexisting health conditions and are more likely to be placed in a long-term care facility.[15] All types of abuse increase the risk of depression and anxiety,[15] and abuse victims may have an increased risk for thoughts of suicide compared with unexposed peers. Given this fact, abuse victims use more behavioral health services than other older adults.[16] Physical abuse victims experience physical pain and may sustain injuries, including fractures, wounds, and head injuries. Most importantly, studies repeatedly have shown victims of abuse have a higher risk of mortality than older adults who have not been victimized.[17] Older people exposed to abuse are more likely to utilize an emergency department (ED) and to require hospitalization,[18] because they are less likely to have a primary care doctor and may suffer from acute injury. Therefore, the direct health care expenditures associated with this phenomenon are significant.

IDENTIFYING ELDER ABUSE AND NEGLECT IN THE EMERGENCY DEPARTMENT
History

When obtaining a history from an older adult, it is important to interview the patient both with and without the caregiver present, especially if there is concern for abuse or neglect. The patient may be less forthcoming with reports of mistreatment if the caregiver remains in the room during the history-taking. If the patient presents to the ED for evaluation of a trauma, the physician should ask the patient directly if they were hit, punched, kicked, pushed, or struck. Patients with cognitive impairment can be poor historians, but studies suggest that even patients with some cognitive deficits can report mistreatment reliably.[19] Emergency practitioners should not rely solely on their history-taking to identify signs of elder abuse and neglect. While obtaining the history, the emergency clinician should be perceptive of any signs of tension between the patient and the caregiver (**Box 1**).

A Critical Role for Other Health Care Team Members

Other members of the care team also can provide valuable data. Emergency medical service (EMS) providers, including paramedics, have the unique advantage of seeing inside a patient's home and can comment on habitability and availability of resources, such as food and medication.[20] These professionals sometimes develop relationships with patients who frequently use their services and can report signs of physical decline or worsening living conditions to the care team in the ED. Physicians should utilize the EMS perspective when evaluating patients with other suggestions of abuse or neglect.

Nursing staff are likely to spend more time with patients and their caregivers in the ED. As such, they can relay their observations of the interactions between these two parties and may pick up on subtle signs of mistreatment. Nurses and patient care technicians also perform a majority of the personal care tasks for patients in the ED and may be better positioned to notice soiled clothing, poor hygiene, nonhealing wounds, or other clues of abuse.[21] By educating ED nursing and support staff about the prevalence of abuse and neglect in this population and informing them of the signs

> **Box 1**
> **Observations from older adult/caregiver interaction that should raise concern for elder abuse or neglect**
>
> - Older adult and caregiver provide conflicting accounts of events
> - Caregiver interrupts/answers for the older adult
> - Older adult seems fearful of or hostile toward caregiver
> - Caregiver seems unengaged/inattentive in caring for the older adult
> - Caregiver seems frustrated, tired, angry, or burdened by the older adult
> - Caregiver seems overwhelmed by the older adult
> - Caregiver seems to lack knowledge of the patient's care needs
> - Evidence that the caregiver and/or older adult may be abusing alcohol or illicit drugs
>
> *Data from* Rosen, Tony, et al. Identifying and initiating intervention for elder abuse and neglect in the emergency department. Clinics in geriatric medicine 2018;34(3): 435-451.

and symptoms, physicians can encourage an open dialogue and improve the chances of detection of mistreatment in the ED. Social workers working in the ED, who are trained to assess for abuse and interpersonal violence and provide resources and referrals, should evaluate older adult patients if any concern for mistreatment exists. Their perspective can inform the level of suspicion and appropriate next steps.

Physical Signs

Physical abuse may be the most amenable form of abuse to detection in the ED, but the diagnosis remains challenging because geriatric patients are prone to unintentional injuries and normal aging processes can mimic abuse. When examining an older person after a trauma, clinicians should look for signs of injury that are not typical of accidental trauma[22] (**Box 2**).

Many patients report their traumatic injuries resulted from "falling" so as not to reveal that injuries actually were caused by abuse. If a patient presents to the ED more than one day after the occurrence of injury, the clinician should consider the possibility of mistreatment.[23]

> **Box 2**
> **Injury patterns concerning for nonaccidental trauma**
>
> - Injuries in the maxillofacial, dental, and neck areas and the upper extremities[5]
> - Injuries to the head and neck without injury to other parts of the body—a fall usually results in other signs of injury to extremities, back, or trunk.[44]
> - Neck injuries—the head and shoulders typically protect the neck from injury in a fall.[44]
> - Ear injuries—ear injuries typically are not seen in falls and are very concerning for nonaccidental trauma.[44]
> - Left-sided facial injuries—many abusers are right-handed and punches or hits affect the left side of the victim's face.[44]
> - Ligature marks[24]
> - Bruises larger than 5 cm or in the shape of objects[38]

Signs of neglect may include dehydration and foul-smelling decubitus ulcers with surrounding maceration. Poor hygiene, dirty/soiled clothing, multiple diapers, or exacerbations of chronic medical conditions that should be well-controlled also may signal neglect.[24]

Any signs of vaginal/penile/perineal/anal trauma or evidence of a sexually transmitted infection in a patient with cognitive impairment who is not sexually active should trigger consideration of an evaluation for possible sexual abuse.

This assessment is made more challenging because normal changes of aging may mimic elder abuse. Unintentional injuries are common and can cause bruising and skin tears. Vasculitis can masquerade as nonaccidental trauma. Anal fissures caused by constipation and vulvar injuries from traumatic urinary catheter placement or lichen sclerosis all can mimic signs of sexual abuse.[24]

Laboratory Tests and Imaging

Abnormalities in laboratory studies can raise red flags for elder abuse and neglect. Laboratory data that may arouse suspicion include hypernatremia, an elevated blood-urea-nitrogen/creatinine ratio and yes add level after hematocrit. Rhabdomyolysis has several mistreatment-related causes in older adults. It can be caused by prolonged immobility because caregivers may be using inappropriate restraints or not repositioning the older adult frequently enough. Severe dehydration or malnutrition or exposure to high heat (ie, no access to air conditioning) also may cause rhabdomyolysis. Therefore, elevated creatine kinase or myoglobinuria should stimulate the ED provider to consider mistreatment as a diagnosis.[25] Additionally, although dehydration is common among the elderly secondary to decreased thirst reflex and dysphagia, it also can be a sign of mistreatment because some caregivers may withhold fluids to decrease urination. Patients with poorly controlled chronic medical conditions also may benefit from additional laboratory testing by the ED if close follow-up with their primary physician cannot be arranged. An elevated hemoglobin A_{1c} in a diabetic patient despite reported adherence to a medication regimen or abnormally low international normalized ratio measurements in an anticoagulated patient reportedly getting scheduled warfarin could signal medication withholding or neglect to the emergency physician.[25] A urine toxicology screen or abnormal thyroid studies also could suggest medication noncompliance in the appropriate patients.[25]

Radiologists are trained to identify fracture patterns or other radiographic signs of child abuse and can do the same for elder abuse. As patterns of elder abuse become better established, emergency physicians can utilize their radiology colleagues to raise red flags for possible nonaccidental trauma. Although more research is needed, currently, radiologists can identify when an injury pattern does not match with proposed injury mechanism or when a patient has new and healed injuries identified on the same studies.[20]

SCREENING

Although common among older adults, abuse is under-recognized; the proportion of ED visits by older adults receiving a diagnosis of elder abuse is at least 2 orders of magnitude lower than the estimated prevalence in the population.[26] Multiple screening tools have been developed to increase detection of this morbid condition.[27] Universal screening of all older patients in the ED could have adverse effects. No screening tool has 100% specificity, and false-positive tests can lead to undesirable results. Psychological distress, family tension, and, in extreme circumstances, a possible change in living situation or even loss of personal autonomy all potentially could occur after a positive screen and report to the authorities.[28] If a caregiver is wrongly accused of abuse, they could become more reluctant to seek indicated medical care in the future. The importance of these issues with screening is poorly understood and deserves more study.[23] Despite the obvious potential to increase detection and initiate intervention, the US Preventive Services Task Force found insufficient evidence that screening for elder abuse in clinical settings reduces harm.[29] These studies also have shed doubt on the proposed benefits of universal screening for elder abuse and neglect and suggest that early detection does not decrease exposure to abuse or physical or mental harm from abuse.[11] Despite the lack of evidence for harm reduction, the American Medical Association and other professional organizations still recommend physicians assess patients for elder abuse, citing an ethical responsibility to attempt to detect this life-threatening condition. Although the data do not prove that using specific screening protocols is superior to having a generally increased threshold of suspicion, screening may help clinicians remember to consider elder abuse and neglect as part of the differential diagnosis. Tools may assist ED providers who are unsure about what questions to ask or signs for which to look. Additionally, the identification of elder abuse victims is important in order to develop and implement effective harm reduction strategies. Common screening scores are included in **Table 2**, including the ED Senior Abuse Identification tool, which was designed specifically for ED use.

Ideally, screening protocols target only the individuals at highest risk for abuse. Doing so would require fewer resources than universal screening and may improve specificity. Unfortunately, no validated protocol currently exists to identify high-risk older adult patients.[27] Research that has sought to identify risk factors for the purpose of targeting screening has not identified specific demographic risk factors that can be

Table 2		
A summary of available screening tools		
Elder Abuse Screening Tool	**Description**	**Clinical Applicability**
Elder Abuse Suspicion Index[45]	Five yes-or-no questions directed to the patient, one question based on the physician observation of the patient's appearance and behavior	Validated but suffers from poor specificity. Lauded for its brevity, this tool could be helpful for screening in the ED.
Elder Assessment Instrument[42]	A nursing assessment that utilizes an interview and physical assessment of the older person	A comprehensive assessment but time intensive
ED Senior AID[23]	A tool designed for use in cognitively intact adults based on a questionnaire and physical assessment	Combines direct questioning with physical examination findings but is designed only for cognitively intact patients.
Vulnerability to Abuse Screening Scale (Schofield and Mishra, 2003)	A series of questions that assess for risks of dependence, dejection, vulnerability, and coercion.	Brief and easy to use, can be self-administered by an older adult

Data from Refs.[2,45–48]

utilized reliably to design targeted screening protocols. Therefore, based on available data, any targeted screening for elder abuse in the ED is likely to miss cases of abuse.

A promising approach to ED screening currently being tested is a two-step process with a universal two-question brief screen ("Has anyone close to you harmed you?" and "Has anyone close to you failed to give you the care that you need?")[27] for all patients followed by a triggered comprehensive screen using the ED Senior Abuse Identification tool for those with a positive brief screen. This approach balances efficiency in a busy ED with not missing potential victims.

Emergency Medical Services Screening

Older patients are four times more likely to use EMS services than younger adults, and EMS providers interact with these patients and their caregivers in their home.[16] Given this rate of utilization, innovative approaches to the diagnosis of elder abuse are needed to increase detection in the prehospital setting. Having EMS providers screen for elder mistreatment as part of their routine protocols may increase detection of mistreatment. The Detection of Elder Mistreatment Through Emergency Care Technicians screening tool incorporates EMS providers' observations of a patient's emotional state, living conditions, physical symptoms, and interactions with caregivers. Although additional study of this tool is required, it is promising, with feasibility of incorporating it into EMS practice already demonstrated.[30]

Screening and Technology

Technology has the potential to streamline and target screening. EDs already overtaxed by clinical responsibilities and budget constraints may utilize the electronic medical record and smart technology, like tablet touchscreen devices, to incorporate elder abuse screening into an ED visit with less burden. Self-screening tools combined with a touchscreen device could be used to reduce the amount of time required of ED staff to execute screening tools. In one study, approximately half of surveyed seniors were willing to use a tablet device to input information, although most did require assistance to complete the tasks in front of them.[31] This likely will improve as technology continues to advance and as seniors continue to interact with these types of devices outside the ED.

At a minimum, the electronic medical record can remind a busy physician to perform an elder abuse screen.[32] Outside of a simple alert reminding clinicians to use a screening tool, the electronic health record may be able to process vast amounts of clinical data to look for signs of elder abuse that are not immediately apparent to clinicians, such as multiple ED visits in a short time period, frequent traumatic injuries, missed primary care doctor appointments, or lapses in refills of chronic medications.[33] This artificial intelligence has the potential to facilitate targeted screening and additional work-up in select patients.[27]

REPORTING

Once elder abuse is suspected, ED providers should report to adult protective services (APS) or law enforcement. Physicians are mandatory reporters in nearly every US state. Unfortunately, under-reporting is rampant and only a small percentage of elder abuse victims are ever referred to external services.[34] Many ED physicians do not report suspected abuse despite mandatory reporting requirements. The barriers to reporting elder abuse are numerous. Clinicians have difficulty distinguishing between accidental injuries and intentional injuries. An assessment for abuse may be time-consuming, and frequently ED physicians may not have enough time to perform a thorough evaluation.[21] Doctors cite a lack of familiarity with state reporting laws. Many also have doubts about the efficacy of reporting, worrying that reporting actually place may a patient at higher risk for mistreatment. They also have concerns about how reporting suspected abuse will affect the doctor-patient relationship.[35] Currently, physician training on the detection and reporting of elder abuse is limited. Available data suggest that elder abuse case simulations and active hands-on learning incorporated into physician training can result in improved knowledge and confidence in their abilities to report suspected cases of mistreatment.[36]

It is critical for ED physicians to report elder mistreatment, because most older adults, even those who are able to, seldom self-report.[37] Many victims of abuse are reliant on their abuser for care and worry about loss of support if they report their abuse. Often, the abuser is a close family member and the victim does not want to get them in trouble.[37]

DISPOSITION

If an emergency clinician suspects elder mistreatment, the treatment plan must include several critical actions. The emergent medical issues must be addressed and clinical findings and mistreatment-related suspicions reported to the appropriate authorities. The physician must also take steps to ensure the patient's safety and make a plan for either admission or safe discharge. While in the ED, severing contact between a patient and an abuser may be necessary if a patient is in immediate danger. This process can be complicated if the abuser also is the patient's medical decision maker or has power of attorney. The use of a multidisciplinary team with social work and hospital administration may be the best approach to this challenging scenario.[20]

If the patient is not at immediate risk for harm and does not require hospitalization, the ED team should develop a plan for safe discharge. A patient's primary care physician can act as a great resource to enact a care plan that includes close follow-up. Case management or social work also can help to organize community resources and offer outpatient support to the patient.

In an important difference between child abuse and elder abuse, many older adult patients may refuse the recommendations of medical providers and choose to leave the ED even if doing so may be unsafe. If a patient is refusing interventions in the ED, the clinician should assess the patient's decisional capacity. If a patient has capacity to make decisions regarding discharge, then they can refuse admission even if it will return them to an abusive situation.[20] Safety education and planning still should be offered. For patients who do not have the capacity to make these decisions, the ED provider should act in their best interest. This may involve attempting to identify non-abusive family members who can make decisions on their behalf and involving the hospital's administration and legal services.

SPECIAL TOPICS
Elder Abuse and COVID-19

The effects of the Corona virus disease- 19 (COVID-19) pandemic are far reaching for older adults and likely will increase the number of people who experience elder abuse or mistreatment. Although no event in modern history directly correlates to the COVID-19 pandemic, past experiences during natural disasters mimic some of the current conditions and likely can be extrapolated to this public health crisis. Data collection during previous disaster events show that elder abuse cases increase when people are confined to their homes and under financial and emotional stress.[38] During natural disasters and this pandemic, access to community services, senior centers, and medical care and interactions with social support structures, family, and friends may be severely limited for victims already at high risk for abuse.[39] Home health aides, on whom many older adults rely for care, may not be able to go to older adults' homes during this pandemic. Factors that increase the risk of elder mistreatment, such as decreased income, unemployment, and increased stress for family caregivers, all are more common. During this pandemic, APS workers who investigate potential abuse cases have been limited in their ability to assess older adults in person, instead having to utilize virtual visits and other nontraditional modes of communication to reach out to at-risk elders. This increases challenges to a system that already is over-burdened. Although older adults in the community are at higher risk for mistreatment during this pandemic, long-term care facility residents also are likely in increased danger. With mandatory visitor restrictions, there is a significant decrease in visibility into these facilities by family members. Family visits are very protective against abuse and neglect in these institutions. State agencies must increase inspections and ensure that facilities are staffed adequately with qualified personnel to protect these vulnerable adults from neglect, resident-to-resident abuse, and staff mistreatment.[40]

Given these increased risks, ED providers should be particularly vigilant in considering elder mistreatment in the differential diagnosis for older adults during COVID-19 outbreaks and their aftermath.

Elder Abuse and Cultural Considerations

Emergency physicians care for patients from all different cultures and ethnicities, and elder mistreatment is a universal problem. One large meta-analysis suggests that globally, 16% of older adults experience some form of elder abuse.[5] The highest prevalence of elder abuse is reported in developed countries,[7] but it is difficult to assess the prevalence of elder abuse in developing countries given a lack of high-quality research on the topic.

In the United States, minority adults may be at higher risk for mistreatment and also are much less likely to report or seek assistance from available services.[34] Although research suggests that 40% of Latinx older adults have experienced elder abuse, only 2% of this mistreatment ever is reported.[41] Many factors prevent Latinx older adults from reporting abuse. Citizenship status and fear of deportation can hinder reports of abuse in undocumented Latinx immigrants, as can a lack of fluency in English. Culturally, Latinx older adults also are more likely to rely on family members for their daily care, increasing their risk of mistreatment but also decreasing their likelihood of self-reporting abuse.[41]

African Americans experience three times as much financial exploitation and four times as much psychological abuse as their white counterparts.[42,43] Possible explanations include socioeconomic factors and cultural differences in family dynamics. African Americans also have higher rates of contact with police and other law enforcement agencies, due in part to systemic racism. As a result, the number of reports to APS may be higher in this population, falsely elevating the reported incidence of elder mistreatment.[42]

SUMMARY

Emergency physicians strive to identify all potentially life-threatening conditions patients may have and to develop comprehensive treatment plans for them to prevent morbidity and mortality. Given the high prevalence of and morbidity and mortality associated with elder abuse and neglect, emergency providers should consider this under-recognized phenomenon when assessing older adult patients. EDs should consider adopting screening protocols. ED providers ethically and legally are obligated to report suspicion of mistreatment to the appropriate investigative agency, and EDs should develop protocols and utilize multidisciplinary teams to ensure patients' safety while in the ED and after discharge.

CLINICS CARE POINTS

- Older adults exposed to abuse are more likely to utilize the ED and to require hospitalization. They experience higher morbidity and mortality than older adults who do not experience mistreatment.

- Validated screening tools exist to detect elder abuse, and future developments in electronic health records may help clinicians to target screening.

- Physicians are mandatory reporters of elder abuse and can utilize other members of their health care team, such as nursing staff, social workers, and paramedics, to identify signs of mistreatment, thereby increasing rates of detection.

- Factors associated with the COVID-19 pandemic, such as stay-at-home orders, likely will increase the number of older adults who experience elder abuse while straining existing investigative agencies, making detection of abuse in the ED even more important.

ACKNOWLEDGMENTS

The authors wish to thank Alyssa Elman for her review of multiple drafts of this article and helpful comments.

DISCLOSURE

The authors have nothing to disclose.

REFERENCES

1. Elder Justice Roadmap. Available at: https://www.justice.gov/file/852856/download. Accessed July 15, 2020.
2. Burnett J, Achenbaum WA, Murphy KP. Prevention and Early Identification of Elder Abuse. Clin Geriatr Med 2014;30(4):743–59.
3. Bond M, Butler KH. Elder abuse and neglect: definitions, epidemiology, and approaches to emergency department screening. Clin Geriatr Med 2013;29(1):257–73.
4. Pillemer K, Burnes D, Riffin C, et al. Elder abuse: global situation, risk factors, and prevention strategies. Gerontologist 2016;56(Suppl 2):S194–205.
5. Yon Y, Mikton CR, Gassoumis ZD, et al. Elder abuse prevalence in community settings: a systematic review and meta-analysis. Lancet Glob Health 2017;5(2):e147–56.
6. Schonfeld L, Larsen RG, Stiles PG, et al. Behavioral health services utilization among older adults identified within a state abuse hotline database. Gerontologist 2006;46(2):193–9.
7. Sooryanarayana R, Choo W, Hairi N. A review on the prevalence and measurement of elder abuse in the community. Trauma Violence Abuse 2013;14(4):316–25.
8. VandeWeerd C, Paveza GJ, Walsh M, et al. Physical mistreatment in persons with Alzheimer's disease. J Aging Res 2013;2013:920324.
9. Wallman KK. Older Americans 2016: Key Indicators of well- being. 2016. Available at: https://agingstats.gov/docs/LatestReport/Older-Americans-2016-Key-Indicators-of-WellBeing.pdf. Accessed July 15, 2020.

10. Kemper P, Komisar HL, Alecxih L. Long-Term Care Over an Uncertain Future: What Can Current Retirees Expect? Inquiry 2005;42(4):335–50.
11. Moyer VA. Screening for intimate partner violence and abuse of elderly and vulnerable adults: U.S. preventive services task force recommendation statement. Ann Intern Med 2013;158(6):478–86.
12. Lachs MS, Teresi JA, Ramirez M, et al. The prevalence of resident-to-resident elder mistreatment in nursing homes. Ann Intern Med 2016;165(4):229–36.
13. Page C, Conner T, Prokhorov A, et al. The effect of care setting on elder abuse: results from a Michigan survey. J Elder Abuse Negl 2009;21(3):239–52.
14. McDonald L, Sheppard C, Hitzig SL, et al. Resident-to-resident abuse: A scoping review. Can J Aging 2015;34(2):215–36.
15. Pillemer K, Connolly MT, Breckman R, et al. Elder mistreatment: Priorities for consideration by the White House Conference on Aging. Gerontologist 2015; 55(2):320–7.
16. Shah MN, Bazarian JJ, Lerner EB, et al. The epidemiology of emergency medical services use by older adults: An analysis of the national hospital ambulatory medical care survey. Acad Emerg Med 2007;14(5):441–7.
17. Lachs MS, Williams CS, O'Brien S, et al. The mortality of elder mistreatment. Jama 1998;280(5):428–32.
18. Dong X, Simon MA. Elder abuse as a risk factor for hospitalization in older persons. JAMA Intern Med 2013;173(10):911.
19. Richmond NL, Zimmerman S, Reeve BB, et al. Ability of older adults to report elder abuse: an emergency department–based cross-sectional study. J Am Geriatr Soc 2020;68(1):170–5.
20. Rosen T, Hargarten S, Flomenbaum NE, et al. Identifying elder abuse in the emergency department: toward a multidisciplinary team-based approach. Ann Emerg Med 2016;68(3):378–82.
21. Rosen T, Stern ME, Elman A, et al. Identifying and initiating intervention for elder abuse and neglect in the emergency department. Clin Geriatr Med 2018;34(3): 435–51.
22. Rosen Tony, LoFaso VM, Bloemen EM, et al. Identifying injury patterns associated with physical elder abuse: analysis of legally adjudicated cases. Ann Emerg Med 2020;76(3):277–9.
23. Beach SR, Carpenter CR, Rosen T, et al. Screening and detection of elder abuse: Research opportunities and lessons learned from emergency geriatric care, intimate partner violence, and child abuse. J Elder Abuse Negl 2016;28(4–5): 185–216.
24. Danesh MJ, Chang AL. The role of the dermatologist in detecting elder abuse and neglect. J Am Acad Dermatol 2015;73(2):285–93.
25. LoFaso VM, Rosen T. Medical and laboratory indicators of elder abuse and neglect. Clin Geriatr Med 2014;30(4):713–28.
26. Evans CS, Hunold KM, Rosen T, et al. Diagnosis of Elder Abuse in U.S. Emergency Departments. J Am Geriatr Soc 2017;65(1):91–7.
27. Rosen T, Platts-Mills TF, Fulmer T. Screening for elder mistreatment in emergency departments: current progress and recommendations for next steps. J Elder Abuse Negl 2020;32(3):295–315.
28. Gallione C, Dal Molin A, Cristina FVB, et al. Screening tools for identification of elder abuse: a systematic review. J Clin Nurs 2017;26(15–16):2154–76.
29. Hoover RM, Polson M. Detecting elder abuse and neglect: assessment and intervention. Am Fam Physician 2014;89(6):453–60.

30. Cannell B, Gonzalez JMR, Livingston M, et al. Pilot testing the detection of elder abuse through emergency care technicians (DETECT) screening tool: results from the DETECT pilot project. J Elder Abuse Negl 2019;31(2):129–45.
31. Brahmandam S, Holland WC, Mangipudi SA, et al. Willingness and ability of older adults in the emergency department to provide clinical information using a tablet computer. J Am Geriatr Soc 2016;64(11):2362–7.
32. Li J, Westbrook J, Callen J, et al. The role of ICT in supporting disruptive innovation: a multi-site qualitative study of nurse practitioners in emergency departments. BMC Med Inform Decis Mak 2012;12(1):27.
33. Platts-Mills T, Zhang Y, Bao Y, et al. Can artificial intelligence help identify elder abuse and neglect? J Elder Abuse Neglect 2020;32(1):97–103.
34. Burnes D, Rizzo VM, Gorroochurn P, et al. Understanding service utilization in cases of elder abuse to inform best practices. J Appl Gerontol 2016;35(10): 1036–57.
35. Rodríguez MA, Wallace SP, Woolf NH, et al. Mandatory reporting of elder abuse: Between a rock and a hard place. Ann Fam Med 2006;4(5):403–9.
36. Alt KL, Nguyen AL, Meurer LN. The effectiveness of educational programs to improve recognition and reporting of elder abuse and neglect: a systematic review of the literature. J Elder Abuse Negl 2011;23(3):213–33.
37. Burnes D, Connolly MT, Hamilton R, et al. The feasibility of goal attainment scaling to measure case resolution in elder abuse and neglect adult protective services intervention. J Elder Abuse Negl 2018;30(3):209–22.
38. Gutman GM, Yon Y. Elder abuse and neglect in disasters: Types, prevalence and research gaps. Int J Disaster Risk Reduct 2014;10:38–47.
39. Elman A, Breckman R, Clark S, et al. Effects of the COVID-19 outbreak on elder mistreatment and response in new york city: initial lessons. J Appl Gerontol 2020; 39(7):690–9.
40. Gardner W, States D, Bagley N. The coronavirus and the risks to the elderly in long-term care. J Aging Soc Policy 2020;32(4–5):310–5. https://doi.org/10. 1080/08959420.2020.1750543.
41. DeLiema M, Gassoumis ZD, Homeier DC, et al. Determining prevalence and correlates of elder abuse using promotores: low-income immigrant latinos report high rates of abuse and neglect. J Am Geriatr Soc 2012;60(7):1333–9.
42. Beach SR, Schulz R, Castle NG, et al. Financial exploitation and psychological mistreatment among older adults: differences between African Americans and Non-African Americans in a Population-Based Survey. Gerontologist 2010; 50(6):744–57.
43. Dong XQ. Elder abuse: systematic review and implications for practice. J Am Geriatr Soc 2015;63(6):1214–38.
44. Rosen T, Stern ME, Mulcare MR, et al. Emergency department provider perspectives on elder abuse and development of a novel ED-based multidisciplinary intervention team. Emerg Med J 2018;35(10):600–7.
45. Yaffe MJ, Wolfson C, Lithwick M, et al. Development and validation of a tool to improve physician identification of elder abuse: The Elder Abuse Suspicion Index (EASI). J Elder Abuse Negl 2008;20(3):276–300.
46. Fulmer T. Elder abuse assessment tool. Dimens Crit Care Nurs 1984;3(4):216–20.
47. Platts-Mills TF, Dayaa JA, Reeve BB, et al. Development of the emergency department senior abuse identification (ED Senior AID) tool. J Elder Abuse Negl 2018;30(4):247–70.
48. Schofield MJ, Mishra GD. Validity of self-report screening scale for elder abuse: Women's Health Australia Study. Gerontologist 2003;43(1):110–20.

Physical Therapy, Occupational Therapy, and Speech Language Pathology in the Emergency Department

Specialty Consult Services to Enhance the Care of Older Adults

Elizabeth A. Pontius, DPT*, Robert S. Anderson Jr, MD

KEYWORDS

- Emergency department • Physical therapy • Occupational therapy
- Speech-language pathology • Geriatrics

KEY POINTS

- Physical therapy (PT), occupational therapy (OT), and speech-language pathology (SLP) can assist in determining a safe discharge plan for older adults with complex disposition problems.
- PT in the emergency department (ED) has been shown to decrease length of stay, admissions, opioid administration, and unnecessary imaging and to increase patient satisfaction.
- SLP in the ED can identify dysphagia in at-risk patients such as those with stroke, aspiration pneumonia, and frailty.

INTRODUCTION

Although Rehabilitation Medicine has long been a pivotal part of inpatient care, it has been slow to take hold in the emergency department (ED) setting. As recently as 2010, Physical Therapy (PT) in the ED was being described as a novel practice.[1] In 2018, Occupational Therapy (OT) in the ED was described as a "nascent field" that is "only beginning."[2] There is a paucity of literature describing Speech Language Pathology (SLP) services in the ED. Given the high volume of older adults in the ED with complex disposition problems, the roles of PT/OT/SLP can be of particular value. Their input regarding whether the patient can be safely discharged home or

Maine Medical Center, 22 Bramhall Street, Portland, ME 04102, USA
* Corresponding author.
E-mail address: PONTIL@mmc.org

Emerg Med Clin N Am 39 (2021) 419–427
https://doi.org/10.1016/j.emc.2021.01.005
0733-8627/21/© 2021 Elsevier Inc. All rights reserved.

needs admission to the hospital is relatively well understood. However, rehabilitation medicine expertise also includes the diagnosis and treatment of gait and balance disorders, musculoskeletal injuries, impaired cognition, and dysphagia. It has been observed that elders sustaining injury from a fall rarely have formal fall risk assessment in the ED. Miller and colleagues[3] found that in older adults presenting with a fall and subsequently discharged home, gait was assessed only 10.2% of the time, balance 4.1%, lower extremity range of motion 4.9%, lower extremity strength 2.0%, cognition 26.1%, vision 2.0%, and ability to perform activities of daily living 7.3%.

Excluding these elements in the evaluation of older adults in the ED is a missed opportunity to prevent additional injuries, decrease ED recidivism, and improve safety and patient/family satisfaction. Consider, for example, the traditional model where one might splint the wrist after a fall, do a "road test," and discharge the patient. Compare with an integrated model where one might also learn that the patient needs additional outpatient help with PT or medication management for a safe discharge from the ED.

BACKGROUND

Integration of PT in the ED setting was described in the literature as far back as the 1990s in the United Kingdom (UK).[4] In the time since then, the international model for PT in the ED has evolved in countries such as Australia, Canada, and the UK where physical therapists (PTs) are fully integrated and work as primary providers, caring for lower acuity patients with musculoskeletal complaints presenting to the ED. In these countries, at some locations, PTs assess and treat patients independently and are able to order and interpret imaging as well as prescribe certain medications.[5,6] Studies have shown that for patients with musculoskeletal disorders, there is often agreement between ED physicians and PTs with respect to care plans.[7] In addition, when patients are seen by PT in the ED, there is an associated reduced length of stay and wait times.[8-10]

PT/OT/SLP services in the United States (US) are still considered novel, and the model of care varies significantly from the international model. In the US, rehabilitation services are secondary consult services, relying on a physician's referral to initiate care. The role of PT in the ED in the US was first described around 2000.[10] The body of literature has grown since that time, examining perceptions, length of stay, readmissions, patient satisfaction, rates of imaging, opioid use, and cost. For example, in 2011 the American Physical Therapy Association (APTA) published "Incorporating Physical Therapy in the Emergency Department: A Toolkit for Practitioners." The APTA "promotes physical therapy as a professional service in the emergency care environment" and at the same time recognized that developing a PT program in the ED is a daunting task. The toolkit provides a roadmap for building a program, but unfortunately, the utilization of PT services in the ED remains limited.

Research on OT in the ED is in its infancy.[2,11] To date, studies have examined OT's perspectives on working in the ED, hospital admission rates, and readmission rates. International studies have shown that patient admissions to the hospital are reduced with the use of OT services.[12-14]

Speech-language pathologists (SLPs) are specialists in dysphagia, and their evaluations can be valuable in determining a safe disposition plan for older adults where oropharyngeal dysphagia is a major concern. Functional oropharyngeal dysphagia affects up to 84% of patients with Alzheimer's disease and more than 50% of elderly institutionalized patients.[15,16] Oropharyngeal dysphagia and aspiration are also prevalent findings in elderly patients with pneumonia, and an SLP assessment should be considered.[17]

ROLE OF PHYSICAL THERAPY

PT practice in the ED has been developed around the world, and the body of literature continues to grow supporting the value of this service. Studies have shown that PT intervention in the ED can lead to decreased wait and treatment times, decreased admission rates, increased patient satisfaction, decreased opioid administration, decreased cost of unnecessary tests and services such as diagnostic imaging, and improved patient function and outcomes.[8,9,14,18-20] A qualitative study by Lebec and colleagues shows that many ED physicians recognize the benefits of PTs in the evaluation of ED patients. Specifically, PTs are seen as having more functional clinical knowledge of musculoskeletal injuries than ED physicians, as reported by the physicians. In addition, ED physicians feel PTs complete clinical tasks that would have otherwise been delegated to patient care technicians, nurses, or other providers; this is seen as time saving and helps with department throughput.[10,21,22]

In the ED setting, PTs commonly manage conditions that affect the lumbar and thoracic spine (39%–43%) and injuries of the neck or cervical spine (12%–18%), hip and/or knee (11%–17%), shoulder (8%–9%), foot/ankle (7%-9%), and hand, wrist, or elbow ($\sim$3%).[23] In addition, PTs are trained in lower extremity and spine bracing as well as neurovestibular assessment and treatment and should be considered as a specialty referral service in these areas as well (**Table 1**).

PTs have the potential to offer considerable improvements in care to older adults who present to the ED after a fall, a common presenting complaint. In one study, nearly 90% of older adults discharged home after a fall did not have a formal gait assessment with more than 95% not having a formal balance assessment.[3] Identifying impairments in gait mechanics such as a foot drop, or impairments in balance such as difficulty in reaching outside the base of support, can guide the therapist in prescribing bracing or assistive devices to decrease the risk of future falls. In one study, targeted referrals to existing community services in isolation did not seem to be effective in preventing the recurrence of falls in a 12-month period.[24] PT services can play an integral role in filling this gap, as it has been shown that patient education provided by a PT in the areas of safety awareness and mobility training is effective in reducing falls for at-risk patients presenting to the ED.[21] A geriatric population presenting to the ED can be better served by PT through emphasis on injury prevention, fall risk assessment, gait training, use of assistive devices, and mobility assessment.[1,18]

ROLE OF OCCUPATIONAL THERAPY

OTs focus on assessing functional ability and cognition and their impact on activities of daily living.[25] Given that only 7.3% of older adults presenting to the ED are assessed for their ability to perform ADLs and 26.1% have their cognition assessed, there is considerable opportunity for OT involvement in the ED. OT referrals in the ED have been shown to be as low as 5.3%.[3] Early studies have shown that OT intervention alone, and as part of a multidisciplinary team, results in a reduced rate of hospital admission.[12-14,26]

OTs recommend interventions and adaptations to address functional and cognitive impairments related to patient education, equipment prescription, and referrals to community resources.[25] It has been demonstrated that even though an older adult may meet the medical criteria for discharge from the ED, a lack of functional capacity

Table 1 Rehabilitation areas of service		
Physical Therapy (PT)	**Occupational Therapy (OT)**	**Speech-Language Pathology (SLP)**
Safety assessment focused on mobility • Discharge recommendation • Falls/fall risk	Safety assessment focused on cognition and activities of daily living • Discharge recommendation • Falls/fall risk • Visual perceptual	Dysphagia/Swallowing • Acute aspiration risk/ pneumonia • Acute stroke
Acute musculoskeletal injuries • Hip • Knee • Ankle • Shoulder • Neck • Back	Cognition • Acute cognitive changes • Formal cognitive assessments	Speech/Language • Acute changes in speech or language
Gait training • Assess need for a device • Training with new device and/or weight-bearing restriction	Splinting and bracing • Wrist and hand splints/braces • Spine bracing • Slings	Cognition • Acute changes impacting linguistics/ communication
Bracing and splinting • Fracture walking boots • Off-loading shoes • Spine bracing		
Peripheral vertigo assessment and treatment • Canalith repositioning maneuvers for benign paroxysmal positional vertigo		

or social supports may make it difficult for them to return to their prior circumstances, resulting in prolonged length of stays and increased risk of ED recidivism.[27] The expertise of an OT can be valuable in determining whether the elderly patient is safe for discharge to home by considering functional status and life situations beyond the immediate medical concern.[11]

Occupational therapists perform independent, in-depth histories that focus on the patient's home environment, prior level of function, and available support. Examinations include upper extremity range of motion, strength, coordination, cognition, functional mobility, and balance. This assessment is then conceptualized with activities of daily living (ADLs) and instrumental activities of daily living (IADLs). Examples of ADLs and IADLs are included in **Table 2**. In addition to evaluating function status, OTs are also trained in upper extremity splinting and the use of adaptive equipment to promote independence (see **Table 1**).

ROLE OF THE SPEECH-LANGUAGE PATHOLOGIST

SLPs can complete an in-depth history and an assessment of a patient's cognition, hearing, communication, oral motor function, and each of the phases of swallowing. SLP is well established in the inpatient care setting and the value of their integration

Table 2	
Examples of activities of daily living and instrumental activities of daily living	
Activities of Daily Living (ADL)	**Instrumental Activities of Daily Living (IADL)**
• Eating	• Medication management
• Toileting	• Meal preparation
• Bathing	• Cleaning and maintaining the house
• Dressing	• Laundry
• Grooming	• Grocery shopping
• Oral hygiene	• Safety procedures and emergency responses

in the ED is growing.[28] Their screening can facilitate referrals for appropriate follow-up in a timely and cost-effective manner.[28]

SLPs are experts at screening individuals for possible swallowing disorders and the differential diagnosis of these disorders. Recognizing dysphagia and recommending follow-up can be useful in preventing aspiration and the associated complications. It has been shown that oropharyngeal dysphagia affects up to 84% of patients with Alzheimer's, 50% of elderly patients living in nursing homes, and 40% of older adults living alone[17] and that dysphagia is a "strong risk factor for pulmonary aspiration, pneumonia and aspiration pneumonitis."[29] This can be an important consideration for ED physicians assessing and treating elders, and an SLP referral may be appropriate if dysphagia is suspected in order to mitigate the risk of aspiration until follow-up after discharge from the ED can occur.[29]

SLPs can identify patients with dysphagia and make specific recommendations with a focus on patient education. Recommendations can include diet consistency, positioning during eating, and follow-up services such as outpatient SLP or specialist consult. In part, SLP areas of service delivery that can be useful to ED physicians are feeding and swallowing to include the oral phase, pharyngeal phase, and esophageal phase and cognition related to attention, memory, problem solving, and executive functioning.[28] SLP areas of service delivery are typically focused on swallowing to assess aspiration risk. In determining whether to consult SLP services, special consideration should be made for elders with neurologic, cognitive, and respiratory impairments (see **Table 1**).

INCORPORATING REHABILITATION MEDICINE INTO THE EMERGENCY DEPARTMENT

It is remarkable that Rehabilitation Medicine is not prominent in the ED compared with inpatient medicine. Imagine asking inpatient physicians or advanced practice providers to perform their own gait and balance evaluations with specific recommendations for the next level of care. Imagine asking them to evaluate ADLs and IADLs. Imagine asking them to become experts in bracing and assistive devices. Imagine asking them to evaluate the phases of swallowing. Yet, every day, physicians or advanced practice providers in the ED are expected to make these critical evaluations based on gestalt or a "road test" without adequate training or expertise. These decisions matter and are linked to satisfaction, safety, and cost.

The authors' own experience incorporating Rehabilitation Medicine in the ED has been an overwhelming success. Initial concerns regarding increasing length of stay were unfounded and mirrored findings that PT/OT/SLP in the ED actually decreased wait times, decreased ED length of stay, and improved workflow.[1,20,30] Barriers to successful implementation also include administration buy in, financial support, physical space limitations, and staffing availability. Rehabilitation administrators should consider alternative staffing patterns to allow for later hours of coverage and expanded availability.

In addition, it is important to appreciate the unique ED environment. For those rehabilitation specialists who can function in the uncertainty of the ED and work in parallel with other providers, it can be a wonderful fit. It is past due that older patients seeking care in the ED are afforded the same expertise as those upstairs.

CASE STUDIES: APPLYING REHABILITATION MEDICINE SERVICES IN EMERGENCY DEPARTMENT

Case 1: Mrs A. presents to the ED after her first fall at home. Her daughter is worried about her living independently and wants her admitted for placement. The trauma workup is negative. The ED provider, because this is a new fall, does a medical workup, which is also negative. PT and OT are consulted for mobility and cognition evaluation and conclude that she is safe for discharge home with outpatient physical therapy. Care management arranges home PT and social work services. The patient and the daughter are reassured and leave the ED satisfied.

Case 2: Mrs B presents to the ED after yet another fall. This is her third visit in 6 months for a fall. On each prior occasion, her trauma and medical workup was negative, and she was discharged home. During this visit, PT/OT/SLP evaluate her and document that she has mobility, functional, and cognitive issues that preclude safe discharge home. The patient is admitted. Importantly, rehabilitation evaluation in the ED lays the foundation for both continued inpatient care and discharge planning.

Case 3: Mrs C presents as a transfer related to cervical spine fracture after a fall. She has been in a rigid field cervical collar for 6 hours. There is a bed shortage, and she will likely be in the ED for at least a few hours. OT is consulted in the ED and places her in the appropriately padded and ventilated long-term collar preventing further pain and skin breakdown. OTs may be trained in the proper evaluation, sizing, and placement of collars.

Case 4: Mr D presents to the ED from home after burning his hand on the stove. Medically, he is "clear" for discharge. However, the nurse feels that he is a little "off" and is worried about him going home safely. SLP and OT evaluate him and discovers issues with executive functioning related to his ability to manage his own medications. His daughter is updated and feels relieved that his memory issues have finally been addressed. She agrees to increase her support with medications, follow-ups, and driving. Resources for community support are provided to her.

Case 5: Mr E presents after a fall. PT is asked to evaluate and fit a fracture walking boot for his distal fibula fracture. During the evaluation, PT notes gait mechanics, motor planning, and perceptual and balance issues that are more consistent with a central nervous system deficit than an ankle fracture. PT suggests neuroimaging to the ED provider and 2 brain tumors are diagnosed. The patient is admitted for neurosurgery.

Case 6: Mr F presents with recurrent peripheral vertigo during a busy shift. The ED provider briefly attempts canalith repositioning maneuvers that are not successful but must keep seeing critically ill patients. In lieu of medications and a period of observation, the provider consults PT who is successful in improving symptoms with additional repositioning maneuvers, and the patient is discharged to home with a referral to outpatient vestibular rehabilitation specialist.

SUMMARY

The specialty consult services of PT/OT/SLP have been shown to improve care delivery in the ED setting. Each discipline offers an area of expertise that can be integrated into disposition planning. PT and OT referrals are especially beneficial for older patients in the case of falls, and their intervention has been shown to mitigate the risk of future falls and reduce hospital admissions. Although a growing area of practice, rehabilitation services are underused in the ED. Successful implementation starts with a change in mindset by appreciating that older adults in the ED face the same challenges as those admitted upstairs.

CLINICS CARE POINTS

- PT/OT intervention in the ED can decrease admission rates.
- PTs provide assessments and education that are effective in reducing falls for at-risk older patients.
- OTs can determine safety around discharge to home with respect to performing activities of daily living.
- PTs can determine safety around discharge to home with respect to mobility and balance.
- SLPs perform swallow assessments to determine the presence of dysphagia and patient education to prevent aspiration.
- PTs are musculoskeletal specialists that can manage conditions affecting the spine and extremities.
- The role of PT/OT/SLP in the ED is novel but makes good clinical sense.

DISCLOSURE

The authors have nothing to disclose.

REFERENCES

1. Fleming-McDonnell D, Czuppon S, Deusinger SS, et al. Physical therapy in the emergency department: development of a novel practice venue. Phys Ther 2010;90(3):420–6.
2. James K, Jones D, Kempenaar L, et al. Occupational therapy and emergency departments: a critical review of the literature. Br J Occup Ther 2016;0(0):1–8.
3. Miller E, Wightman E, Rumbolt K, et al. Management of fall-related injuries in the elderly: a retrospective chart review of patients presenting to the emergency department of a community-based teaching hospital. Physiother Can 2009; 61(1):26–37.
4. Ferreira GE, Traeger AC, O'Keeffe M, et al. Staff and patients have mostly positive perceptions of physiotherapists working in emergency departments: a systematic review. J Physiother 2018;64(4):229–36.
5. McClellan CM, Greenwood R, Benger JR. Effect of an extended scope physiotherapy service on patient satisfaction and the outcome of soft tissue injuries in an adult emergency department. Emerg Med J 2006;23(5):384–7.
6. Sutton M, Govier A, Prince S, et al. Primary-contact physiotherapists manage a minor trauma caseload in the emergency department without misdiagnoses or adverse events: an observational study. J Physiother 2015;61(2):77–80.
7. Matifat E, Perreault K, Roy J-S, et al. Concordance between physiotherapists and physicians for care of patients with musculoskeletal disorders presenting to the emergency department. BMC Emerg Med 2019;19(67):1–10.

8. Taylor NF, Norman E, Roddy L, et al. Primary contact physiotherapy in emergency departments can reduce length of stay for patients with peripheral musculoskeletal injuries compared with secondary contact physiotherapy: a prospective non-randomised controlled trial. Physiotherapy 2011;97(2):107–14.

9. Bird S, Thompson C, Williams KE. Primary contact physiotherapy services reduce waiting and treatment times for patients presenting with musculoskeletal conditions in Australian emergency departments: an observational study. J Physiother 2016;62(4):209–14.

10. Lebec MT, Jogodka CE. The physical therapist as a musculoskeletal specialist in the emergency department. J Orthop Sports Phys Ther 2009;39(3):221–9.

11. Spang L, Holmqvist K. Occupational therapy practice in emergency care: occupational therapists' perspectives. Scand J Occup Ther 2015;22(5):345–54.

12. Carlill G, Gash E, Hawkins G. Preventing unnecessary hospital admissions: an occupational therapy and social work service in an accident and emergency department. Br J Occup Ther 2002;65(10):440–5.

13. Morphet J, Griffiths DL, Crawford K, et al. Using transprofessional care in the emergency department to reduce patient admissions: a retrospective audit of medical histories. J Interprof Care 2016;30(2):226–31.

14. Arendts G, Fitzhardinge S, Pronk K, et al. The impact of early emergency department allied health intervention on admission rates in older people: a non-randomized clinical study. BMC Geriatr 2012;12(8):1–6.

15. Ekberg O, Hamdy S, Woisard V, et al. Social and psychological burden of dysphagia: its impact on diagnosis and treatment. Dysphagia 2002;17(2):139–46.

16. Lin LC, Wu SC, Chen HS, et al. Prevalence of impaired swallowing in institutionalized older people in Taiwan. J Am Geriatr Soc 2002;50(6):1118–23.

17. Rofes L, Arreola V, Romea M, et al. Pathophysiology of oropharyngeal dysphagia in the frail elderly. Neurogastroenterol Motil 2010;22(8):851.e230.

18. Kesteloot L, Lebec MT. Physical therapist consultation in the emergency department: a multiple case report describing three Arizona programs. J Acute Care Phys Ther 2012;3(3):224–31.

19. Watson WT, Marshall ES, Fosbinder D. Elderly patients' perceptions of care in the emergency department. J Emerg Nurs 1999;25(2):88–92.

20. Pugh A, Roper K, Magel J, et al. Dedicated emergency department physical therapy is associated with reduced imaging, opioid administration, and length of stay: a prospective observational study. PLoS One 2020;15(4). e0231476-12.

21. Lebec MT, Cernohous S, Tenbarge L, et al. Emergency department physical therapy service: a pilot study examining physician perceptions. Internet J Allied Health Sci Pract 2010;8(1):1.

22. DiCaprio MR, Covey A, Bernstein J. Curricular requirements for musculoskeletal medicine in american medical schools. J Bone Joint Surg Am 2003;85-A(3):565–7.

23. Ciccarella S, et al. Incorporating physical therapist practice in the emergency department: a toolkit for practitioners. American Physical Therapy Association website. 2012. Available at: https://fptcu.com/Gep%20Files/Emergency%20PT/Reading%205%20EmergencyDepartment_Toolkit%20for%20PT.pdf. Accessed May 12, 2016.

24. Russell MA, Hill KD, Day LM, et al. A randomized controlled trial of a multifactorial falls prevention intervention for older fallers presenting to emergency departments. J Am Geriatr Soc 2010;58(12):2265–74.

25. Lloyd C, Hilder J, Williams PL. Emergency department presentations of people who are homeless: the role of occupational therapy. Br J Occup Ther 2017; 80(9):533–8.
26. Smith T, Rees V. An audit of referrals to occupational therapy for older adults attending an accident and emergency department. Br J Occup Ther 2004; 67(4):153–8.
27. Manzano-Santaella A. From bed-blocking to delayed discharges: precursors and interpretations of a contested concept. Health Serv Manage Res 2010;23(3): 121–7.
28. Ad Hoc Committee. Scope of practice in speech-language pathology. American Speech-Language-Hearing Association website. 2016. Available at: https://www. asha.org/policy/SP2016-00343/. Accessed June 25, 2020.
29. Meals C, Roy S, Medvedev G, et al. Identifying the risk of swallowing-related pulmonary complications in older patients with hip fracture. Orthopedics 2016;39(1): e93–7.
30. Kim HS, Strickland KJ, Mullen KA, et al. Physical therapy in the emergency department: a new opportunity for collaborative care. Am J Emerg Med 2018; 36(8):1492–6.

Applying Geriatric Principles to Transitions of Care in the Emergency Department

Kimberly Bambach, MD, Lauren T. Southerland, MD*

KEYWORDS

- Transitions of care • Care transfer • Geriatric assessment • Geriatrics
- Emergency medicine • Safe discharge

KEY POINTS

- Transitions of care represent times at which older adults are particularly vulnerable to adverse events, such as medication errors, difficulty recovering from the illness or injury, and miscommunication due to fragmented care.
- Familiarization with the variety of care settings that older adults inhabit can help facilitate a safe disposition by understanding the level of care and adjuncts that are available.
- The Institute for Healthcare Improvement 4-Ms model helps clinicians develop a safe discharge plan. This involves understanding medications, mentation, mobility, and what matters most to the patient as well as safety and social support.
- Goals of care conversations are about what matters most to the patient, which informs the level of care desired.
- Communication is key to safe dispositions, and ED physicians can take steps to ensure that changes to the patient care plans are understood by the patient, caregivers, and other members of the medical team.

INTRODUCTION

Transitions of care occur every time an older adult moves from one physical care setting to another or when a new provider assumes care. Transitions of care are frequent for older adults, who often have multiple comorbidities requiring an interdisciplinary team of providers across multiple care settings (**Fig. 1**). Such transitions often are unplanned and occur when either an exacerbation of an underlying illness or an acute illness or injury results in a visit to the emergency department (ED). This may be due to frailty, where an older person is functioning well but does not have the physical or psychosocial reserve to compensate for an additional injury or illness, or due to

Department of Emergency Medicine, The Ohio State University Wexner Medical Center, 376 West 10th Avenue, Columbus, OH 43210, USA
* Corresponding author. 753 Prior Hall, 376 West 10 Avenue, Columbus, OH 43210.
E-mail address: Lauren.Southerland@osumc.edu
Twitter: @kimbambach (K.B.); @LSGeriatricEM (L.T.S.)

Emerg Med Clin N Am 39 (2021) 429–442
https://doi.org/10.1016/j.emc.2021.01.006
0733-8627/21/© 2021 Elsevier Inc. All rights reserved.

emed.theclinics.com

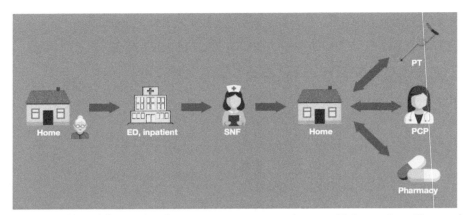

Fig. 1. An older adult entering the ED can expect to experience multiple care transitions and care providers. Systems issues, such as limited Medicare funding for SNF costs after hospitalization, can lead to premature discharges to home without appropriate medications, therapy and handoffs to primary care in place. PCP, primary care physician; PT, physical therapy.

the severity of the underlying medical condition. Fragmentation of outpatient care between multiple specialist providers has resulted in the ED becoming an important hub at the center of geriatric care. The ED visit may result in discharge back to the community with a new care plan, discharge to a new care setting, or hospital admission.

Adverse events with transitions to or from the ED are well documented. Adverse events during transitions can be life-threatening or life-altering for older adults and their loved ones, leading to a decline in independence and functional status.[1] Within 3 months of an ED visit, approximately one-third of older adults experience an adverse outcome.[2] Many of these adverse events are medication interactions or side effects. More than a third of patients (38%) prescribed medications from the ED have potential drug-drug interactions on pharmacist review.[3] Prescribing from the ED is complicated by the fact that patient self-report of medications is poor, with older patients taking on average 3.8 more medications than they report.[4] Additionally, emergency providers may feel medication reconciliation is too difficult or not in their scope of practice. Further barriers are created by health systems, because outpatient or clinic electronic health record (EHR) systems often are inaccessible to the ED provider. This is an example of how system-level, provider-level, and patient-level factors all can interact to complicate transitions of care (**Table 1**). Patient factors contribute to the complexity of decision making and communication at the time of discharge or admission. Systems constraints include limited time in the ED for comprehensive geriatric assessments and the cognitive load of caring for multiple, acutely ill patients.[5] Fragmentation of a patient's health care team also plays a large role in how information is lost during transitions. Information that is critical to providing optimal care may be miscommunicated or communicated inadequately to other members of their interdisciplinary team and outpatient providers.[6] Insurance issues, social services availability, and stress on family caregivers also play a role in adverse events with transitions of care.

How then can emergency clinicians ensure safe transitions of care? One critical issue that is amenable to intervention by the ED team is communication with the patient. Communication with patients and ensuring understanding of diagnosis and care in this population are difficult. Only a fifth of older adults discharged from EDs can

Table 1
System-level, provider-level, and patient-level factors that can complicate safe discharges, collated from qualitative staff and patient studies[5,27–29]

System Factors	Provider Factors	Patient Factors
Insurance issues: precertification for medications or home health or nursing facility placement	Patient load	Complex interacting comorbidities
Barriers to access to outpatient resources	Implicit biases	Polypharmacy
No communication between EHR systems	Lack of training	Cognitive impairment
Minimal face-to-face time with the patient and heavy charting requirements	Perception that it takes too much time	Low health literacy or educational level
Multiple handoffs and multiple providers	Focus on acute issue only in the ED leads to disregarding chronic issues	Lack of social support
Reduced services due to time of day or weekend transitions	Low engagement with community partners	Cultural preferences on communication and family involvement
Lack of in person or face-to-face handoffs	Difficulty tailoring instructions to individuals	Communication difficulties (eg, sensory impairment and language barriers)
Poor integration of transitions of care services	Minimal planning time for discharge from the ED compared with inpatient time	
Lack of inpatient-outpatient continuity of providers	Limited training in transitional care principles	
ED crowding and/or inadequate staffing		

state their diagnosis, as opposed to 70% to 80% of younger adult ED patients.[7,8] Communication barriers to patients include cognitive impairment, language and sensory barriers, small print instructions, and cultural differences on engagement in health care. In 1 study comparing understanding of return instructions in older adults with varying degrees of cognitive impairment (dementia, delirium, and normal cognition), understanding ranged from 10% to 49%, based on the level of cognitive impairment.[9] This suggests that, at best, only half of older adults discharged understand critical discharge instructions. Emergency clinicians are in a unique position to minimize risk to the patient at care transitions by improving communication and using cognitive screening and strategies, such as teach-back, to assess patient understanding.

THE IMPACT OF CARE SETTINGS

There are myriad possible care settings that a patient may be coming from or transitioning to as well as additional services that can be of assistance in these different settings. Understanding the capabilities, advantages, and disadvantages of different care settings is essential to determining the appropriate level of care and best transition for patients (**Fig. 2**). Settings range from aging independently in the community to nursing facilities (skilled nursing facility [SNF]) with 24-hour medical support. The information required at discharge is similar no matter the living situation: medication information, appointments scheduled or needing to be scheduled, any treatments, wound care or therapies needed, and the level of assistance required with ambulation, toileting, and feeding.[10] Many providers assume that home caregivers have been trained to provide services, such as gastric tube care or incontinence care, but home caregivers often are appreciative of further details regarding this care. The ability to discharge a patient

Aging in Place

Older adults live independently in their own homes or with a family member or caregiver.

Assisted Living

Typically a community of small apartments that allow older adults to live predominantly independently but provide a range of services, such as laundry, housekeeping, and community dining.

Skilled Nursing Facility

Commonly referred to as a nursing home, SNFs provide long and short term care. Long-term care includes nursing, dietary, medical, and social services. Short-term care is often utilized for subacute rehabilitation.

Acute Rehabilitation Center

ARCs provide intensive therapy and exercise after an acute illness or injury, but admissions are typically short in duration.

Long Term Acute Care Hospital

Medically complex patients requiring 24-hour care, such as patients requiring long-term mechanical ventilation who no longer require inpatient hospital services, may be admitted to an LTACH.

Home Health Agency

Offer a variety of care services for homebound patients, including nursing care, physical therapy, occupational therapy, social work, and more.

Hospice

Supportive care focusing on comfort and quality of life for terminally ill patients with a life expectancy <6 months.

Fig. 2. Older adults may inhabit a variety of care settings that change their ability to obtain assistance in the areas of mobility, medications, and ADLs. Assisted-living facilities can greatly vary in what they provide for health care services, and a call to the facility can help clarify what resources are available to a patient returning from the ED. ARCs, acute rehabilitation centers; LTACH, long term acute care hospital; SNFs, skilled nursing facilities.

to home with home health rather than admission to an SNF often is desired by patients, but this can create a burden on caregivers and has been associated with more ED revisits in the short term.[11] The social support, abilities, and availability of caregivers must be clear and discussing alternative options in the event of caregiver burnout is very helpful.

Another frequent care transition that can lead to need for emergency care is SNF discharge to home. SNFs are pressured to discharge patients to home care, resulting in unexpected challenges for patients who often end up in the ED when family is unable to care for them.[12] System factors, such as insurance payments, may contribute to precipitous care transitions. Patients on Medicare may be unable to afford the $170.50 daily copay (2019 rates) for skilled nursing care after the 20 days of 100% cost coverage elapse, resulting in premature discharges to home.[13] In 1 study, 25% of older adults discharged from a SNF where in the ED within 30 days, compared with 12.6% when a specialized pharmacist/geriatrician discharge intervention was done in the SNF prior to discharge.[14] This illustrates how a lack of attention during transitions still can end up with ED providers caring for these patients and attempting to resolve complicated home care needs and care transition issues.

Another alternative to hospital or SNF admission is Hospital in the Home, a care model for providing acute or subacute care for conditions, such as cellulitis, chronic obstructive pulmonary disease (COPD) exacerbation, a congestive heart failure (CHF) exacerbation, that usually require admission. The Hospital in the Home model has been shown to be feasible and efficacious as well as cost-effective.[15] Patients also are more at ease and may be more active in their own home settings, mitigating the risks of functional decline and delirium seen with normal hospital admissions. Consider, for example, an older adult with COVID-19 stable on 2 L of supplemental oxygen and requiring assistance with activities of daily living (ADLs) due to their illness. This patient may be a candidate for Hospital in the Home and receive in-home nursing care with frequent assessment of vitals and assistance with ADLs while avoiding inpatient admission.

Considering caregiver burden and well-being is crucial to ensuring that older adults under their care receives adequate support. Respite care for older adults at an SNF or at an adult day care is an adjunct utilized to provide respite to caregivers on the order of days to weeks. Caregivers also may benefit from support groups and other community resources. If an older adult with care needs is in the ED for an issue that is subacute or chronic, the underlying reason may be caregiver stress rather than a health issue for the patient. Identifying and addressing this can improve both the patient's and the caregiver's health.

CHOOSING THE APPROPRIATE CARE SETTING

Multiple risk screening tools have been developed to risk-stratify older adults for adverse health events after an ED visit, but none has shown the necessary levels of sensitivity and specificity.[16,17] This likely is due to the fact that there is a plethora of nonmedical and nonquantifiable criteria not included in these scoring systems that influence care decisions. Every patient has a certain level of medical needs that determines the lowest level of care required. For example, a patient who medically needs intensive care needs intensive care regardless of socioeconomic status, home safety, or cognition. On the opposite side of the spectrum, a patient whose medical needs require only outpatient care may require observation or inpatient floor care if they lack social support. Conversely, a patient who medically requires a high level of care may be best discharged to home if what matters most to the patient is not quantity, but rather quality, of life.

One model of geriatric care from the Institute for Healthcare Improvement and John A. Hartford Foundation uses the 4-Ms model: what matters, medications, mentation, and mobility.[18] Although this model was designed for clinics and inpatient settings, the model also is germaine to the ED visit. For the ED, the authors recommend including an S to this model: safety and social support. There also are several validated screening tools that can aid with assessment (**Table 2**).

1. What matters most? Person-centered and family-centered care is essential for all patients, but especially older adults making difficult decisions about their care. This conversation can start by asking patients and caregivers what they are most concerned about and why. This helps guide the conversation on what the physician can offer. It is important to think creatively. Options, such as hospital at home, overnight observation for further assessment and care coordination, and ED-to-hospice transitions need to be considered in addition to the traditional admit versus discharge decision. This is a type of goals of care conversation that involves the clinician learning about the patient as a person. Exploring the free resources at https://www.vitaltalk.org/ can help in learning how to map out what is most important to the patient, discussing patient goals with a surrogate, and more.

2. Medications: a full medication review includes which medications are taken and how and when they are taken, including over-the-counter medications or supplements. Medication review in the ED by a pharmacist identifies errors and medication interactions in 68% of patients, with a mean number of discrepancies of 3 per patient.[19] Common classes of medications known for interactions include proton pump inhibitors, anticoagulants, and selective serotonin reuptake inhibitors.[20] If a trained medication reviewer or pharmacist is not available in the ED, referral for outpatient follow-up with a pharmacist or polypharmacy clinic should be considered. This ED-to-outpatient review strategy led to an absolute 9% reduction in proportion of patients requiring admission to the hospital in the 4 months after an ED visit.[4]

3. Mentation: evaluation of mentation requires understanding a patient's baseline cognitive status as well as screening for delirium and cognitive changes with validated tools during the ED visit.[21] Currently, ED providers rarely formally screen for cognitive changes.[22,23] Ignoring cognitive limitations leads to difficulty understanding discharge instructions, which can result in return ED visits, medication misuse, or inability to care for the illness or injury properly at home. Subtle delirium also often is noted only with testing. Mentation is worsened by sensory impairment, such as lack of hearing aids or reading glasses, so, if possible, temporary-use items should be stocked in the ED and hospital to help better assess cognition in the setting of sensory impairment.

Table 2
Formal, validated assessment tools and training for the 4-Ms model in the emergency department setting

Category	Assessment Tools
What matters most?	Brief negotiated interview model, VitalTalk model, Education in Palliative and End-Of-Life Care for Emergency Medicine (EPEC-EM)[30]
Medications	Online medication interaction checkers
Mentation	Short Blessed Test, Brief Alzheimer Screen, Mini-Mental State Examination, Montreal Cognitive Assessment, 4AT
Mobility	TUG, 4 Stage Balance Test, Sit to Stand Test

4. Mobility: safe mobility requires an understanding of what assistive devices patients require, what they have available, and their home living situation. Can they get in and out of the house safely, or are they newly homebound? Will this illness require temporary support? Some EDs have access to physical therapists for gait assessments and equipment training but most do not. ED nurses often can provide insightful information on gait and self-care ability as they are in the room and assisting with toileting and transfers. Mobility can be assessed using the Timed Up and Go (TUG) test, a validated tool accounting for both static and dynamic balance.[24] This is performed by timing the patient when asked to perform the following: stand up from a chair, walk 3 m at their normal pace, turn, and walk back to the chair and sit down (**Fig. 3**). Patients can use their baseline assistive devices. Individuals with a TUG test greater than 13.5 seconds are in a high-risk category for falls. For EDs that do not have the space for this test or when patients need to remain on telemetry or other monitors, the 4 Stage Balance Test is preferred (**Fig. 4**). This can be done at the bedside and involves having the patient stand with progressively more difficult stances.

5. Safety and social support: the patient's home safety and social support should be considered. Safety includes considering the possibility of elder abuse and neglect as well as caregivers' abilities to provide the support needed. Often, a caregiver has as many chronic health issues as the patient in question. Assisting them in setting up home meal delivery (eg, Meals on Wheels), home health aides or nursing, or a home safety assessment by a community paramedic team or the local area agency on aging can make the difference between a supportive community dwelling adult and further functional decline.

One limitation to applying the 4-Ms model in the ED is clinician time. A team approach can alleviate some of this burden. For example, a social worker or case manager can discuss mobility and safety/social support. A physical therapist or ED nurse can administer mobility testing. A pharmacy technician or pharmacist can assist by verifying medications. This multidisciplinary approach is common in the inpatient setting, and case managers, social workers, and nurses in the ED can assist with gathering information to form a holistic care plan. Palliative medicine consultation can

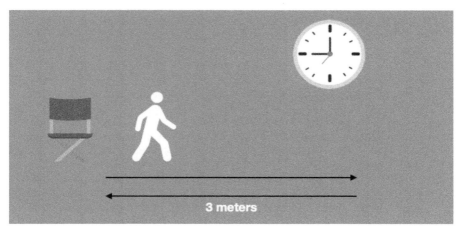

Fig. 3. The TUG test is used to assess mobility. A time of greater than 13.5 seconds signifies abnormal mobility and high risk for falling.

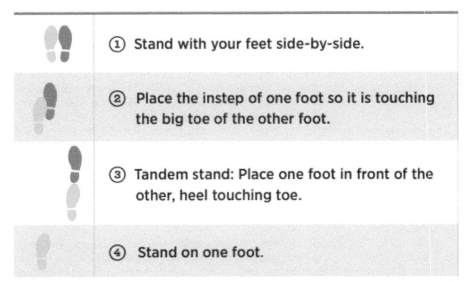

1. Stand with your feet side-by-side.

2. Place the instep of one foot so it is touching the big toe of the other foot.

3. Tandem stand: Place one foot in front of the other, heel touching toe.

4. Stand on one foot.

Fig. 4. The 4 Stage Balance Test is a test of static balance and to assesses mobility differently from the TUG but is very quick and able to be done at the bedside in the ED. Supportive devices, such as a walker, may be used to move into the appropriate stance. The ability to hold the tandem gait for greater than 10 seconds demonstrates good balance. (*Adapted from* CDC STEADI Guidelines, https://www.cdc.gov/steadi/pdf/STEADI-Assessment-4Stage-508.pdf.)

assist with determining what matters most and increases the likelihood a patient is discharged to the community.[25] If a patient has a complicated social situation or may need intensive intervention by case management, physical therapists, or pharmacists, an observation unit can be used for this holistic multidisciplinary assessment.[26]

Older adults can encounter significant challenges functioning at home with relatively minor illnesses. For example, a distal radius fracture is treated almost exclusively with a splint and referral to orthopedics in younger adults. But for older adults, a conversation about increased fall risk, self-care at home, and early physical therapy to avoid muscle atrophy in that arm all are essential. An older patient already may have limited range of motion or be unable to manage splint care if they live alone. Another example of a common ailment addressed on ED visit is a mild COPD exacerbation. An older adult with a COPD exacerbation is sent home with appropriate treatments and a new patient appointment with a pulmonologist. The patient, however, was not screened for cognitive deficits and was unable to drive to the pulmonology clinic, a new and unfamiliar environment, and missed his appointment. He was never started on a long-acting preventative inhaler and was back in the ED with another exacerbation 2 months later. This type of cycle can repeat indefinitely, and the patient often is labeled "noncompliant" when in fact the patient has cognitive or transportation issues that would have been identified if the 4-Ms model were used prior to discharge.

Once the disposition decision has been made by taking the 4-Ms model into account, communication is key to ensure a successful transition. If the patient is discharged back home, clear written and verbal instructions should be provided to the patient and caregivers. Most EHRs allow for large font printing for discharge instructions to ensure legibility. Return precautions also are an important component of discharge counseling. A brief call or message to the patient's primary care provider can ensure that changes to the care plan are communicated directly and appropriate follow-up is in place. If the patient is discharged back to a facility, such as an SNF, a verbal handoff with the patient's nurse can ensure their care team is aware of any medication changes, abnormal laboratory results, procedures, and follow-up needed. SNF nurses identify poor-quality discharge communication as a major barrier to safe and effective transitions.[10] SNFs rely heavily on discharge materials, so complete and accurate discharge information, including wound care, medications, and upcoming appointments, are crucial. SNFs often have central pharmacies, and calling before discharge can ensure the patient is able to obtain all prescribed medications. If the patient is admitted, communicating directly with the inpatient team can avoid potentially dangerous omissions.

CASE STUDIES: APPLYING THE 4-MS MODEL TO EMERGENCY DEPARTMENT CASES

Case 1: Mrs Z is an 82-year-old woman with diet-controlled diabetes, hypertension, and osteoarthritis. She presents to the ED with left-sided flank pain and vomiting and is found to have an uncomplicated renal stone, 4 mm in size. Her urine is concentrated but does not show signs of infection. She is treated with an intravenous (IV) fluid bolus, ondansetron for nausea, and ketorolac for pain. She now is able to tolerate a few sips of juice. What is the appropriate disposition?

1. What matters most? She would like to be home if at all possible because she has 2 cats at home and does not have anyone in the area to feed them if she is gone for a long time.
2. Medications: a full medication review reveals that she is not on any QT-prolonging drugs so ondansetron is reasonable for nausea. She does, however, take celecoxib daily for arthritis pain, which is a nonsteroidal anti-inflammatory medication (NSAID). Adding an additional NSAID to this could cause significant and potentially dangerous side effects.
3. Mentation: she scores a 7 on the Short Blessed Test, signifying some mild cognitive impairment mainly with short-term recall. She is oriented fully.
4. Mobility: Mrs Z is able to ambulate well with her cane, which is what she uses at home for her arthritis pain.
5. Safety and social support: Mrs Z lives in her own 2-story home. She has a daughter who lives an hour away and visits more than weekly but is unable to come daily.

Discussion: The physician know that Mrs Z is likely to pass the stone without trouble at home but are concerned based on her memory issues, so the physician obtains her permission to speak with her daughter. The daughter cannot stay with Mrs Z but understands that she will need more support this week and arranges for family and friends to check in by phone or in person several times a day to encourage her to drink fluids and check her symptoms. The physician put her on acetaminophen instead of NSAIDs and arrange for a referral to a geriatric assessment clinic for further cognitive testing. Both the patient and her daughter are very happy with this plan. The physician send a brief message to the patient's urologist to facilitate an outpatient appointment as well and ensure that she and her daughter are aware of the next steps in follow-up.

What if Mrs Z lived in a senior assisted-living complex? Depending on the resources of the facility, the facility may be able to provide daily wellness checks, monitor medications, or even check her vitals to assess for fever daily. Assisted-living complexes vary greatly in the assistance they can provide post–ED visit. It is important to have clear instructions on the level of monitoring needed, sometimes written as a prescription or "doctor's orders." Speaking to a staff member at the facility also is helpful. If the patient presents from a long-term care facility, staff from the facility can be a valuable source of collateral information. Because staff often do not accompany the patient to the ED, calling the facility for a verbal handoff regarding any changes to a patient's care plan can prevent errors. The physician also can ensure that written discharge instructions are clear and complete to reinforce the changes.

Case 2: Mr Y is a 75-year-old man who presents to the ED for chest pain after eating dinner. He had a cardiac catheterization last year, which showed diffuse coronary artery disease not amenable to cardiac stenting, which is being medically managed. Medical evaluation, including serial electrocardiograms, basic laboratory tests, a chest radiograph, D-dimer, and 2 troponins all are reassuring. He is eating and drinking well and says he gets these pains frequently. His initial blood pressure was high but, after giving him his home evening blood pressure medication, it comes back down to 130/80 mmHg. What is the appropriate disposition?

1. What matters most? Mr Y says the most important thing to him is to "keep on going" because he is a "tough old guy" and thinks his health is good.
2. Medications: when asked if he takes all his medications, Mr Y answers affirmatively. But he cannot tell the physician the names of all his medications. When pressed, he also cannot say how many he takes in the morning or evening. He just takes "whatever comes in those packets they send." He admits to drinking daily but does not say how much.
3. Mentation: Mr Y is circuitous to his answers. He confabulates when he does not know the day of the week or the date ("I'm retired, I don't need to know that anymore!"). A Brief Alzheimer Screen reveals that his short-term recall is 1/3 and his fluency is diminished.
4. Mobility: Mr Y says he gets around fine in his house without any assistive devices, but, when pressed, he holds onto furniture and the walls for support. In the ED, he has no difficulty getting out of the bed but then has an unsteady gait.
5. Safety and social support: Mr Y lives alone in an apartment. He does not drive but does take the bus or walks to the nearby corner store and pharmacy. He has family but they live several states away.

Discussion: Many physicians, before going through the 4-Ms model, would discharge Mr Y back to his living situation. With this additional knowledge, however, it is clear that Mr Y is not able to take his medications appropriately and has significant cognitive impairment. He is drinking daily and may not be caring for himself well. He has no social support structure. He would benefit from full cognitive assessment and arranging for resources, such as a home health nurse, to fill and monitor his pillboxes; a home safety check; a system to call for help if he falls; a physical therapy evaluation and recommendation for gait assistance; and a complete cognitive assessment to evaluate his ability to make health care decisions. An observation stay would allow the time needed to complete these evaluations and ensure that he is safe to go home. Given his cognitive issues, he is unlikely to be able to arrange all of this from home by himself. A brief call to his inpatient team ensures that they understand that his admission is not due simply to his chief complaint of chest pain work-up but rather to concerns regarding his fall risk, cognitive impairment, and need for additional resources at home.

Case 3: Mr X is an 89-year-old man with stage 4 metastatic small cell lung cancer, presenting with worsening cough and fever. He is cachectic and ill appearing and at baseline uses 2 L of supplemental oxygen. In triage, he requires 3 L of oxygen via nasal cannula to keep his pulse oximeter level greater than 90%. He is febrile and chest radiograph demonstrates a postobstructive pneumonia. What is the appropriate disposition?

1. What matters most? Mr X says the most important thing to him is to spend the remaining time he has surrounded by his family at home. When asked, he states that he does not want to be admitted to the hospital, even if the pneumonia is treatable, because every time he comes in it results in at least a 2-week stay. With his permission, his son joins the discussion and supports his father in his wishes. They would like to pursue home hospice and have been considering this even prior to this ED visit because his health has declined in the past couple of weeks.
2. Medications: a full review of his medications is performed by the ED pharmacist. The physician comes to the decision with the patient that he would like to treat the pneumonia at home for palliation. To avoid interactions with his other medications, Levofloxacin is not an option. The hospice team is able to do IV ceftriaxone at home.
3. Mentation: Mr X scores 30/30 on a Mini-Mental State Examination. He displays no signs of cognitive impairment and clearly understands the risks and benefits of both inpatient admission and home hospice care. Because he clearly understands the medical decisions and options presented to him, he has medical decision-making capacity.
4. Mobility: Mr X has very limited mobility at home and can ambulate only a few steps with assistance due to his deconditioning and frailty. He mainly uses a wheelchair and walker. Hospice will help with arranging durable medical equipment, such as hospital bed and bedside commode.
5. Safety and social support: he lives with his son. His son cooks meals for him, assists him with the ADLs, and is his sole source of social support. This has taken a toll on his son as well, causing considerable stress. He would welcome additional assistance provided by hospice nurses to help treat his father's pain and shortness of breath and home health aides to assist with other activities, such as bathing and dressing. The ED social worker begins making arrangements for home hospice. The home hospice agency also is able to provide his son with additional resources for emotional and spiritual support.

Discussion: If care had not been taken to address what matters most to Mr X, he may have been admitted to the hospital, which is not consistent with his goals of care. By enlisting the help of the ED social worker, Mr X is able to return back home with additional support services, including medical equipment, nursing care, and home health, all through a home hospice agency. The needs of his son, who is his sole source of support, also were addressed during the visit.

SUMMARY

Caring for older adults in the ED presents unique challenges and transitions are inherently risky. ED providers can play a crucial role in preventing adverse events by utilizing the 4-Ms model and providing clear communication.

CLINICS CARE POINTS

- Common adverse events after a transition of care include medication interactions, injurious falls, and ED revisits or rehospitalizations.
- Clear communication with the patient, caregiver, and outpatient care team (both from the facility if the patient is not community dwelling and the medical team) requires dedicated time to answer questions at discharge and verbal and written handoffs. At best, fewer than 50% of older adults understand their discharge instructions and diagnosis.

- The Institute for Healthcare Improvement 4-Ms model can be adapted to the ED setting and recommends assessing what matters most, medications, mentation, and mobility. In the ED, add an S for assessing safety (concerns for elder abuse and home safety) and social support.
- Alternatives to hospital admission can include a short observation stay for multidisciplinary geriatric assessment, hospital-at-home programs, and hospice care.

DISCLOSURE

L.T. Southerland is funded to investigate geriatric EDs through NIH K23AG06128401. Reference to specific commercial products, manufacturers, companies, or trademarks does not constitute its endorsement or recommendation by the US Government, Department of Health and Human Services, or Centers for Disease Control and Prevention.

REFERENCES

1. Nagurney JM, Fleischman W, Han L, et al. Emergency department visits without hospitalization are associated with functional decline in older persons. Ann Emerg Med 2017;69:426–33.
2. Hastings SN, Oddone EZ, Fillenbaum G, et al. Frequency and predictors of adverse health outcomes in older Medicare beneficiaries discharged from the emergency department. Med Care 2008;46:771–7.
3. Jawaro T, Bridgeman PJ, Mele J, et al. Descriptive study of drug-drug interactions attributed to prescriptions written upon discharge from the emergency department. Am J Emerg Med 2019;37:924–7.
4. Briggs S, Pearce R, Dilworth S, et al. Clinical pharmacist review: a randomised controlled trial. Emerg Med Australas 2015;27:419–26.
5. Lennox A, Braaf S, Smit V, et al. Caring for older patients in the emergency department: Health professionals' perspectives from Australia - The Safe Elderly Emergency Discharge project. Emerg Med Australas 2019;31(1):83–9.
6. Apker J, Mallak LA, Gibson SC. Communicating in the "gray zone": perceptions about emergency physician hospitalist handoffs and patient safety. Acad Emerg Med 2007;14:884–94.
7. Leamy K, Thompson J, Mitra B. Awareness of diagnosis and follow up care after discharge from the Emergency Department. Australas Emerg Care 2019;22: 221–6.
8. Hastings SN, Barrett A, Weinberger M, et al. Older patients' understanding of emergency department discharge information and its relationship with adverse outcomes. J Patient Saf 2011;7:19–25.
9. Han JH, Bryce SN, Ely EW, et al. The effect of cognitive impairment on the accuracy of the presenting complaint and discharge instruction comprehension in older emergency department patients. Ann Emerg Med 2011;57: 662–71.e2.
10. King BJ, Gilmore-Bykovskyi AL, Roiland RA, et al. The consequences of poor communication during transitions from hospital to skilled nursing facility: a qualitative study. J Am Geriatr Soc 2013;61:1095–102.
11. Werner RM, Coe NB, Qi M, et al. Patient outcomes after hospital discharge to home with home health care vs to a skilled nursing facility. JAMA Intern Med 2019;179:617–23.

12. Tyler DA, McHugh JP, Shield RR, et al. Challenges and consequences of reduced skilled nursing facility lengths of stay. Health Serv Res 2018;53:4848–62.

13. Werner RM, Konetzka RT, Qi M, et al. The impact of Medicare copayments for skilled nursing facilities on length of stay, outcomes, and costs. Health Serv Res 2019;54:1184–92.

14. Reidt SL, Holtan HS, Larson TA, et al. Interprofessional collaboration to improve discharge from skilled nursing facility to home: preliminary data on postdischarge hospitalizations and emergency department visits. J Am Geriatr Soc 2016;64: 1895–9.

15. Caplan GA, Sulaiman NS, Mangin DA, et al. A meta-analysis of "hospital in the home". Med J Aust 2012;197:512–9.

16. Carpenter CR, Shelton E, Fowler S, et al. Risk factors and screening instruments to predict adverse outcomes for undifferentiated older emergency department patients: a systematic review and meta-analysis. Acad Emerg Med 2015; 22:1–21.

17. Apostolo J, Cooke R, Bobrowicz-Campos E, et al. Predicting risk and outcomes for frail older adults: an umbrella review of frailty screening tools. JBI Database System Rev Implement Rep 2017;15:1154–208.

18. Pelton LJ, Fulmer T, Hendrich A, Mate K. Creating age-friendly health systems. Healthcare Executive. 2017 Nov;32(6):62-63. Available at : http://www.ihi.org/resources/Pages/Publications/Age-Friendly-Health-Systems-Meeting-Needs-of-Older-Adults.aspx.

19. Choi YJ, Kim H. Effect of pharmacy-led medication reconciliation in emergency departments: A systematic review and meta-analysis. J Clin Pharm Ther 2019; 44:932–45.

20. Merel SE, Paauw DS. Common drug side effects and drug-drug interactions in elderly adults in primary care. J Am Geriatr Soc 2017;65:1578–85.

21. Carpenter CR, Bassett ER, Fischer GM, et al. Four sensitive screening tools to detect cognitive dysfunction in geriatric emergency department patients: brief Alzheimer's Screen, Short Blessed Test, Ottawa 3DY, and the caregiver-completed AD8. Acad Emerg Med 2011;18:374–84.

22. Kennelly SP, Morley D, Coughlan T, et al. Knowledge, skills and attitudes of doctors towards assessing cognition in older patients in the emergency department. Postgrad Med J 2013;89:137–41.

23. Taylor A, Broadbent M, Wallis M, et al. The use of functional and cognitive assessment in the emergency department to inform decision making: A scoping review. Australas Emerg Care 2018;21:13–22.

24. Barry E, Galvin R, Keogh C, et al. Is the Timed Up and Go test a useful predictor of risk of falls in community dwelling older adults: a systematic review and meta-analysis. BMC Geriatr 2014;14:14.

25. Scott M, Shaver N, Lapenskie J, et al. Does inpatient palliative care consultation impact outcomes following hospital discharge? A narrative systematic review. Palliat Med 2020;34:5–15.

26. Southerland LT, Vargas AJ, Nagaraj L, et al. An emergency department observation unit is a feasible setting for multidisciplinary geriatric assessments in compliance with the geriatric emergency department guidelines. Acad Emerg Med 2018;25:76–82.

27. Tobiano G, Chaboyer W, Teasdale T, et al. Patient engagement in admission and discharge medication communication: A systematic mixed studies review. Int J Nurs Stud 2019;95:87–102.

28. Lee JS, Napoles A, Mutha S, et al. Hospital discharge preparedness for patients with limited English proficiency: A mixed methods study of bedside interpreter-phones. Patient Educ Couns 2018;101:25–32.

29. Scott AM, Li J, Oyewole-Eletu S, et al. Understanding Facilitators and Barriers to Care Transitions: Insights from Project ACHIEVE Site Visits. Jt Comm J Qual Patient Saf 2017;43:433–47.

30. Jain N, Bernacki RE. Goals of care conversations in serious illness: a practical guide. Med Clin North Am 2020;104:375–89.

Clinical Relevance and Considerations of Palliative Care in Older Adults

Leah Bright, DO[a],*, Bonnie Marr, MD[b]

KEYWORDS

- Palliative care • Emergency medicine • Older adults

KEY POINTS

- The geriatric population is more likely to have serious and chronic illnesses that benefit from palliative care involvement.
- Recognition of disease processes amenable to palliative care should be standard practice for emergency medicine physicians.
- Understanding the unmet needs of the geriatric population amenable to palliative care can change the trajectory of care in a positive manner.

INTRODUCTION AND EPIDEMIOLOGY

Emergency physicians routinely care for patients with serious illness. Geriatric patients are more likely to have life-limiting illnesses and also suffer from a significant burden of chronic disease.[1] Since its recognition as an official subspecialty of emergency medicine (EM), palliative care (PC) has become better appreciated and its importance with respect to caring for chronically ill persons recognized.

As the population in the United States continues to age, with baby boomers now retiring at a rate of 10,000 individuals per day, a corresponding increase in Medicare costs, especially among patients with chronic disease, has increased substantially.[2] This concomitant increase in older adults, patients with chronic disease, and associated costs creates a health care system likely to benefit from the further involvement and consideration of palliative care.

Furthermore, given that emergency departments (EDs) are seen as the safety net in any health care system, many older adults with exacerbation of chronic disease are seen in this setting. Often these patients, who increasingly have challenges accessing primary care, never return to their baseline after these exacerbations.[3] Moreover,

[a] Emergency Medicine Department, Johns Hopkins Hospital, 1830 East Monument Street, Baltimore, MD 21287, USA; [b] The Johns Hopkins Hospital, 600 N. Wolfe Street, Section of Palliative Medicine, Blalock 359, Baltimore, MD 21287, USA
* Corresponding author.
E-mail address: lbright5@jhmi.edu

Emerg Med Clin N Am 39 (2021) 443–452
https://doi.org/10.1016/j.emc.2021.01.007
0733-8627/21/© 2021 Elsevier Inc. All rights reserved.

emed.theclinics.com

these ED visits increase toward the end of life.[4] Approximately 15% of people younger than 84 years old visit the ED in the last 6 months of life, while 75% of people older than 84 year old visit the ED in the last 6 months of life, with half of these patients presenting during their last month of life.[1,4,5] For these reasons, it is imperative that PC practices and interventions be considered a standard part of any EM physician's armamentarium.

Despite the rather recent recognition of PC in the ED, its value in addressing the needs of the geriatric population in this setting has been demonstrated in the literature.[6] Early PC intervention has been shown to decrease depression, improve quality of life, and extend life expectancy by almost 3 months.[7] It also has been shown to decrease length of hospital stay.[8] It is recognized not all EDs may have PC consultants available; the involvement of the primary care physician (PCP), outpatient PC referral, virtual PC consultations, and social work consultation may be a more feasible alternative.

Incorporating PC into one's practice in the busy environment of the ED may be challenging; however, it is important to recognize that EM physicians are often caring for patients at a pivotal point in the trajectory of a chronic disease. These encounters offer EM physicians the opportunity to intervene and introduce the support PC can offer patients and their families in the setting of serious illness. Therefore, the EM clinician has to be facile at rapidly assessing for potential PC needs within the geriatric population.

It is important to distinguish PC from hospice care. PC focuses on specialized medical care for people living with a serious illness with the goal of improving quality of life for both the patient and the family.[6] PC involvement can begin at any phase of a serious illness, including at the time of diagnosis. Hospice, on the other hand, is care in the last phase of a life-ending illness. The role of PC in treating the patient and the family as a unit is especially important in geriatric patients, for whom there is often significant caregiver involvement and fatigue. In addition, older adults are more likely to have polypharmacy and under-recognized symptoms requiring careful symptom management. Early involvement of PC should be considered a cornerstone in the management of the older adults with chronic diseases presenting to the ED.[6] **Fig. 1** illustrates the difference in disease trajectory and continuum of support between early and late PC intervention.

INTERVENTIONS AND CONSIDERATIONS
Recognizing Opportunities for Palliative Care Involvement

PC is often associated with hospice, when in actuality, hospice is only a small part of the spectrum of PC. The World Health Organization describes PC as "an approach that improves the quality of life of patients and their families facing the problem associated with life-threatening illness, through the prevention and relief of suffering by means of early identification and impeccable assessment and treatment of pain and other problems, physical, psychosocial and spiritual."[9] Life-threatening illnesses include not only cancer but also congestive heart failure, end-stage liver disease and renal disease, advanced chronic obstructive pulmonary disease (COPD), and advanced neurocognitive diseases such as Alzheimer disease and Parkinson disease. Recognizing that these chronic conditions, which are often debilitating and negatively impact quality of life, are amenable to PC is paramount. The geriatric population is likely to have at least one of these chronic medical conditions, as modern medicine has been able to prolong lifespan projections with medical management.[10] However, extended quantity of life does not always correlate with ongoing quality of life. This is where awareness of PC is crucial in EM. George and colleagues[11] published a PC

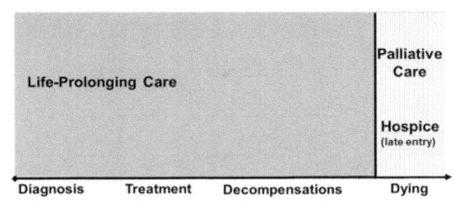

Current Paradigm: Disease Trajectory with **Late** Palliative Care Intervention

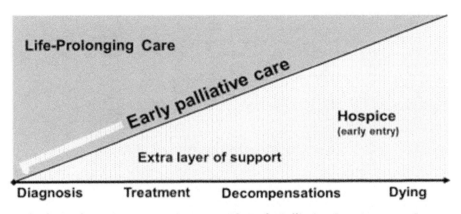

Ideal Paradigm: Disease Trajectory with **Early** Palliative Care Intervention

Fig. 1. Reconceptualizing palliative care as a continuum of support. (*Reproduced from*: Wang DH. Beyond Code Status: Palliative Care Begins in the Emergency Department. *Ann Emerg Med.* 2017;69(4):437-43.)

screening tool specific to EM (**Fig. 2**). This tool can be used as a general guide to identify potential PC needs in ED patients and demonstrates the breadth of disease conditions where PC may be beneficial.

Another useful tool in the ED is the tool offered by the Center to Advance Palliative Care.[12] The tool identifies unmet palliative needs similar to the one by George and colleagues, such as frequent visits/bounce backs, uncontrolled symptoms, functional decline, and the surprise question. It also adds complex care requirement as a potential PC need.[12]

A Road Map to Palliative Care Screening Tools for the Older Adult

Most ED clinicians are likely able to identify the presentations related to unmet PC consultations, but do not necessarily view them as opportunities to include PC. The following outline will provide a road map of these opportunities and demonstrate

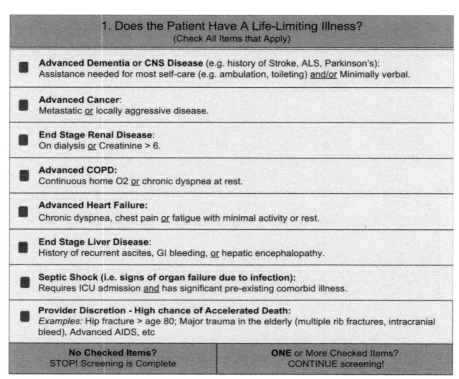

1. Does the Patient Have A Life-Limiting Illness?
(Check All Items that Apply)

- **Advanced Dementia or CNS Disease** (e.g. history of Stroke, ALS, Parkinson's):
  Assistance needed for most self-care (e.g. ambulation, toileting) and/or Minimally verbal.

- **Advanced Cancer:**
  Metastatic or locally aggressive disease.

- **End Stage Renal Disease:**
  On dialysis or Creatinine > 6.

- **Advanced COPD:**
  Continuous home O2 or chronic dyspnea at rest.

- **Advanced Heart Failure:**
  Chronic dyspnea, chest pain or fatigue with minimal activity or rest.

- **End Stage Liver Disease:**
  History of recurrent ascites, GI bleeding, or hepatic encephalopathy.

- **Septic Shock (i.e. signs of organ failure due to infection):**
  Requires ICU admission and has significant pre-existing comorbid illness.

- **Provider Discretion - High chance of Accelerated Death:**
  Examples: Hip fracture > age 80; Major trauma in the elderly (multiple rib fractures, intracranial bleed), Advanced AIDS, etc

No Checked Items?	**ONE** or More Checked Items?
STOP! Screening is Complete	CONTINUE screening!

2. Does the Patient Have TWO or More Unmet Palliative Care Needs?
(Check All the Apply)

- **Frequent Visits:**
  2 or more ED visits or hospital admissions in the past 6 months.

- **Uncontrolled Symptoms:**
  Visit prompted by uncontrol symptom: e.g. pain, dyspnea, depression, fatigue, etc.

- **Functional Decline:**
  e.g. loss of mobility, frequent falls, decrease PO, skin breakdown, etc.

- **Uncertainty about Goals-of-Care and/or Caregiver Distress**
  Caregiver cannot meet long-term needs; Uncertainty/distress about goals-of-care.

- **Surprise Question:**
  You would not be surprised if this patient died within 12 months.

Less than TWO checked Items?	**TWO or more checked Items?**
STOP! Screening is Negative	PC Referral Recommended!

Fig. 2. Palliative care screening tool for emergency medicine. (*Reproduced from*: George N, Barrett N, McPeake L, Goett R, Anderson K, Baird J. Content Validation of a Novel Screening Tool to Identify Emergency Department Patients with Significant Palliative Care Needs. Acad Emerg Med. 2015;22(7):823-837.)

how this intersection between PC and EM can lead to collaboration and improvement in patient care overall.

Category 1: Frequent Visits

Two or more visits to the ED within the last 6 months can be indicative of uncontrolled symptoms and/or a medical care plan that is only temporizing the patient for brief periods as an outpatient.[4] Review of symptom management, including meticulous review for polypharmacy in the geriatric population, and evaluation of goals of care (GOC) may address underlying issues related to these presentations. PC consultation or referral can support the ED clinician in this effort. Repeat presentations also present opportunities to collaborate with the patient's PCP and specialists in a unified care plan. PC specializes in symptom management and the communication inherent to complex medical decision making and therefore is uniquely equipped to help address the underlying reasons behind bounce-back presentations for patients with serious illness.

Category 2: Uncontrolled Symptoms

Management of uncontrolled symptoms is an opportunity to address the symptom causing distress to the patient put in perspective how this acute exacerbation may be linked to the underlying trajectory of a serious illness. An example of this process is end-stage COPD, when patients present for acute shortness of breath, but continue to be oxygen- and steroid-dependent upon discharge with potential for concurrent impact to quality of life. **Fig. 3** demonstrates the disease trajectory seen with organ

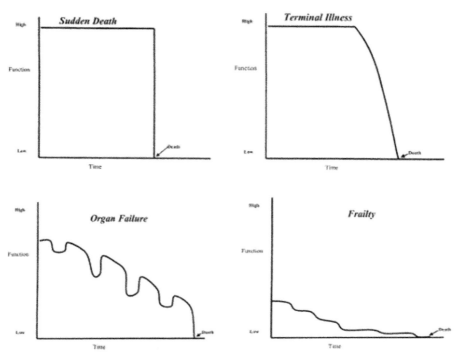

Fig. 3. Proposed trajectories of dying. (*Reproduced from*: L Lunney JR, Lynn J, Hogan C. Profiles of older Medicare decedents. *J Am Geriatr Soc.* 2002;50(6):1108-1112.)

failure, where the patient may improve from an exacerbation, but never return to his or her prior baseline.[13] Symptom management using medication can be complicated by polypharmacy and resulting medication effects, as well as the possibility of compromised renal and hepatic function and/or decreased cerebral perfusion. Therefore, appropriate drug selection, judicious prescribing, and monitoring for adverse effects are of particular importance.[14] An ED presentation for an uncontrolled symptom may also be an opportunity for collaboration with the patient and his or her family as well as the patient's PCP to explore GOC and identify a plan moving forward for future management of exacerbations or anticipated disease sequelae.[15] In addition to engaging pharmacist support when appropriate and available, EM physicians should consider a PC consultation where available. PC can assist with management of uncontrolled symptoms and polypharmacy, with expertise in utilizing medications in the setting of compromised end-organ function and with reviewing GOC and streamlining coordination of care across settings. Additionally, institutional policies and what is available on formulary may restrict what options are available to ED physicians; partnering with the ED pharmacist or available pharmacy support is generally advised. Interventional anesthesia or consultation services devoted to pain management may also provide additional support when appropriate, especially if PC consultation is not readily available. Finally, symptom management is complex and nuanced, with many important factors regarding the patient that should be taken into consideration.

Category 3: Functional Decline

Assessment of functional status and evaluating for functional decline are essential components of geriatric medicine and relate to the concept of frailty. The frailty syndrome has been described in different ways in the literature, but generally refers to a set of phenotypic characteristics that are more likely to be present in an older adult who is vulnerable to poor outcomes, frequent hospitalization, and overall mortality.[16,17] **Fig. 3** illustrates the functional status for the frail individual, which starts out as low with ongoing losses over time until death. Resources within the ED may assist with further evaluation if frailty or independent functional capacity concerns exist. Specifically, social workers may be helpful in the evaluation of dependence on caregivers and understanding the home environment and any safety concerns. Physical therapy and occupational therapy, if available, also offer insight into patient's ability to complete activities of daily living (ADLs) and instrumental activities of daily living (IADLs). Insight into these factors may guide GOC discussions and help the physician understand possible outcomes of the current ED presentation. Understanding a patient's baseline functional status and frailty is even more important when treatment options are considered high risk with unfavorable outcomes, making shared decision making even more of a priority.[18] Reviewing GOC with prioritization of a patient's personal definition of what quality of life means to him or her may facilitate discussions regarding disposition planning and referral to hospice when appropriate. PC teams often are multidisciplinary and may include a social worker, chaplain, nurses, physicians, nonphysician practitioners, pharmacists, and case managers, as well as insight or support from therapy experts, making these teams ideal for the evaluation of functional decline.

Category 4: Uncertainty about goals of care and caregiver distress

The ED often witnesses life-changing events, and critical discussions take place under time-limited circumstances on a more frequent basis in the ED than in other health care environments. The EM physician should feel confident about working to establish a treatment plan that aligns with a patient's GOC. If the patient is unable to participate in the discussion, many communication tools exist to assist health care practitioners in broaching GOC discussions with surrogate decision-makers for health care, including from the Centers to Advance Palliative Care[19] and VitalTalk. Individual states have varying laws and policies for obtaining emergent consent of which the physician must be aware. Complex communication needs surrounding GOC are an indication for a PC consultation, which helps begin the process of engaging with the patient and/or his or her family in exploration of GOC.

Caregiver distress is a significant indicator for PC involvement. According to the Centers to Advance Palliative Care, improving the quality of life for both the patient and the family is an important goal for PC.[19] There are many different terms used to

Table 1
Palliative care resources

Resource Name	Contents and Use	Link
Palliative Care Fast Facts	App for mobile phones and resources on a Web site Categories include medical management of various medical conditions for PC and tips for difficult topic-specific discussions	https://www.mypcnow.org/fast-facts/
Center to Advance Palliative Care (CAPC) Web site	Categories include tools for dementia care, opioid prescribing tools, and more CME credit available for members of enrolled institutions Some of the content requires registration/institutional enrollment	Clinical tools: https://www.capc.org/toolkits/clinical-tools-delivering-high-quality-care/ Online courses: https://www.capc.org/training/ Integrating Palliative Practices in the Emergency Department Toolkit: https://www.capc.org/toolkits/integrating-palliative-care-practices-in-the-emergency-department/
CAPC COVID-19 Web site[a]	Resources specific to emergency care of COVID patients, including symptom management, coping in a crisis, and communication	https://www.capc.org/toolkits/covid-19-response-resources/
Vital Talk©	Resource for communication skills and guides, such as how to conduct a family conference, disclose serious news, and address goals of care	https://www.vitaltalk.org/resources/

Abbreviations: CME, continuous medical education; COVID, coronavirus disease.
[a] This site has ongoing updates as new information becomes available.

describe the experience of caregivers of a chronically ill or disabled individual for an indeterminate amount of time.[18] These terms, such as caregiver fatigue, have variable definitions in the literature and can include the physical, emotional, and social dimensions of this experience, including sense of duty.[20] At times, the circumstances and challenges of caregiving may lead to hospital admission for social reasons to allow for a safe disposition. A PC consultation can be considered to offer support to the patient and family as well as explore GOC as appropriate.[20] If not available, the interdisciplinary ED team, including social work, can participate in evaluation of caregiver distress and offer specific guidance related to this need.

Category 5: Suprise question/increasing complexity

The surprise question refers to whether the health care practitioner would be surprised if the patient died within 12 months, as mentioned in step 2 of the palliative screening tool in **Fig. 2**. Despite its inclusion in several palliative care screening tools,[11,12] a systematic review and meta-analysis by Downar and colleagues[5] found it does not perform well as a predictive tool for death, especially in noncancer illness. The surprise question is not recommended as a stand-alone prognostic tool; however, it does encourage a broader perspective beyond the acute presentation at hand to assess for unmet PC needs and may allow for consideration of hospice. An estimated prognosis of 6 months or less in the setting of terminal illness can be supported by evidence of progression of disease, increasing clinical complexity, and declining functional status, and, together with the patient's GOC, helps demonstrate potential eligibility for hospice.[21] Hospice eligibility can be explored with the patient's primary physician of record, the medical director of the hospice of the patient's choice, resources available from Medicare, and the expertise of local social work and case management support. Early consideration of hospice (when appropriate) is further supported by the Choosing Wisely campaign from the American College of Emergency Physicians, which states: "Don't delay engaging available palliative and hospice care services in the emergency department for patients likely to benefit."[5] Overall, recognizing the downward trajectory of a chronic illness and increasing complexity encourage the active assessment of PC and hospice needs in the ED and building this intersection in the patient's overall care earlier in their course.

SUMMARY

Though PC has not historically been within the purview of EM, recognition of the PC needs of the geriatric population should be part of standard practice and will be of increasing importance as older adults will represent an increasing percentage of the patients cared for in the ED based on current projections.[10] EM is in a unique position to facilitate early PC intervention, and thereby influence the overall trajectory of care for these patients. Integrating PC into EM practice starts with an understanding of the disease processes amenable to PC. Understanding the often unmet needs in the older population is also critical: frequent visits to the ED for chronic disease exacerbation, challenges of uncontrolled symptoms, functional decline, and the uncertainty around GOC.[11,12] These criteria can serve as a roadmap for the EM physician to guide partnership with the PC team in the management of complex patients in order to optimize their care and quality of life. **Table 1** lists some additional PC resources available to EM physicians that can be used for additional guidance.

CLINICS CARE POINTS

- PC referral or interventions should be considered in older adults suffering from symptoms of longstanding chronic disease, and not only at the end of life.
- Interdisciplinary PC teams, including social workers, physical/occupational therapists, and nurse case managers, should be engaged to provide an extra layer of support to chronically ill patients and their families.
- Caregiver burden should be considered by EM physicians when treating older adults dependent on support for IADLs and ADLs, especially at the time of discharge.
- GOC discussions can and should be conducted in the ED. Various tools are available to EM physicians to assist with these difficult but important conversations.

DISCLOSURE

The authors have nothing to disclose.

REFERENCES

1. Grudzen CR, Richardson LD, Morrison M, et al. Palliative care needs of seriously ill, older adults presenting to the emergency department. Acad Emerg Med 2010; 17(11):1253–7.
2. Meier DE. Palliative care facts and stats. Center to Advance Palliative Care (CAPC). 2014. Available at: https://media.capc.org/filer_public/68/bc/68bc93c7-14ad-4741-9830-8691729618d0/capc_press-kit.pdf. Accessed June 3, 2020.
3. Kerns C. The problem with U.S. health care isn't a shortage of doctors. Harvard Business Review. 2020. Available at: https://hbr.org/2020/03/the-problem-with-u-s-health-care-isnt-a-shortage-of-doctors. Accessed June 3, 2020.
4. Smith AK, McCarthy E, Weber E, et al. Half of older Americans seen in emergency department in last month of life; most admitted to hospital, and many die there. Health Aff (Millwood) 2012;31(6):1277–85.
5. Downar J, Goldman R, Pinto R, et al. The "surprise question" for predicting death in seriously ill patients: a systematic review and meta-analysis. CMAJ 2017; 189(13):E484–93.
6. Don't delay engaging available palliative and hospice care services in the emergency department for patients likely to benefit. In: Choosing Wisely; an Initiative of the ABIM Foundation. American College of Emergency Medicine; 2013. Available at: https://www.choosingwisely.org/clinician-lists/american-college-emergency-physicians-delaying-palliative-and-hospice-care-services-in-emergency-department/. Accessed September 9, 2020.
7. Temel JS, Greer JA, Muzikansky A, et al. Early palliative care for patients with metastatic non-small-cell lung cancer. N Engl J Med 2010;363(8):733–42.
8. Wu FM, Newman JM, Lasher A, et al. Effects of initiating palliative care consultation in the emergency department on inpatient length of stay. J Palliat Med 2013; 16(11):1362–7.
9. WHO definition of palliative care.. Available at: https://www.who.int/cancer/palliative/definition/en/. Accessed September 3, 2020.
10. Gornick ME, Warren JL, Eggers PW, et al. Thirty years of Medicare: impact on the covered population. Health Care Financ Rev 1996;18(2):179–237.

11. George N, Barrett N, McPeake L, et al. Content validation of a novel screening tool to identify emergency department patients with significant palliative care needs. Acad Emerg Med 2015;22(7):823–37.

12. Quest TE, Bryant EN, Waugh D, et al. Palliative care ED screening tool A technical assistance resource from the IPAL-EM project. Available at: https://www.capc.org/toolkits/integrating-palliative-care-practices-in-the-emergency-department/. Accessed June 2, 2020.

13. Lunney JR, Lynn J, Hogan C. Profiles of older Medicare decedents. JAGS 2002; 50(6):1108–12.

14. Caroline Ha M. Geriatric gems and palliative pearls; palliative: pain management. Available at: https://www.uth.tmc.edu/hgec/GemsAndPearls/index.html. Accessed June 25, 2020.

15. Ouchi K, George N, Schuur JD, et al. Goals-of-care conversations for older adults with serious illness in the emergency department: challenges and opportunities. Ann Emerg Med 2019;74(2):276–84.

16. Lazris A. Geriatric palliative care. Prim Care Clin 2019;46(3):447–59.

17. Xue Q. The frailty syndrome: Definition and natural history. Clin Geriatr Med 2011; 27(1):1–15.

18. Cooper Z, Koritsanszky L, Cauley CE, et al. Recommendations for best communication practices to facilitate goal-concordant care for seriously ill older patients with emergency surgical conditions. Ann Surg 2016;263(1):1–2, 3,4,5,6.

19. Centers to Advance Palliative Care. Patient and family resources. Available at: https://www.capc.org/about/patient-and-family-resources/. Accessed June 20, 2020.

20. Beydoun J, Nasrallah L, Sabrah T, et al. Towards a definition of caregiver fatigue: a concept analysis. Adv Nurs Sci 2019;42(4):297–306.

21. The Official U.S. Government Site for Medicare. Hospice care. Available at: https://www.medicare.gov/coverage/hospice-care. Accessed June 20, 2020.

Moving?

Make sure your subscription moves with you!

To notify us of your new address, find your **Clinics Account Number** (located on your mailing label above your name), and contact customer service at:

Email: journalscustomerservice-usa@elsevier.com

800-654-2452 (subscribers in the U.S. & Canada)
314-447-8871 (subscribers outside of the U.S. & Canada)

Fax number: 314-447-8029

Elsevier Health Sciences Division
Subscription Customer Service
3251 Riverport Lane
Maryland Heights, MO 63043

*To ensure uninterrupted delivery of your subscription, please notify us at least 4 weeks in advance of move.